The Daily Telegraph

Encyclopedia of Vitamins, Minerals and Herbal Supplements

DR SARAH BREWER is a recognized expert on sensible supplementation and was voted Health Journalist of the Year by the Health Food Manufacturers' Association. She is a regular correspondent for *The Daily Telegraph*, *Top Santé*, *Real Health & Beauty*, *Sugar*, *Let's Live* and *Slimming World* and the author of over 20 popular health books. She is currently formulating her own consumer range of supplements, Trilogy.

The Daily Telegraph

Encyclopedia of Vitamins, Minerals and Herbal Supplements

Dr Sarah Brewer

ROBINSON
London

Constable & Robinson Ltd.
3 The Lanchesters
162 Fulham Palace Road
London W6 9ER
www.constablerobinson.com

First published in the UK by Robinson
an imprint of Constable & Robinson Ltd 2002

ISBN 1-84119-184-1

Edited and designed by Grapevine Publishing Services
Printed and bound in the EU

Contents

*This book is dedicated to my wonderful family,
who willingly provided invaluable back-up
and support during those long hours of
research and writing*

Acknowledgements

I would like to thank everyone who has been so helpful in providing research papers and information on the many invaluable nutritional supplements covered in this book.

How to use this book

The first part of this book looks at individual vitamins, minerals, herbs and other supplements. If you want to know more about a particular supplement, most of your questions should be answered here.

The second part of this book looks at a number of common health problems and tells you a little about them, their causes and symptoms plus the main treatments and supplements that are likely to help. Once you have looked up a condition, and selected a few possible remedies, you can then check these out in the first part of the book to choose those that are most likely to suit you.

Doses
The doses given in this book are only meant to be indicative of those in common use. Always follow the manufacturer's instructions as doses will depend on the strength of individual products.

Pregnancy
Never take any supplements during pregnancy or breastfeeding, unless they are especially designed for use at this time (e.g. pregnancy vitamin and mineral blends) or have been recommended by a doctor or qualified medical herbalist.

IMPORTANT NOTES

- This book is not intended to be a substitute for medical advice or treatment. Any person with a condition requiring medical attention should consult a qualified medical practitioner or suitable therapist.

- All suggested doses are for adults only; specialist advice should be sought for supplementation in children.

- Where not otherwise stated, supplements may be taken for an unlimited period, until symptoms improve.

- Where no side effects are mentioned, no serious ones have been reported at standard doses.

- Some herbal supplements may interact with prescribed drugs. Always check with a pharmacist or doctor before combining herbs with drugs.

- Some herbal medicines may cause bleeding, heart problems or low blood sugar in patients undergoing surgery. Always tell your doctor what supplements you are taking as they may need to be stopped before an operation.

Introduction

An almost bewildering range of vitamin, mineral and herbal supplements is now available in chemists, supermarkets and healthfood shops. Unfortunately, legislation dictates that full information about the benefits of these supplements cannot be given on their packaging as this would constitute a health claim. As a result, people who would like to take supplements to improve a particular aspect of their health and well-being often find it difficult to select those supplements most likely to suit them.

This book aims to tell readers everything they need to know about the main vitamin, mineral and herbal supplements available, their benefits, research evidence to back their use, and any possible side effects, as well as an indication as to who should not take them.

Why take a vitamin and mineral supplement?

In an ideal world, we would get all the vitamins, minerals and essential fatty acids we need from our food. In reality, however, very few of us achieve this. Three quarters of women and almost nine out of ten men eat fewer than the recommended five servings of fruit and vegetables per day. In addition, over two thirds of people do not eat oily fish on a regular basis even though one or two portions per week are important for their essential fatty acid content. Similarly, over 90 per cent of people do not eat the recommended three servings of wholegrains a day.

Even when we do eat reasonable amounts of healthy foods, their nutritional content is depleted compared with

What is a serving?

Aim to eat at least five, and preferably eight servings of fruit and vegetables per day.

A serving is basically the amount you are happy to eat in one sitting – the more the better. Typically, this would amount to a glass of fruit juice, a generous helping of green or root vegetables (excluding potatoes), a large mixed salad, 1 large beef tomato or 2 medium tomatoes, a handful of grapes, cherries or berries, and a single item of apple, orange, kiwi, peach, pear, nectarine, or banana. A serving of larger items may amount to ½ grapefruit, ½ ogen melon, ½ mango, ½ papaya, while for smaller and dried fruits, it could amount to 2–4 dates, figs, satsumas, passion fruit, apricots, plums or prunes. The phrase to hang on to is 'at least' – ideally we would all benefit from eating 8–10 servings of fruit, vegetables or salads per day, but some people, especially those with digestive problems, may find this difficult. Plant-based foods are important sources of vitamins, minerals, antioxidants, fibre and non-nutrient substances known as phytochemicals that help to protect against a variety of common conditions, including coronary heart disease and cancer.

how it was just a few decades ago. Apart from genetic manipulation aimed at producing fruit and vegetables especially for their colour, uniform size, and their capacity to look good for longer (at the expense of flavour and nutrients), intensive farming practices often mean that the soils in which crops are grown, and on which livestock are reared, are deficient in vital trace elements. The most startling example is selenium – intakes have dropped significantly over the last 25 years, and in Britain have almost halved from 60mcg in 1974 to just 34 mcg per day in 1994. Intakes of essential fatty acids (EFAs – found in nuts, seeds and fish) are also low with an estimated eight out of ten adults deficient in them. Deficiency of EFAs during pregnancy is now implicated in the development of dyslexia, attention deficit hyperactivity disorder and even schizophrenia in the resultant offspring.

Taking an A to Z-style vitamin and mineral supplement providing around 100 per cent of the recommended daily amount (RDA) of as many vitamins and minerals as possible, plus an EFA supplement (e.g. evening primrose, flaxseed, hempseed or fish oils) acts as a nutritional safety net, and is becoming an increasingly wise investment for all adults. (*See also* **RDAs**, page 272.)

As you get older, your need for particular vitamins and minerals will change and the amount of nutrients that can be absorbed from your intestines will decrease. It is therefore a good idea to take a vitamin and mineral supplement designed for your age group and several are now specially formulated for those in later life. Research involving 96 older people showed that those taking multivitamins for one year had better immune function, mounted a better response to influenza vaccination, and had half as many days ill with infections compared with those not taking multivitamin supplements (23 days in the year versus 48).

Unless otherwise stated on the packaging, vitamin and mineral supplements should be taken immediately after food and washed down with water or juice. Some can make you feel sick or cause indigestion if taken on an empty stomach. Never wash them down with coffee or tea, as these may interfere with absorption. Coffee, for example, can reduce iron absorption from the gut by up to 80 per cent if drunk within an hour of a meal. It also reduces uptake of zinc and is associated with increased excretion of magnesium, calcium and other minerals. Against this, however, is the fact that caffeine is a potent stimulator of gastric acid secretion (which will assist absorption of some micro-nutrients). It is also a rich source of vitamin B3 (niacin) although drinking coffee in excess depletes vitamin B levels generally.

Where you have to take two or more capsules of the same preparation, it is a good idea to spread these out over the day in order to maximize absorption and cause less fluctuation in blood levels. If you take a one-a-day vitamin and mineral supplement that is not time-released, it is usually better to take it after your evening meal rather than with breakfast. This is because repair processes and mineral flux in your body is greatest at night when growth hormone is secreted. You are also less likely to drink coffee in the evening if it keeps you awake so there is less likely to be a problem with iron absorption.

Herbal remedies

Herbalism, or phytotherapy – the use of plant extracts for healing – is now one of the most exciting areas of medical research. Different parts of different plants are used – roots, stems, flowers, leaves, bark, sap, fruit or seeds depending on which has the highest concentration of a particular active ingredient. Herbal remedies can have powerful effects – between 30 and 40 per cent of prescription drugs are in fact derived from plant origins. In most cases, herbal supplements contain a blend of constituents that have evolved together over thousands of years to achieve a synergistic balance which tends to have a gentler effect than that of pharmaceutical extracts containing only one or two isolated active ingredients. The risk of side effects with herbal remedies is therefore relatively low.

The herbal and other supplements included in this book are my own selection, and comprise those I find most helpful, have most experience with, or which are backed by a long tradition of use and/or convincing research findings. Many other traditional herbal remedies are available, and their exclusion from this book does not mean that they are unhelpful. It merely indicates that I have not yet become fully acquainted with them, or that I choose to use other remedies for their particular indications. The growing data bank of research into herbal and other supplements will no doubt mean that other remedies will be included in future editions of this book.

Standardized herbal extracts?

Herbal extracts are prepared in ways designed to concentrate the active components of the herb. Tinctures are made by soaking herbs in an alcoholic base and may be described as, for example, a 1:10 extract, which means that 10 per cent of the tincture is made up of the herbal base, while 90 per cent is solvent. Traditional herbalists tend to prefer using tinctures. Personally, I prefer solid extracts which tend to be easier to use, and are more likely to contain therapeutic levels of ingredients.

Solid extracts are prepared by removing the solvent (e.g. alcohol) used to extract the active components from the original herbal base. The residual solids are then dried and powdered to make tablets or capsules. Solid extracts are described according to their concentration so that, for example, a 10:1 extract means that ten parts crude herb was used to make one part of the extract. The more concentrated the extract, theoretically the stronger it is, although more volatile components may have become lost so that the

Doses

A milligram (µg) is one thousandth of a gram, while a microgram (mcg or mg) is one millionth of a gram. 1 g therefore equals 1000 mg, and 1mg equals 1000 mcg. This can lead to some confusion, as a product containing (for example) 1 g vitamin C contains the same amount as one claiming 1000 mg vitamin C, while a product containing 400 mcg folic acid provides the same amount as one listing 0.4 mg folic acid, although one value may sound more than another. International units (IU) were used to measure biological activity of vitamins A, D and E before the pure compounds were isolated and quantified. Although these are considered obsolete by some, they are still in wide usage. This makes it even more difficult to compare one product with another. For vitamin A, 3 IU are equivalent to 1 mcg retinol, for vitamin D, 1 mcg is equivalent to 40 IU and for vitamin E, 1mg (or 1000 mcg) is approximately equivalent to 1.5 IU. For the EC recommended daily amounts (RDAs) of each of these three vitamins, the equivalents are therefore:

Vitamin A: 800 mcg	**= 2400 IU**
Vitamin D: 5 mcg	**= 200 IU**
Vitamin E: 10 mg	**= 15 IU**

concentration does not accurately reflect its activity. Because of this, it is best to use a standardized preparation.

As the quality of different batches of raw material can vary significantly, standardization helps to ensure consistency. Although only one or two ingredients may be assayed to ensure a standardized concentration, this does not, in any way, discount the synergy that occurs between the multitude of other components present in a preparation, but whose concentration has not been exactly determined.

Standardization is merely a tool that reassures both prescriber and consumer that their selected product delivers an effective dose.

My preference for standardized extracts also comes from their widespread medical use in Europe and their ability to provide good, scientific evidence for their efficacy. Standardized remedies are more likely to be backed by good quality, randomized, double-blind, placebo-controlled trials. Unfortunately, this does mean you get what you pay for, and many cheap, non-standardized herbal preparations contain very little active ingredient and are consequently of little benefit to the user. Where possible, buy the best supplements you can afford – those offering a year's supply of a herbal supplement for a fraction of the cost of the brand leaders should be regarded with suspicion. They may be made from the wrong part of the plant (such as leaves rather than berries), contain a very low concentration of herbs, and therefore provide very little of the beneficial, active ingredients.

I hope you find this book invaluable and I wish all readers a future that is as healthy and natural as possible.

Sarah Brewer
e-mail: DrSarah@medilance.com

PS My own range of vitamin, mineral, essential fatty acid and herbal supplements is available in shops, providing a simple three-step approach to supplementation.

Table showing the scientific evaluation of the range of safe intake levels of vitamins and minerals

Nutrient	Unit	Upper safe level Long-term consumption	Upper limit Short-term consumption
Vitamin A (retinol)	µg	3,000	7,500
Vitamin D	µg	20	50
Vitamin E	µg	800	None established
ß carotene	mg	25	None established
Thiamin	mg	50	None established
Riboflavin	mg	200	None established
Nicotinamide	mg	1,500	3,000
Nicotinic acid	mg	500 (250 slow release)	1,000 (500 slow release)
Pyridoxine	mg	200	200
Folic acid	µg	1,000	None established
Vitamin B12	µg	3,000	None established
Biotin	µg	2,500	None established
Pantothenic acid	mg	1,000	None established
Vitamin C	mg	1,000	None established
Calcium	mg	1,500	>2,500
Phosphorus	mg	1,100	1,900
Magnesium	mg	700	None established
Chromium	µg	200	None established
Copper	mg	8	None established
Iodine	µg	1,000	None established
Iron	mg	20	80
Manganese	mg	20	None established
Molybdenum	µg	300	10,000
Selenium	µg	200	750
Zinc	mg	30	50

In this table the data for consumption (Long-term – Upper safe level and Short-term – Upper Limit) refers to total intake from all food sources and not to supplementation alone.

Courtesy of Dr Derek Shrimpton, European Federation of Health Product Manufacturers Associations

PART 1:

A–Z
OF
SUPPLEMENTS

A

Vitamin A is a fat-soluble vitamin that is stored in the liver. It can be obtained either as pre-formed vitamin A (retinol – which is only found in foods from animal sources such as animal fat, meat, liver, kidney, fish oil (especially fish liver oil), eggs, milk and dairy products) or as carotenoids, which are yellow-orange pigments derived from plant sources, some of which can be converted into vitamin A in the body.

Benefits

Vitamin A has a number of important functions in the body, including that of a powerful antioxidant. It binds to special receptors inside cells and regulates the way in which genes are read to produce a number of proteins, including many important enzyme systems. As so many genes are controlled by this hormone-like action of vitamin A, it is essential for normal growth and development, sexual health and fertility. It maintains healthy skin, teeth, bones and mucous membranes such as those lining the eyes, nose, throat and gums. It is also important in the healing of sores, wounds, or burns.

Vitamin A plays an important role in maintaining immunity and strengthening resistance. It is needed in higher amounts during times of infection and is involved in the production of immune cells needed to line the mucus membranes of the respiratory and intestinal tracts – two of the body's front lines against infection. Because of its role in immunity, optimum intakes of vitamin A help to protect against viral infections such as sore throats, the common cold, influenza, warts, conjunctivitis, cold sores, acute bronchitis and possibly shingles. It is also thought to have a protective action against inflammatory bowel disease, peptic ulcers, Candida yeast infections and may play a role in reducing allergies.

In the eye, vitamin A is converted into a pigment known as visual purple (rhodopsin). When exposed to light, this pigment absorbs photon energy which induces a change that stimulates nerve endings in the back of the eye (retina) to trigger sensory messages. These are relayed to the brain for interpretation by the visual cortex to form visual images. This was one of the first functions of vitamin A to be recognized – hence its common name of retinol.

Vitamin A derivatives are now available on prescription to treat severe forms of acne, psoriasis and sun damage (photo-ageing) including wrinkles. It may be also helpful in diabetes, by promoting the action of insulin hormone to provide better control of blood glucose levels and in people with chronic lung disease.

As vitamin A is such a powerful antioxidant in both the water soluble (as carotenoids) and fat soluble (as retinol) phases of the body, several studies have suggested that natural dietary intakes of vitamin A and betacarotene are important in reducing the risk of coronary heart disease and a number of cancers, including breast, lung, skin cancer (melanoma) and possibly leukaemia.

Dose

Ideally, an adult needs around 800 mcg (2664 IU) vitamin A daily (EC RDA).

If vitamin A supplements are used, they are best limited to less than 1500 mcg (5000 IU) a day although intakes of up to 3000 mcg (10,000 IU) are considered safe.

New guidelines for safe levels of vitamin A issued by the National Academy of Sciences Institute of Medicine in the USA state that adults should not consume more than

3000 mcg (10,000 IU) vitamin A each day. Even so, nutritional supplements with mega levels (e.g. 25,000 IU of vitamin A) are available, which is worrying as excess vitamin A is toxic (see below).

Children should ideally take a supplement providing vitamins A, D and E (at doses appropriate for their age) up until at least the age of five unless their diet is known to provide sufficient amounts of these important micro-nutrients.

Deficiency

Vitamin A deficiency is uncommon in developed countries, but relatively common in poorer parts of the world. One of the first signs of lack of vitamin A is loss of sensitivity to green light, followed by difficulty in adapting to dim light (night blindness), hence the old adage that 'carrots help you see in the dark'.

More severe deficiency leads to dry, burning, itchy eyes, hardening of the cornea (the transparent part of the front of the eye) followed by corneal ulceration – a condition known as xerophthalmia. Lack of vitamin A also increases the risk of cataracts. It is estimated that as many as half a million people worldwide go blind from vitamin A deficiency each year.

Other symptoms of vitamin A deficiency include increased susceptibility to infection, scaly skin with raised, pimply hair follicles and flaky scalp; dull, brittle hair, inflamed gums and mucous membranes, loss of appetite and possibly kidney stones.

Pregnant women and those planning a baby should not take more than 1500 mcg (5000 IU) vitamin A daily as higher doses may cause birth defects. Also to be avoided is cod liver oil as this contains high quantities of vitamin A.

The safest way to obtain vitamin A is in the form of natural carotenoids.

Supplements containing vitamin A are best taken with food as dietary fat aids absorption. It is most effective taken in conjunction with other antioxidants such as vitamins C, E, carotenoids and mineral selenium and zinc.

Vitamin A is easily destroyed by exposure to light.

Symptoms of vitamin A poisoning

It is important not to exceed recommended doses of any supplement containing vitamin A. It has a narrow therapeutic window and intakes of just double the recommended daily amount may cause problems – especially during pregnancy.

Cases of vitamin A toxicity are usually associated with taking supplements at doses above 30,000 mcg (100,000 IU) daily.

As it is fat soluble, vitamin A enters the central nervous system more easily than most other vitamins and excess causes symptoms of retinol poisoning which include liver and nerve damage, headache, irritability, blurred vision, nausea, weakness, fatigue, dry skin, hair loss, itchy eyes, bone and joint pain, bone loss, bleeding gums and skin sores. In the long term, excess vitamin A may increase the risk of liver cirrhosis. Avoid eating polar bear liver, which is said to contain so much retinol that just 100g of it can be lethal!

Excess vitamin A is also known to cause developmental defects and, in a study of over 22,700 pregnant women, those with total intakes (from both food and supplements) of more than 15,000 IU (4500 mcg) of pre-formed vitamin A (retinol) daily were three or four times more likely to deliver a baby with congenital defects than those whose intakes

> 1 International Unit (IU) Vitamin A = 0.3 mcg retinol
> 1mcg vitamin A = 3.33 IU

were 5000 IU (1500 mcg) daily. In those women whose vitamin A intake came mainly from supplements, those obtaining 10,000 IU (3000 mcg) daily were four to five times more likely to deliver a baby with congenital abnormalities. The researchers concluded that, among the women taking more than 10,000 IU vitamin A per day, one infant in 57 had abnormalities due to the supplement. The most dangerous time to take excess vitamin A during pregnancy seems to be within the first seven weeks.

It is preferable for pregnant women to take supplements that are specifically designed for pregnancy. These usually contain either no, or low levels of vitamin A, mainly in the form of carotenoids. It is also recommended that pregnant women avoid eating liver and liver products during pregnancy because of their high vitamin A content.

Carotenoids are a useful way to obtain vitamin A, as excess pre-formed retinol is toxic, especially during pregnancy.

See also **Carotenoids**

Adaptogens

An adaptogen is a tonic substance that strengthens, normalizes and regulates all the body's systems.

Benefits

Adaptogens have wide-ranging benefits and boost immunity through several different actions rather than one specific effect. An adaptogen can strengthen, normalize and regulate your body systems. Some have been shown to bring blood sugar, blood pressure, cholesterol and hormone levels back to normal and to counter the effects of stress or disrupted biorhythms. This helps you to adapt to a wide variety of new or stressful situations, mostly by supporting the action of the adrenal glands so that their weight is maintained and they do not become exhausted during prolonged exposure to stress.

Research suggests that adaptogens work by boosting the creation of energy in body cells by making the uptake of oxygen and processing of cell wastes more efficient. This encourages cell growth and increases cell survival. Supplements with adaptogenic properties also contain vitamins, minerals and unique plant chemicals whose complex role in disease prevention is still being unravelled.

Adaptogens seem to work best as an energy stimulant if fatigue is not directly due to excess physical exertion but to an underlying problem such as poor or irregular diet, hormone imbalance, stress or excess consumption of coffee, nicotine or alcohol. Lifestyle changes to redress the balance (e.g. stopping or cutting back on smoking) are also important to re-energize the body. When adaptogens are used together with vitamin C (at least 500 mg a day) and the B complex (50–100 mg daily in divided doses), results are often improved.

Important herbal adaptogens include:

Ashwagandha
Astragalus

Black cohosh
Dong quai
Gotu kola
Gynostemma (Jiaogulan)
Korean and American ginsengs
Maca
Maitake
Pfaffia
Reishi
Rhodiola
Schisandra
Siberian ginseng
Yerba maté

African prune
(Pygeum africanum)

The bark of the evergreen African plum tree is a popular treatment for benign prostatic hyperplasia (enlargement known as BPH) in continental Europe.

Benefits

Extracts of *Pygeum* have anti-inflammatory actions and can stop irritable bladder symptoms by damping down over-reactivity of the bladder muscle. When 18 men with sexual difficulties due to symptoms of either BPH or prostatitis, took *Pygeum africanum* extracts (200 mg daily) for 60 days, all showed significant improvement in urinary symptoms and sexual activity, and swelling of the gland around the urethra was also reduced.

In a multi-centre study involving 85 men with prostatism, 100 mg per day of *Pygeum africanum* was given for two months. Night-time frequency (nocturia) was reduced by 32 per cent and average urinary flow rates and urinary volume also significantly improved, lasting throughout the following month without treatment.

In a double-blind study (where the identity of those receiving the test supplement is concealed from both administrators and subjects until after the study is completed) involving 134 men with BPH, half received a combination of *Pygeum* plus nettle at standard dose, while the other half received half the normal daily dose. After a month, urinary flow, residual urine and nocturia were significantly reduced in both groups and the researchers concluded that half doses were just as safe and effective as the full recommended dose. Some earlier trials did not produce impressive results, however.

Dose
100–200 mg a day.

Agaricus bisporus

Agaricus bispour is an edible mushroom. Extracts have been developed in Japan to treat bad breath (halitosis) due to a variety of causes including plaque build-up, and odours released from the intestines. It contains enzymes that destroy malodorous sulphur compounds present in plaque, in some foods and those produced by bacterial fermentation in the large bowel. Studies show a significant reduction in the concentration of malodorous substances such as methyl mercaptan within 15 to 30 minutes of taking the supplement. Blood levels of ammonia are also reduced. It is effective for some metabolic conditions in which strong body odours are produced, and can also improve the smell of bowel motions.

Dose
Typically 400 mg after meals, three times daily.
400 mg is enough to eliminate the smell caused by eating 7 g raw garlic.

Agnus castus
(Vitex agnus castus)

Agnus castus – also known as the chaste tree – is native to the Mediterranean and west Asia. Its fruits were traditionally used by monks to reduce sex drive and help them to remain celibate, hence its name.

Benefits
One cause of low sex drive is raised levels of prolactin hormone which has a powerful libido-lowering effect. In low doses, agnus castus extracts increase prolactin levels and, in men, also inhibit the action of testosterone. In higher doses, however, it starts to reduce prolactin secretion in women and can therefore have a beneficial prosexual action in those with raised levels of this hormone.

Agnus castus also has a progesterone-like action in women. It has been shown to decrease secretion of follicle stimulating hormone (FSH) and increase production of lutinizing hormone (LH) probably indirectly as a result of reducing prolactin secretion. LH stimulates ovarian secretion of progesterone, so chaste tree berry indirectly boosts progesterone levels and is valuable in treating premenstrual syndrome. It also helps to regulate the menstrual cycle by tending to shorten a long cycle and vice versa.

Extracts from agnus castus berries help to neutralize the excess testosterone hormone occurring in PCOS (polycystic ovary syndrome) and may reduce acne and excess hair.

Agnus castus is slow acting. It takes an average of 25 days for symptoms to start improving and up to six months to achieve the full effect.

A recent study of 170 women with PMS showed that all symptoms improved by more than 50 per cent in those taking agnus castus, compared with the same improvement in just 24 per cent of those taking a placebo. The greatest improvement was seen in the reduction of irritability, mood alteration, anger, headache and breast fullness.

Other studies found agnus castus to be effective in relieving physical symptoms such as headaches, sore breasts, bloating and fatigue and psychological changes such as increased appetite, sweet cravings, nervousness/restlessness, anxiety, depression, mood swings and lack of concentration in 90 per cent of cases.

Agnus castus has also been found to be successful in increasing fertility where difficulty in conceiving is linked with low progesterone levels during the second (luteal) phase of the menstrual cycle (from ovulation to the onset of menstruation). In one study of 45 women with this form of infertility, seven became pregnant during the three-month trial while low progesterone levels were restored to normal in 25. Treatment should be stopped as soon as pregnancy is suspected.

Another benefit of agnus castus is its capacity to treat menopausal symptoms (especially hot flushes and night sweats) which are indirectly linked with increased levels of FSH.

Traditionally agnus castus has been used to promote breast milk flow, even though it reduces levels of the milk-stimulating hormone, prolactin. This is because, although prolactin stimulates the initial production of breast milk after childbirth, levels naturally return to normal pre-pregnancy levels within eight days of delivery. While continued suckling maintains levels at first, they do still decline, so that by three months after the birth, milk secretion in breast-feeding mothers continues despite prolactin levels being within the normal range. Studies involving 100 nursing mothers found that those given agnus castus extracts rather than a placebo had increased milk flow and ease of milk release. Effects took several weeks to develop and this delay suggests that another action is involved, rather than any effects on prolactin hormone secretion itself. No problems were reported with the safety of agnus castus for breast-fed infants.

Dose

Tablets: 500 mg a day.

Extracts standardized to contain 0.5 per cent agnuside: 175–225 mg a day. Agnus castus is usually taken as a single daily dose first thing in the morning. It is slow acting and can take up to 25 days to show effects. The average length of treatment is six months.

Excess

Excess agnus castus can cause a crawling sensation on the skin (like ants) known as formication.

Contraindications

● Agnus castus is not recommended during pregnancy, neither should it be taken at the same time as other hormone treatments, such as HRT and hormonal methods of contraception.

● As agnus castus is thought to have an anti-androgen effect in men, it is not recommended for use in males, although traditionally it has been given to treat male impotence, premature ejaculation, prostatitis and lack of sexual sensations.

Aloe vera

Native to Africa, aloe vera is a succulent plant with lance-shaped, fleshy leaves. There are over 200 different species, of which only three or four are used medicinally, the most useful being Aloe vera Barbadensis. From its fleshy leaves a gel containing a unique mix of vitamins, amino acids, enzymes and minerals may be squeezed, valued for its healing properties for over 6000 years.

Aloe vera juice can be made from fresh liquid extract (gel) or from powdered aloe. The fresh gel has to be stabilized within hours of harvesting to prevent oxidation and inactivation. When selecting a product, aim for one made from 100 per cent pure aloe vera. Its strength needs to be at least 40 per cent by volume to be effective and should ideally approach 95–100 per cent. You may find it more palatable to choose a product containing a little natural fruit juice (e.g. grape, apple) to improve the flavour.

Benefits

Aloe vera may be taken internally or externally. The juice contains vitamins, minerals and 20 amino acids (including 7 essential amino acids) so it has excellent nutritional properties. The gel also contains substances that:

- have useful anti-inflammatory and anti-itching properties (anthraquinones and natural plant steroids)
- hasten wound healing (fibroblast growth factor)
- are powerful antioxidants (vitamins C, E, betacarotene)
- are cleansing and antiseptic with certain antibacterial, anti-viral and anti-fungal properties (saponins and anthraquinones)
- are soothing and analgesic (salicylic acid, bradykininase and the anthraquinones aloin and emodin).

Taken internally, aloe vera juice appears to boost immunity, and is helpful for people with chronic fatigue syndrome and rheumatoid arthritis. It is also used for a variety of intestinal problems, including indigestion, constipation, irritable bowel syndrome (IBS), diverticulosis and for inflammatory conditions such as ulcerative colitis and Crohn's disease.

Externally, aloe vera gel helps to treat sunburn, cracked or sore lips, cold sores, eczema, psoriasis, rosacea, acne, shingles, ulcers, burns, scars, rashes, bites and stings. It may even interfere with the formation of age spots and help those that are already present to fade. As it stimulates dilation of blood capillaries, it improves local circulation, reaches the site of inflammation more quickly and stimulates tissue regeneration when wounds are shallow. By coating the skin in a moisture-rich film, it also prevents damaged skin from drying out. However, it should not be applied to infected deep wounds (e.g. surgical ones) as there is evidence to suggest that it may lengthen their healing time. It is helpful for treating gum disease (gingivitis and periodontitis) when applied as a dental paste, and some dentists use it to help flush mercury from the body during planned mercury amalgam removal.

A double-blind study of 60 adults with psoriasis found that an ointment containing aloe vera gel (surprisingly, just 0.5 per cent, although 100 per cent gel could be used) applied three times a day healed over 80 per cent of plaques within four weeks as compared with only 8 per cent using a placebo.

Some aloe vera products contain the bitter aloe 'latex' extracted from the inner yellow leaves of the plant. This has a powerful cathartic effect and taking too much will cause a brisk laxative response due to the presence of chemicals known as anthraquinones (e.g. aloin which has a bitter taste). These stimulate contraction of smooth muscle fibres lining the bowel and it usually works within 8–12 hours. This can be a desirable effect. Many products claim to be aloin and emodin free, but independent laboratory tests on leading brands in the USA found high levels of aloin in juices claimed to be aloin-free. Ideally, a product that is stamped with an IASC-certified seal (from the International Aloe Science Council) should be selected; this shows that it has been produced according to recommended guidelines.

Dose

If taking the aloe latex for its laxative effect, start with a small dose of gel (e.g. 1 teaspoon) and work up to around 1–2 tablespoons per day to find the dose that suits you best. Aloe vera juice may be taken more liberally (e.g. 50–100 ml, three times daily).

Side effects

Some women using aloe vera notice that it increases their menstrual flow, but no serious side effects have been reported at standard doses. Some people develop a mild itching rash due to allergy when applying aloe vera gel on the skin; in such cases treatment should be discontinued.

Contraindications

- Taking aloe vera by mouth should be avoided in pregnancy as the anthraquinones it may contain can stimulate uterine contractions which could result in miscarriage.
- It should also be avoided when breast-feeding. If aloin enters breast milk it can trigger stomach cramps and diarrhoea in infants.

Alpha-lipoic acid

Alpha-lipoic acid is a vitamin-like substance that acts as a co-enzyme with B group vitamins to speed up certain metabolic reactions needed for energy production. It is also a powerful antioxidant that helps to regenerate other important antioxidants such as vitamins C and E. The body produces small quantities of alpha-lipoic acid, and some is also obtained from the diet (e.g. in spinach, meats) as well as in supplements containing brewer's yeast.

Benefits

Alpha-lipoic acid is mainly used to boost energy levels, and to treat conditions in which nerve damage is causing symptoms of tingling, numbness or discomfort, such as in diabetic neuropathy. By improving cell function, it also seems to improve the body's use of insulin and to improve diabetic control, but should only be taken by diabetics under medical supervision as blood glucose levels may need frequent monitoring to prevent hypoglycemia.

Alpha-lipoic acid improves liver function, and is used to treat hepatitis, cirrhosis and other liver diseases including toxic damage e.g. due to mushroom poisoning.

It may also improve symptoms of chronic fatigue syndrome, long-term memory loss and psoriasis.

Dose

As an antioxidant, alpha-lipoic acid is usually taken in doses of 50–100 mg a day. For therapeutic use, higher doses of 100–200 mg three times a day may be recommended.

Side effects

Mild skin rashes or gastrointestinal side effects may rarely occur.

Amino acids

Amino acids are the building blocks for proteins, formed when they are linked together to make a chain. Chains in which between two and ten amino acids are linked together are known as peptides; those with 10–100 amino acids tend to be called polypeptides, while chains of over 100 amino acids fold into complex three-dimensional shapes known as proteins.

How does the body use proteins?

When digested, dietary proteins are broken down to release their amino acid building blocks. This process starts in the stomach, where an enzyme (pepsin) divides the bonds between certain amino acid chains to form short peptide chains. Once in the small intestine, these are further attacked by enzymes released from the intestinal wall and pancreas. Chains of double and triple amino acids are absorbed into cells lining the gut and cleaved to release single amino acids into the bloodstream. These are then used as building blocks to make over 50,000 different proteins and polypeptides needed by the human body.

Over 50 per cent of the body's dry weight is made up of protein. Some proteins play a structural role (e.g. collagen), some regulate metabolic reactions (enzymes) while others are vital for immunity (antibodies). These are constantly broken down and re-formed – mostly during sleep under the control of growth hormone – at a rate of around 80–100 g per day. Most muscle protein is renewed every six months – 98 per cent of the body's proteins are renewed within one year. Protein metabolism produces a poisonous by-product, ammonia. This is converted into urea in the liver and transported to the kidneys for excretion in urine.

Over 20 amino acids are important for human health. Of these, ten cannot be synthesized in the body in amounts needed by the metabolism and must therefore come from the diet. These are known as the nutritionally essential amino acids. They are:

- arginine – essential during childhood and sometimes in adulthood
- histidine – essential during childhood and sometimes in adulthood

- isoleucine
- leucine
- lysine
- methionine
- phenylalanine
- threonine
- tryptophan
- valine.

In addition, tyrosine is synthesized from phenylalanine, which is essential, and cysteine is synthesized from methionine, which is also essential.

The non-essential amino acids which can be made in the body include:

- alanine
- asparagine
- aspartic acid
- glutamic acid
- glutamine
- glycine
- proline
- serine
- taurine.

Protein in the diet

Dietary protein can be divided into two groups: first-class proteins, which contain significant quantities of all the essential amino acids (e.g. animal meat, fish, eggs, dairy products) and second-class proteins, which contain some essential amino acids but not all (e.g. vegetables, rice, beans, nuts). Second-class proteins need to be mixed and matched by eating as wide a variety of foods as possible. For example, the essential amino acid missing from haricot beans is found in bread. Hence, combining cereals with pulses or seeds and nuts provides a balanced amino acid intake. Vegetarians can also obtain a balanced protein intake by eating a combination of five parts rice to one part beans.

The average adult needs to obtain around 56 g of protein per day from his food, and those taking part in competitive sports will need more than this. For example, an athlete training for two hours a day will need to obtain 1.1–1.4 g protein per kilogram of body weight per day, depending on the intensity of exercise. Weight-lifters in training may need as much as 2–3.5 g protein per kilogram of body weight a day.

Protein supplements are available for athletes as intact proteins, partially digested (hydrolysed) peptides or free amino acids. Some research suggests that the hydrolysates (dipeptides and tripeptides) may be the best options for bulking up muscle as they are most readily absorbed and utilized in the body.

Amino acid supplements are absorbed most effectively if taken between meals (two hours before or after eating). If using an individual amino acid for more than two weeks, it is best taken with a mixed amino acid complex to guard against amino acid imbalances. Individual amino acid supplements should not normally be taken for more than 12 weeks except under the supervision of a doctor or nutritionist.

Dose

Doses vary considerably; always check the labels.

Angelica – European
(Angelica archangelica)

European angelica is an important component of Bénédictine and Chartreuse liqueurs. Its root contains aromatic essential oils and unique substances such as angelic acid and angelicin.

Benefits

Angelica root is used as an expectorant for coughs and colds, as a bitter tonic (often combined with gentian) to improve appetite and aid digestion, to relieve feelings of fullness or flatulence and as an anti-spasmodic to relax smooth muscle cells in the gastrointestinal and respiratory tracts. In laboratory studies, essential oils from angelica root were also found to have anti-fungal activity.

Dose

Dried root: 1–2 g, three times a day.

Side effects

Possible side effects include:

- an increase in uterine contraction, similar to that occurring with Chinese angelica (*dong quai*)
- photosensitization of skin so avoid excessive exposure to sunlight when taking it.

Contraindications

Angelica root should not be used during pregnancy.

Antioxidants

An antioxidant is a protective substance that helps to neutralize damaging oxidation reactions in the body. Most oxidations are triggered by free radicals – unstable molecular fragments that carry a negative electrical charge in the form of a spare electron. Free radicals try to lose this charge by colliding with other molecules and cell structures in an attempt to either pass on the spare electron, or to pinch a positive charge with which to neutralize it. This chemical process is known as oxidation and one of the best known examples is when iron oxidizes to form rust.

We need a certain amount of free radical activity in the body for certain metabolic and immune processes. Excess, however, will trigger harmful chain reactions in which spare electrical charges are shunted from one chemical to another, damaging proteins, fats, cell membranes and genetic material. When genetic material is damaged, mutations can occur and this is thought to be the main mechanism that triggers cancer. Oxidation of harmful LDL-cholesterol in the circulation creates changes that cause scavenger cells (macrophages) to recognize the fat as foreign. These cells try to remove the oxidized fat by engulfing it, and quickly become over-laden to form bloated 'foam' cells. These leave the circulation by squeezing between cells lining the artery wall where they become trapped and accumulate to form fatty plaques known as atheroma. Lack of antioxidants is now thought by many researchers to be the underlying cause of hardening and furring up of the arteries (atherosclerosis) in this way.

Each body cell undergoes an estimated 10,000 free radical oxidations per day. These oxidations have been linked with a number of degenerative problems and diseases, including hardening and furring up of the arteries, coronary heart disease, cataracts, macular degeneration of the eye, arthritis, premature ageing of the skin and cancer.

Why do we need antioxidants?

Antioxidants are the main defence against free radical attack. They work by quickly mopping up and neutralizing negative charges on free radicals before they can trigger a chain reaction. Several essential vitamins and minerals act as antioxidants. Of these, the most important are:

- vitamin A and betacarotene
- vitamin C
- vitamin E
- selenium.

Lesser antioxidants that are also important include:

- riboflavin
- copper
- manganese
- zinc.

Other antioxidants are also available in supplement form e.g. pine bark extracts, co-enzyme Q10, carotenoids such as lutein and lycopene, cat's claw, alpha-lipoic acid and reishi, plus bilberry, ginkgo, green tea or grapeseed extracts.

Free radicals are generated in a number of ways, including normal metabolic reactions, burning excess body fat while losing weight, exposure to environmental pollutants, during energy production processes when exercising, smoking cigarettes, drinking alcohol, inhaling exhaust fumes, exposure to environmental pollution, x-rays or UVA sunlight and when taking certain drugs – especially antibiotics or paracetamol. Smokers and people with diabetes generate more than usual.

You cannot avoid generating a certain number of free radicals, as some are important for health, but you can minimize the damage caused by excess through ensuring that your intake of antioxidants is high. Many antioxidant supplements are now available to help quench free radicals and protect against their harmful effects. A free radical urine test is also available to help monitor how many free radicals you generate.

Although diet should always come first, many experts now agree that food cannot supply the optimum quantities of antioxidants needed. Surveys suggest that the majority of people do not obtain all the vitamins C, E and carotenoids they need from their food.

Researchers have analysed blood levels of antioxidants in large numbers of people and followed them up to see how many developed coronary heart disease and cancer. Those with the least risk of these diseases are those with the highest circulating levels of protective antioxidants. Recommended daily intakes of antioxidants such as vitamin C were defined as a means of preventing deficiencies such as scurvy, and modern evidence suggests that we might benefit from higher intakes. The daily intake of antioxidant vitamins needed to obtain the same high blood levels as the 20 per cent of people with the lowest risk of coronary heart disease and cancer is as follows:

- vitamin C – 150–250 mg/day
- vitamin E – 50–100 mg/day
- mixed carotenoids – 15 mg/day
- selenium 100 mcg/day.

Those people who smoke, have diabetes, or who are on a slimming diet probably need twice as many antioxidants as other people.

Several important studies have found the following:

● Rats fed on a high antioxidant diet lived, on average, for 18 per cent longer than those not given antioxidants.

● Vitamin C can reduce the amount of harmful LDL-cholesterol that seeps into artery walls by a massive 93 per cent; vitamin E can reduce it by at least 45 per cent.

● The risk of angina among 6000 middle-aged male volunteers was found to be three times higher in those with low levels of vitamins E, C and betacarotene.

● Among 87,000 female nurses and 40,000 male doctors the risk of coronary heart disease was reduced by up to 50 per cent in women and 25 per cent in men taking vitamin E supplements for two years or more.

● Those with the highest intakes of natural betacarotene have a lower risk of coronary heart disease – 22 per cent lower in females and 25 per cent lower in males.

● A ten-year study in California, involving 11,000 people, showed that a high intake of vitamin C lowers the risk of coronary heart disease in men by a dramatic 40 per cent and their risk of dying was 35 per cent lower. Women had a 25 per cent lower risk of heart disease.

● People with the highest antioxidant intake have the lowest risk of cancers affecting the mouth, throat, larynx, oesophagus, stomach, lung, breast, bladder, colon, rectum, cervix, endometrium or prostate gland.

- People who take vitamin C supplements or who eat a diet rich in both vitamins C and A have up to a 45 per cent decreased risk of developing cataracts than those whose diet is poor in vitamin C. Spinach seems to be one of the most protective foods.

One study caused confusion when it was found that smokers taking supplements of vitamin E and betacarotene (singly or together) did not have a lower risk of developing coronary heart disease – and perhaps had a higher risk of developing lung cancer. This contrasted sharply with other trials showing positive effects from taking antioxidant vitamins. However, apart from the fact that the hardened smokers had a high risk of lung cancer before they even started taking the supplements, the lack of additional protection was probably because no vitamin C supplements were taken. Vitamins C and E work together: C is needed to regenerate E after it has performed its antioxidant function. If inadequate amounts of vitamin C are present, vitamin E is not regenerated, and in fact acts as a free radical itself. High dose vitamin E supplements should therefore be taken together with vitamin C.

Single carotenoids such as betacarotene are probably not a good idea either, and it is now considered better to take supplements containing mixed carotenoids instead – which is how they are found in nature.

Arginine

L-arginine is an amino acid that can be synthesized in the body but may become essential for adults under stress or for those who are recovering from injury or surgery. It must then come from the diet, and can be found in many protein foods such as nuts, seeds, pulses, beetroot, onions, grapes, rice, egg yolk and red meat.

Benefits

L-arginine plays an important role in the metabolism of dietary protein, during which ammonia is formed and must be detoxified and converted into urea in the liver.

It also increases the body's levels of a nerve communication chemical (neurotransmitter) called nitric oxide (NO). NO is essential for a number of physiological processes, including increasing blood flow to the penis for normal erectile function and sexual arousal. It also helps to regulate blood pressure, improves circulatory tone and muscle metabolism.

High-dose L-arginine may be helpful for people with congestive heart failure by reducing symptoms, increasing the distance they are able to walk and improving the flow of blood through the arteries. It is also used to reduce an abnormally raised cholesterol level, hardening and furring up of the arteries (atherosclerosis), coronary heart disease and angina. In one study, people with angina who took L-arginine three times a day increased the amount of exercise they could take at moderate intensity without having to stop because of chest pain.

L-arginine stimulates production of insulin in the pancreas and has been shown to improve blood glucose control in people with non-insulin-dependent diabetes.

It also stimulates production of growth hormone and anti-diuretic hormone (vasopressin) in the pituitary gland. It is involved in collagen synthesis and wound healing and is therefore needed during recovery from surgery, injuries and burns. It boosts production and activity of T-lymphocytes to improve immunity against certain infectious diseases and may also play a role in preventing cancer.

Many researchers believe that L-arginine is one of the best all-round prosexual supplements for men. By boosting blood flow to the penis, it produces bigger, firmer erections more frequently and may also improve sensitivity. It is helpful both for men whose sexual function is normal and for those who have erectile difficulties. In one small trial, 15 men with erectile dysfunction took placebo pills for two weeks, then took 2.8 g L-arginine. None of those taking placebo noticed an effect but 6 noticed increased erections while receiving L-arginine. It is also beneficial for women as it is said to improve sexual stamina in both men and women.

L-arginine is also important for sperm health. Seminal fluids contain as much as 80 per cent arginine which helps to improve the quality and motility of sperm. Sperm count can sometimes be increased in men with an unexplained low sperm count and infertility by taking 4–8 g of L-arginine daily.

L-arginine is also believed to play a role in improving learning and memory.

It can take between two and six weeks for L-arginine to achieve its optimum (accumulative) effect.

Dose

500 mg-2 g a day. Some nutritionists advise doses of up to 4 g a day. When taken for its beneficial sexual actions, it

should ideally be taken one hour before sex. Some men require doses of 6 g to achieve a noticeable effect, but this may cause an unwanted side effect of diarrhoea.

In clinical studies, much higher doses (e.g. 6–12 g daily) have been used to treat certain conditions such as coronary heart disease. Doses of above 20 g are not generally recommended.

L-arginine is usually taken on an empty stomach before retiring (as growth hormone is mainly released at night). Supplements in which arginine is chelated with manganese are most easily absorbed.

Side effects

Side effects are uncommon, but high doses may lead to reversible thickening and coarsening of the skin with long term use according to some sources. Those prone to *Herpes simplex* infections (cold sores) are advised not to take L-arginine supplements without balancing them with equal intakes of the amino acid, lysine. Some evidence has suggested that L-arginine helps replication of herpes viruses and may stimulate a recurrence although this is not proven. This effect can be neutralized by lysine which suppresses the growth of viruses.

Contraindications

L-arginine should not be taken:
- during pregnancy
- while breast-feeding
- by children
- by anyone with reduced kidney or liver function
- by those with auto-immune conditions (e.g. rheumatoid arthritis, glomerulonephritis) except under medical supervision (studies in rats have suggested that a low-

arginine diet is more beneficial for immune function in these cases).

Those with schizophrenia should not take very high doses as it may make symptoms worse.

Artichoke
(Cynara scolymus)

Globe artichoke is a perennial herb native to the Mediterranean. Its leaves contain several unique substances such as cynarin, cynaropicrin, cynaroside, plus antioxidant flavonoids such as luteolin. Although it is the fleshy flower that is eaten as a delicacy, it is the leaves that contain the most active ingredients.

Benefits
Globe artichoke is related to the milk thistle and has similar liver regenerating and protective properties. It is used to:
- increase bile secretion and improve digestion of dietary fats
- protect liver cells from toxins – especially alcohol
- reduce blood cholesterol levels and offer protection against atherosclerosis
- stimulate appetite.

A number of studies have shown that artichoke leaf extracts can successfully reduce the effects of excess alcohol, lower cholesterol levels, increase bile secretion and significantly improve digestive symptoms such as bloating, flatulence, nausea and abdominal pain due to intestinal spasm. It usually works quickly, within 15 to 20 minutes. Artichoke extracts also have powerful antioxidant properties and a mild diuretic action which may enhance its anti-bloating effects.

Bile is a yellow-green fluid made in the liver and stored in the gall bladder until needed. When food leaves the stomach and enters the first section of the small intestines (duodenum) this triggers a reflex contraction of the gall bladder which squirts bile into the duodenum where it mixes with food. Bile contains salts and acids that break down fat globules into smaller particles (emulsification) so they can be absorbed and processed more easily.

In one randomized, placebo-controlled trial involving 20 men with acute or chronic symptoms, 320 mg artichoke extracts were shown to increase bile secretion by over 127 per cent after 30 minutes, 151 per cent after 60 minutes and 94 per cent after 90 minutes.

Bloating, spasm and impaired gastrointestinal function are symptoms of irritable bowel syndrome (IBS) and, among 279 people with dyspeptic syndrome who also had symptoms compatible with IBS, 96 per cent found that standardized *Cynara* artichoke supplements were as effective, if not better, than previous treatments they had taken. Overall, IBS symptoms were reduced by 71 per cent within an average of 10 days although a third of those tested noticed an effect within one week. During the six-week study, only three people developed adverse effects that were thought to be associated with artichoke leaf extracts. These were hunger in one person and transient increase in flatulence in two.

A study involving over 550 people has shown that taking artichoke extracts for six weeks can reduce nausea by 82 per cent, vomiting by 88 per cent, bloating by 66 per cent, abdominal pain by 76 per cent, constipation by 71 per cent, fat intolerance by 59 per cent and swelling of the lower legs by 46 per cent.

Similar studies have shown artichoke leaf extracts can lower cholesterol levels by 11.5 per cent and triglyceride levels by 12.5 per cent. After six months treatment there was also an increase in the beneficial, protective HDL-cholesterol level of 6.3 per cent, while for those whose total cholesterol levels were very high, the harmful LDL-cholesterol was reduced by an impressive 20.8 per cent. This was mostly due to the effects of cynaroside and luteolin on blocking synthesis of excess cholesterol in the liver. Importantly, this cholesterol-blocking action does not reduce production of necessary amounts of cholesterol however, as may occur with prescription-only synthetic lipid blockers.

Because artichoke contains insulin, the rate at which glucose is produced after eating is slowed so that large swings in blood levels do not occur. This is especially helpful for people with diabetes.

Dose
Dried leaf: 2 g, three times a day.
Extracts: 320 mg capsules, 1–6 capsules a day, with food.
Tincture: 6 ml, three times a day.

Contraindications
● Do not use globe artichoke if there is obstruction of bile ducts or jaundice.
● In case of gallstones, use only after consulting a physician.

Ashwagandha
(Withania somnifera)

Ashwagandha – also known as winter cherry or Indian ginseng – is a small evergreen shrub native to India, the Mediterranean and Middle East. Its dried root contains iron and a series of unique steroidal lactones known as withanolides.

Benefits

Ashwagandha is used as a restorative tonic in Ayurvedic medicine, to improve resistance to stress. It is a powerful adaptogen whose properties are well researched, and may be superior to those of Korean ginseng for improving mental acuity, reaction time and physical performance in healthy people.

Studies suggest, for example, that ashwagandha can prevent the depletion of vitamin C and cortisol (an adrenal hormone) during times of stress, as well as preventing stress-related gastrointestinal ulcers. Other studies have shown that it can increase haemoglobin levels and that it also has anti-inflammatory properties. It may also be used to reduce greying of hair.

Ashwagandha reduces anxiety and promotes serenity and deep sleep, especially in those suffering from overwork or nervous exhaustion. It is also said to strengthen muscles, tendons, bones, improve concentration, boost immunity and energy levels. It is a renowned aphrodisiac that can improve sexual performance (especially during convalescence) and it is sometimes used to treat impotence. Although it may be used in both men and women, its prosexual actions are probably best reserved for use in men.

Dose

Capsules standardized to contain 2–5 mg with anolides: 150–300 mg.

Because Ashwagandha is somewhat difficult to digest, it is often taken with ginger, warm milk, honey or hot water.

Astragalus
(*Astragalus membranaceus*)

Astragalus (also known as Chinese milkvetch) is an herbaceous perennial native to northern China, Japan, Korea and Tibet. Its root has been used as a traditional Chinese herbal remedy for over 2000 years to balance the life-force energy known as Qi. The medicinal creamy-white root is harvested from plants that are four to seven years old and it has a sweet taste similar to liquorice, so that it is sometimes used in cooking.

Benefits

Astragalus is classed as an adaptogen, helping to support adrenal gland function during times of physical stress, to improve physical endurance as well as being an immune enhancer. It acts as an antioxidant and has antibacterial, anti-viral and anti-fungal actions which are widely used to both treat and prevent respiratory infections (colds, flu, bronchitis, sinusitis) and urinary tract infections. It also has mild diuretic properties and can lower blood pressure.

Astragalus contains a variety of unique substances such as astragalosides that have been shown to improve all aspects of immune function. It can increase proliferation of T-lymphocytes (cells that regulate immune responses), boost the activity of phagocytic (cell-eating) white blood cells, it increases the activity of natural killer cells (which wipe out infected or abnormal body cells) and improves antibody synthesis. It also stimulates production of the powerful anti-viral substance, interferon. It is taken by many people with HIV for its immunosupportive actions.

As astragalus also increases production of red blood cells (to improve oxygen carriage in the circulation) it is often used to treat anaemia.

In people undergoing treatment for cancer, astragalus is used to protect adrenal gland function, improve tolerance to chemotherapy, reduce bone marrow suppression and to minimize any gastrointestinal side effects. It is also helpful in protecting against the free radicals generated during both chemotherapy and radiotherapy.

In those with coronary heart disease, astragalus has protective effects on the cardiovascular system, reducing platelet aggregation, reducing oxidative damage and improving abnormal myocardial electric activity. Studies involving patients with ischemic heart disease found that it was at least as effective in strengthening heart muscle contraction, correcting abnormal electrical activity and dilating blood vessels and in preventing angina pain as a commonly prescribed drug (nifedipine). If taken within a day of a heart attack, similar protective effects are achieved with improved pumping function of the left side of the heart.

Other uses include stimulating sperm motility, improving healing of wounds and peptic ulcers and reducing excessive perspiration (including night sweats). It is also used for its protective actions in inflammation of the liver (e.g. chronic hepatitis) or kidneys (nephritis). It is often recommended to diabetes sufferers for reducing complications such as high blood pressure and poor wound healing.

Dose

For general use, 200–400 mg a day. Astragalus is usually taken for two to three weeks and then alternated with another immune booster such as echinacea or cat's claw. If taken for a respiratory or urinary infection, the dose is usually doubled.

Choose extracts that are standardized to 0.5 per cent glucosides and 70 per cent polysaccharides.

It is often used together with Korean ginseng or echinacea.

Contraindications

● Traditionally, astragalus is best avoided if you have a fever or if you suffer from skin disorders.
● Avoid during pregnancy and breast-feeding except under specialist advice.

B1

Vitamin B1, also known as thiamin or thiamine, is a water-soluble vitamin that is essential for the production of energy from glucose, for transmission of electrical messages in nerve and muscle cells, including the heart, and for the production of red blood cells. It is also needed for the synthesis of some important amino acids and it plays a role in digestion.

Foods containing vitamin B1 include whole grains, oats, soy flour, pasta, meat – especially pork and duck – seafood, nuts and pulses. Brewer's yeast and yeast extracts are also good sources.

Thiamin is easily lost by food processing e.g. chopping, mincing, liquidizing, canning and preserving. Boiling reduces the thiamin content of foods by half as it is so water soluble. It is also destroyed by high temperatures and adding baking powder. Toasting bread can lose almost a third of its thiamin content.

In general, the more carbohydrate you eat, the more thiamin you need. As vitamin B1 is water soluble, it is easily lost from the body through the kidneys and most people only have sufficient stores to last one month.

Benefits

People taking diuretics often lose enough thiamin in their urine to cause thiamin deficiency, and supplements can improve symptoms such as tiredness that may result.

Vitamin B1 also has a beneficial effect on mood, helping you feel more calm, agreeable, clear-headed, elated and energetic. People with low levels of thiamin are less likely to feel composed or self-confident and more likely to suffer from depression than those with higher levels. Even young female students who were not lacking in vitamin B1 were shown to have increased energy levels and alertness, as well as improved mood from taking 50 mg thiamin, while those taking a placebo did not notice a significant benefit.

Many people over the age of 55 have low intakes of thiamin – supplements may help them to increase feelings of general well-being, reduce fatigue and boost appetite. In one trial, 10 mg helped people over the age of 65 to enjoy better quality sleep, increased energy levels and lower blood pressure than those taking a placebo.

Thiamin is especially helpful for symptoms of tingling (pins and needles) and numbness that can occur in some forms of nerve disorder (neuropathy) such as that occurring in diabetes. It has also been used to improve indigestion and to help reduce emotional or psychological symptoms occurring with alcohol withdrawal.

Deficiency

In underdeveloped countries, thiamin deficiency is common especially where the main dietary staple is polished rather than brown rice. This causes a disease known as 'beri-beri', meaning 'extreme weakness'. Dry beri-beri produces heaviness, weakness, numbness and pins and needles in the legs, while wet beri-beri causes severe fluid retention. In those with a high alcohol intake, lack of thiamin is associated with Wernicke-Korsakoff syndrome which, if left untreated, leads to irreversible dementia.

Dose

1–50 mg – usually as part of a B group complex.

The EC RDA for thiamin is 1.4 mg. It is non-toxic as any excess is readily lost in the urine. A regular dietary supply is therefore essential, otherwise deficiency quickly occurs. People drinking large amounts of coffee or tea – which destroy the vitamin – may become thiamin deficient. Other common causes of thiamin deficiency include stress – which quickly uses up available thiamin stores – and drinking too much alcohol, which interferes with thiamin metabolism.

B2

Vitamin B2 – also known as riboflavin – is a water-soluble vitamin that plays an important role in metabolizing proteins, fats and carbohydrate and in the production of energy, thyroid hormones and red blood cells.

Benefits

Vitamin B2 acts as an antioxidant, and helps to maintain immunity as it is involved in the production of antibodies. Riboflavin helps to keep skin, hair, eyes, eye lenses and mucus membranes healthy. It also seems to be important for brain function, as people with good intakes of riboflavin are more likely to show high scores in tests of mental functioning than those with low levels.

As it is water soluble, riboflavin cannot be stored in the body, and a regular dietary intake is essential. Food sources include yeast extract, whole grains, eggs, dairy products, green leafy vegetables and pulses. Although milk is a rich source, its riboflavin content is quickly destroyed when exposed to light so milk sold in cartons contains a higher amount than that sold in bottles. Fortified cereals are another good source, and children who eat them for breakfast are less likely to have inadequate intakes of riboflavin compared with those who do not eat fortified cereals.

Vitamin B2 is often included in nutritional supplements designed to improve the symptoms of pre-menstrual syndrome as it is needed to convert vitamin B6 into its active form. It may also help to reduce migraine attacks, including those associated with menstruation, and is often recommended to reduce the facial redness that occurs in rosacea.

Riboflavin may provide some protection against certain congenital abnormalities (neural tube defects e.g. spina bifida) during early pregnancy in addition to that given by folic acid and vitamin B12.

Riboflavin is needed to protect the eye lens from free radical attack and, in a study involving around 3250 people, those taking supplements of vitamins B2 and B3 were 44 per cent less likely to develop lens opacities (cataracts) than those not taking them.

Older people with low riboflavin levels may have reduced immunity due to sub-optimal antibody production and are also at higher risk of developing cataracts.

People with chronic fatigue syndrome often benefit from taking B group supplements and preliminary research suggests their level of B vitamin activity – including that of riboflavin – is low. Vitamin B2 deficiency may be a cause of recurrent aphthous mouth ulcers in some people.

Other signs that may be due to lack of riboflavin include eyes that are bloodshot, red, tired and which feel gritty or sensitive; cataracts, sores and cracks at the corner of the mouth, a red, inflamed tongue and lips, hair loss, a scaly eczema-like skin rash (seborrhoeic dermatitis), especially on the face and nose as well as trembling, dizziness, difficulty sleeping and poor concentration or memory.

Dose

1.3–50 mg.

For some conditions such as migraine, much higher doses of up to 200–400 mg daily may be prescribed.

The EC RDA for riboflavin is 1.6 mg.

People who are physically active need more riboflavin than those who take little regular exercise. Recent studies also suggest that metabolism changes with age, so older people need to obtain more B2 from their diet to maintain blood levels of this vitamin.

Excess

Excess will be excreted in the urine, and when taking supplements containing riboflavin, urine colour becomes noticeably more yellow.

B3

Vitamin B3 is a water-soluble vitamin, also known as niacin, which exists in two forms: nicotinic acid or nicotinamide.

Niacin is obtained from a number of dietary sources, including whole grains, nuts, meat and poultry, oily fish, eggs, dairy products, dried fruit and yeast extract. Children who eat fortified cereals for breakfast are more likely to have adequate intakes of niacin than those who do not.

Vitamin B3 can also be made in the body in small amounts from the essential amino acid tryptophan (60 mg tryptophan produces 1 mg niacin). Because of this, many foods and supplements may describe their vitamin B3 content in the form of 'niacin equivalents' which are equal to the amount of nicotinamide and nicotinic acid they contain plus one-sixtieth of their tryptophan content. Eggs and cheese are some of the richest dietary sources of tryptophan.

Benefits

Niacin is important for healthy growth and development. Like other B group vitamins, it plays an important role in metabolism, enzyme function and energy production. It is essential for releasing energy from muscle sugar stores (glycogen) and for the uptake and use of oxygen in cells. Niacin works together with vitamins B1 (thiamin) and B2 (riboflavin) for these tasks, and also works on its own to maintain healthy skin, nerves, intestines and intellectual function. In one study involving around 3250 people, those taking supplements of vitamins B2 and B3 were 44 per cent less likely to develop lens opacities (cataracts) than those not taking them.

Niacin also combines with the mineral chromium to form the Glucose Tolerance Factor (GTF). This is essential for the action of the hormone, insulin, in controlling the way glucose is taken up into body cells. Lack of either chromium or niacin is associated with impaired glucose tolerance which may lead to diabetes.

Because niacin is important for the processing of fatty acids released from body fat stores, it is used medicinally to lower abnormally high cholesterol levels. In particular, it lowers levels of harmful LDL-cholesterol and triglycerides, while raising levels of beneficial HDL-cholesterol. At high doses (under medical supervision) it has been shown to reduce the risk of both non-fatal and fatal heart attacks.

Vitamin B3 is a fast-acting aphrodisiac in its pure form. It widens blood vessels and produces a so-called niacin flush similar to the sexual flush. It improves blood flow to the penis and also stimulates secretion of histamine – a chemical that naturally helps to intensify sensations during orgasm. It should not be taken in high doses, however, as this can cause toxic side effects.

Niacin has proved helpful in treating depression, reducing symptoms due to both osteoarthritis and rheumatoid arthritis and has been shown to reduce blood levels of thyroid hormones without causing symptoms of underactivity. These findings are under further investigation as a possible treatment for arthritis and thyroid disorders. Further studies are also under way to investigate niacin's ability to improve glucose control and reduce the risk of insulin-dependent (Type 1) diabetes, and to investigate a possible protective role against cancer.

Deficiency

Lack of vitamin B3 produces a rare deficiency disease known as pellagra which classically produces symptoms of dermatitis, diarrhoea and dementia. This occurs in parts of Africa where the diet contains large quantities of maize whose niacin is in a non-useable form of niacytin. In central America, maize for cooking tortillas is soaked overnight in calcium hydroxide which releases the niacin content.

Dose

The EC RDA for niacin is 18 mg. People who are physically active need more niacin than those with a sedentary lifestyle. When used for medicinal purposes, higher doses of 50 mg niacin a day may be taken. Doses as high as 1500 mg nicotinamide may be prescribed daily for certain medical disorders. Therapeutic use of high-dose niacin usually needs regular blood liver function tests.

Side effects

High-dose niacin (especially in the form of nicotinic acid) can produce a red flush and warming of the skin similar to blushing. People who blush easily seem to be more sensitive to this effect. For those who are very sensitive, a low dose of aspirin (75–300 mg) taken half an hour before the dose of niacin can reduce this effect.

Excess

Symptoms of niacin toxicity can occur at very high doses, including thickening and darkening of patches of skin (acanthosis nigricans), palpitations, worsening of pre-existing conditions such as diabetes and peptic ulceration. Gout and liver inflammation (hepatitis) can also be triggered.

Contraindications

Niacin should not be taken by sufferers of diabetes, low blood pressure, gout, liver disease, glaucoma or peptic ulcers except under medical advice.

Niacin has been shown to increase absorption of dietary zinc and iron from the gut.

B5

Vitamin B5, or pantothenic acid, is a water-soluble vitamin widely found in foods such as whole grains, beans, vegetables, nuts, eggs, meats and yeast extract. One of the richest supplementary sources is royal jelly. Despite its wide distribution in foods, many people do not obtain optimum levels of pantothenic acid, as it is easily destroyed by food processing and by deep freezing.

Benefits

Like other B group vitamins, pantothenic acid is vital for many energy-yielding metabolic reactions involving carbohydrates, fats and protein. It is particularly significant in the synthesis of glucose and fatty acids which are both important fuels for muscle cells and may even improve athletic performance. It has also been suggested that supplements containing pantothenic acid may help during weight-loss diets by ensuring that fatty acids released from body fat stores are fully broken down. This will reduce the formation of ketones so that hunger pangs and weakness are reduced.

Vitamin B5 can stimulate cell growth in healing tissues by increasing the number and speed of cells moving into wounds, increasing the rate at which these cells divide and improving protein synthesis. This encourages stronger scar tissue formation, helps to rejuvenate ageing skin and to reduce skin mottling.

Its boost to healing processes may also explain why vitamin B5 derivatives (calcium pantothenate and pantotheine) are effective in treating viral hepatitis A. When given to 156 patients with this relatively common infection, their liver function tests improved and blood antibody levels increased as did the activity of white blood cells. Pantotheine produced the most pronounced therapeutic effect.

Vitamin B5 plays a role in the production of adrenal gland hormones during times of stress and in maintaining a healthy nervous system. It is also taken to reduce nasal congestion, increase resistance to stress, to help overcome chronic fatigue and indigestion and as an aid in giving up smoking.

Some researchers believe that there is a link between acne and a lack of pantothenic acid. It is also added to many shampoos and conditioners and is said to improve hair colour and lustre and to reduce grey hairs, although there is little evidence to support this. It has been shown to reduce hair loss and to thicken hair structure in some women, however.

Deficiency

Symptoms that may be caused by a lack of vitamin B5 include weakness and fatigue, headache, difficulty in coping with stress, poor muscle co-ordination and muscle cramps, numbness and tingling sensations, loss of appetite, nausea, indigestion, abdominal cramps, painful and burning feet, increased susceptibility to infection, poor wound healing, difficulty in sleeping and depression.

Dose

An intake of around 4–7 mg is believed to be adequate, although doses of up to 1 g daily may be taken to treat problems such as chronic fatigue.

The EC RDA for vitamin B5 is 6 mg. Some studies suggest extra B5 is needed to maintain blood levels of this vitamin as you get older.

B6

Vitamin B6 is not just one vitamin, but a group of water-soluble compounds including pyridoxine, pyridoxal and pyridoxamine, which are all converted to the most active form, pyridoxine, in the body. As it is water soluble, it is readily lost in the urine, so regular intakes are essential. Food sources of vitamin B6 include whole grains, liver, meat, oily fish, soy products, bananas, nuts (especially walnuts), green leafy vegetables, avocado and egg yolk. Yeast extract and royal jelly are also good sources.

Benefits

Pyridoxine is an essential co-factor for the action of over 60 enzymes involved in the synthesis of genetic material, amino acids, proteins and the metabolism of carbohydrate and essential fatty acids. It is especially important for the health of rapidly dividing cells such as those found in the gut, skin, hair follicles and marrow as well as those involved in immunity. It increases production of antibodies and the number and activity of T4–helper lymphocytes. It is therefore undergoing investigation in the treatment of infectious diseases including AIDS, as well as cancer.

Vitamin B6 is involved in the synthesis of some brain chemicals (neurotransmitters) that pass messages from one brain cell to another and pass impulses down nerve endings, and many people with depression may have vitamin B6 deficiency. It is also involved in regulating the function of sex hormones which may explain why it is often helpful in the treatment of pre-menstrual syndrome.

An analysis of nine trials involving over 900 women has confirmed that high doses of up to 100 mg vitamin B6 daily can help to reduce symptoms in women with pre-menstrual syndrome, including premenstrual depression.

Recent research provides preliminary evidence that people with chronic fatigue syndrome are lacking in some B group vitamins, including vitamin B6. Taking supplements may therefore help people with long-term tiredness.

Vitamin B6 is needed for the production of hydrochloric acid in the stomach so that calcium can be absorbed. It is also necessary for cross-linking collagen (bone matrix material) and for breaking down homocysteine – an amino acid which in excess is linked with osteoporosis and heart disease. A raised blood level of the amino acid, homocysteine, is now recognized as an important risk factor for developing coronary heart disease and stroke. Homocysteine is formed in the body from the breakdown of the dietary amino acid methionine. Normally, its level is tightly controlled by three different enzymes that convert homocysteine to cysteine – a safe end product used by cells for growth. When certain B vitamins are lacking, including vitamin B6, this conversion cannot occur so efficiently and potentially harmful levels of homocysteine build up in the circulation. Taking supplements of B group vitamins (folic acid plus vitamins B6 and B12) has been shown to lower homocysteine levels where they are raised – especially in older people. Results from following over 600 women for 14 years shows that those with the highest intakes of folic acid and vitamin B6 had the lowest risk of coronary heart disease after other factors such as smoking and intakes of alcohol, fat and vitamin E were taken into account.

Vitamin B6 supplements may protect against kidney stones as it decreases the production of a chemical, oxalate, that is found in many kidney stones. It can also help to improve asthma by reducing the severity and frequency of attacks.

Deficiency

Lack of vitamin B6 can cause carpal tunnel syndrome, recurrent mouth ulcers (aphthous ulceration), split lips, red, inflamed tongue, burning skin, anaemia, headache and symptoms similar to those occurring in PMS such as anxiety, irritability, mild depression, bloating and tender breasts. Some studies suggest that as many as one in five women is deficient in B6.

Dose

Supplements range from 1–100 mg depending on what they are being used for. Higher doses (within this range) are suggested for PMS. Do not take high doses for more than a few months without seeking medical advice. There have been some suggestions that prolonged high doses may cause reversible nerve symptoms such as pins and needles, but this is not conclusive.

The EC RDA for vitamin B6 is 2 mg. In general, the more protein you eat, the more vitamin B6 you need.

Taken at a dose of 25 mg daily for five days, vitamin B6 can help to relieve the severity of nausea due to morning sickness in early pregnancy but a doctor should be consulted before taking them.

Vitamin B6 supplements (20 mg daily for 3 months) can improve memory in older people.

B12

Vitamin B12, also known as cobalamin, is a water-soluble substance that contains cobalt – the only known requirement for this metal in the human body. Unlike most water-soluble vitamins, B12 can be stored in the liver with enough stocks to last for several years.

Food sources of vitamin B12 include liver, kidney, oily fish – especially sardines – red meats, white fish, eggs and dairy products. Vegetarians, especially vegans, are at risk of vitamin B12 deficiency since it is only found in animal-based foods. No natural plant products contain consistent amounts of vitamin B12 with the possible exception of blue-green algae and there is some controversy over whether the

B12 they contain is in an active form. Vitamin B12 is, however, also made by bacteria, and supplements containing B12 derived from bacterial cultures are available that are ethically acceptable to most vegetarians.

Vitamin B12 is absorbed in the lower part of the small intestine, but only if a special carrier protein, intrinsic factor, is present. Intrinsic factor is made in the stomach and vitamin B12 deficiency can develop due to lack of intrinsic factor, lack of acid production in the stomach or due to inflammatory conditions of the small intestine such as Crohn's disease.

Benefits

Vitamin B12 is needed together with another vitamin, folic acid, when new genetic material (DNA) is made during cell division. It is most needed by cells with a rapid turnover such as those lining the gut (shed every three days on average), cells in hair follicles and in the marrow, which is continually producing new red blood cells.

Vitamin B12 also plays a role in the formation of healthy nerve sheaths (myelin) needed for the transmission of electrical signals down nerve endings and may be helpful for treating pins and needles, neuropathy, tinnitus and multiple sclerosis. It is also needed for healthy immunity, appetite and for healing during convalescence.

Together with folic acid, vitamin B12 seems to protect against some congenital developmental disorders (neural tube defects) such as spina bifida.

A raised blood level of the amino acid, homocysteine, is now recognized as an important risk factor for developing coronary heart disease and stroke. Homocysteine is formed in the body from the breakdown of the dietary amino acid, methionine. Normally, its level is tightly controlled by three different enzymes that convert homocysteine to cysteine – a safe end product used by cells for growth. When certain B vitamins are lacking, including vitamin B12, this conversion cannot occur so efficiently and potentially harmful levels of homocysteine build up in the circulation. Taking supplements of B group vitamins (folic acid plus vitamins B6 and B12) has been shown to lower raised homocysteine levels – especially in older people.

Deficiency

Low vitamin B12 levels are common in the elderly both because of reduced dietary intake and reduced absorption from the gut (malabsorption) linked with reduced production of hydrochloric acid in the stomach.

Lack of vitamin B12 causes production of cells that are larger than they should be. In the case of red blood cells, this leads to a particular form of anaemia known as pernicious anaemia. As this creeps up slowly, symptoms are often not recognized until it is advanced. If deficiency is not corrected, nerves in the spinal cord can be damaged leading to a rare condition known as sub-acute, combined degeneration of the cord.

Other symptoms that may be due to vitamin B12 deficiency include a smooth, sore tongue, tiredness, exhaustion, menstrual disorders, numbness, tingling, trembling, clumsiness, difficulty walking, especially in the dark when you can't see where you are going, poor memory, lack of concentration, confusion and depression. Because the symptoms are so variable, vitamin B12 deficiency should be considered in all spinal cord, nerve and psychiatric disorders. Many people who are lacking in B12 do not develop obvious symptoms for several years, however.

Research suggests that lack of vitamin B12 can be associated with infection of the stomach with *Helicobacter pylori*, a motile form of bacteria that burrows into the stomach lining to trigger inflammation. Although it doesn't cause symptoms in everyone, virtually all patients with duodenal ulcers are infected, plus three quarters of those with gastric ulcers. *H. pylori* infection is also associated with an increased risk of gastric cancer.

B12 is needed to make antibodies after vaccination, or infections and, in people who are HIV positive, those with the highest levels of B12 seem to progress to AIDS more slowly than those whose levels are low.

Dose

Doses vary from 1 mcg daily (in A to Z-style formulas) to as much as 1000 mcg (1 mg) for treating specific conditions such as tinnitus or multiple sclerosis. Although vitamin B12 supplements to treat pernicious anaemia are traditionally given as regular injections, it can be given orally in very high dose (e.g. 2 mg=2000 mcg a day). Research is also currently looking at giving it by absorption through the mucus membranes of the mouth (e.g. under the tongue) or nose.

The EC RDA for vitamin B12 is 1 mcg.

Vitamin B12 supplements are best taken together with folic acid (folate) supplements.

Excess

As excess B12 is excreted in the urine, there are no known toxic side effects from high doses.

Bee products

The four main bee products used as health supplements are:

● bee pollen
● royal jelly
● propolis
● manuka honey.

Bee pollen

Pollen is an ultra-fine dust made up of sex cells produced on the anthers of male flowers. When foraging for nectar, bees visit as many as 1500 blossoms during their life. The collected pollen is compressed into granules – known as bee pollen – and transported back to the hive. Each granule contains as many as 5 million live pollen grains and is stored in honeycomb cells as 'beebread', to feed young, developing bees.

Bee pollen is rich in B-complex vitamins, essential fatty acids, and also contains 28 minerals, 22 amino acids and thousands of enzymes and co-enzymes.

Benefits

Unfortunately, little research has been carried out into the beneficial effects of bee pollen although it is widely used as a nutritious tonic. Some evidence suggests it is helpful for reducing allergic symptoms such as sneezing, runny nose, watering eyes and nasal congestion. This may act by desensitizing the immune system, and bee pollen collected from your local environment seems to be most effective in this respect.

Bee pollen needs to be freeze-dried to preserve its nutrients intact.

Dose
Start with a few granules daily, and if no allergic symptoms develop (e.g. wheezing, rash, headache, itching), increase the dose to 250 mg–2g daily for at least one month.

Contraindications
Bee pollen should be avoided if you are allergic to bee products or to pollen, especially if you have asthma or are allergic to bee stings.

Royal jelly

Royal jelly is a milky-white substance – also known as bee's milk – secreted in the salivary glands of worker honey bees. It is a highly concentrated food given to all larvae for the first three days of their lives. After that, they're nourished on a diet of honey, pollen, and water except for the larva destined to become a queen bee which continues to receive royal jelly. It is such a nutritious and potent energy source that the queen bee grows to be 50 per cent larger than other genetically identical female bees and lives for nearly 40 times longer.

Benefits
Royal jelly is one of the richest natural sources of vitamin B5 (pantothenic acid), and also contains other B vitamins as well as vitamins A, C, D and E, 20 amino acids, essential fatty acids, minerals such as potassium, calcium, zinc, iron and manganese plus acetylcholine – a neurotransmitter needed to transmit messages from one nerve cell to another.

It also contains a powerful antibiotic that has been named royalisin. It is effective against gram-positive bacteria (e.g. *Staphylococci, Streptococci*) and may be effective when applied to skin although it is largely inactivated by stomach enzymes when taken by mouth.

In the laboratory, royal jelly seems to have an anti-tumour effect against a type of cancer cell known as sarcoma.

Royal jelly is traditionally taken to boost energy levels and mental alertness, and to combat stress, fatigue and insomnia. As a tonic, it boosts feelings of well-being, increases vitality, improves the complexion and helps to maintain healthy skin, hair and nails.

Royal jelly may help to protect against hardening and furring up of the arteries (atherosclerosis) by lowering total blood fats and abnormal cholesterol levels. In studies, doses of 50–100 mg royal jelly per day decreased total serum cholesterol levels by 14 per cent and total serum lipids by 10 per cent – possibly by increasing cholesterol excretion in the bile and decreasing its reabsorption in the gastrointestinal tract so that less enters the circulation.

Dose
Typically 50–100 mg a day.

Royal jelly must be blended with honey or freeze-dried to preserve its active ingredients. It is best kept refrigerated and taken on an empty stomach.

Contraindications
Royal jelly has been known to trigger severe asthma attacks in some people with asthma so do not take if you are allergic to bee products, or if you suffer from asthma or other allergic conditions.

Propolis

Propolis is a yellow-brown sticky resin – sometimes known as bee glue – that is made by some species of bees from wax mixed with the resinous sap of a variety of trees (e.g. beech, birch, chestnut, conifers). More than 180 compounds have been identified in propolis, many of which have anti-inflammatory, antioxidant and anti-cancer properties.

Bees use propolis as a cement to repair cracks and crevices in the hive and in honeycombs. It is also placed around hive entrances to help keep infections at bay. Given that a typical hive contains 50,000 bees, has a temperature of up to 95 degrees and 90 per cent humidity – perfect conditions for the growth of moulds, mildew and bacteria – it is remarkably effective.

Benefits

Propolis is a rich source of B group vitamins and also contains bioflavonoids – at a concentration 500 times greater than that in oranges – that help to improve the absorption and action of vitamin C.

Propolis works against bacteria by preventing bacterial cell division and by breaking down bacterial walls and cytoplasm. It is especially active against the bacteria that cause upper respiratory tract and skin infections, including strains that are resistant to penicillin.

Propolis has been used for over 2000 years as an antiseptic salve to hasten wound healing, overcome sore throats and as a supplement to boost energy levels and treat stomach ulcers. It helps to overcome infections of the skin, ear, nose, mouth and sinuses, and is frequently taken to boost immunity against colds and flu in winter.

One constituent of propolis, caffeic acid phenethyl ester, has been shown to have anti-cancer, anti-inflammatory and immune-boosting properties. It has also been shown to increase regeneration of tissues, including bone. It may also prevent unwanted blood clots and can help to lower high blood pressure.

Dose
250–500 mg a day. For acute infections, higher doses may be taken (e.g. four to eight 400–600 mg capsules a day for two weeks).

As propolis is not water soluble, it is usually extracted in alcohol and made into a tincture. It is also available as chewing gum, chips, lozenges, and powdered in capsules.

Contraindications
Propolis should not be taken by anyone who has an allergy to bee products. It causes allergic reactions in between 1 and 7 per cent of those taking it, including contact dermatitis in people with eczema.

Manuka honey

Manuka honey is made by bees feeding on nectar from the flower of the manuka, or New Zealand tea tree.

Benefits
It has unique antibacterial properties that are often effective in eradicating *Helicobacter pylori*, a bacterium which infects the stomachs of at least half the population, and is associated with peptic ulcers. Of all the honeys tested against *Helicobacter*, manuka honey was the only one able to cure the infection, even when diluted to a 5 per cent solution.

Manuka honey is sometimes also applied to wounds to help treat or prevent infections. Honeys absorb fluid due to their high concentration of natural sugars. This osmotic effect makes it difficult for bacteria to thrive. Manuka honey also releases natural antiseptics, hydrogen peroxide and gluconic acid which inhibit many common skin bacteria, especially *Staphylococcus aureas*.

Manuka honey contains an additional natural antibiotic known as the unique Manuka factor (UMF). Those with a rating of at least UMF 10 are as effective against the skin bacterium *Staphylococcus aureas* as a 10 per cent phenol solution.

Dose

To help eradicate *H. pylori*: usually taken on an empty stomach at a dose of four teaspoons, four times a day, for eight weeks. This provides around 80 kcals per dose and there are no guarantees it will work.

For use on the skin as an antiseptic, the honey is applied (e.g. to leg ulcers) on absorbent dressings under medical supervision, to draw fluid out of the infected area. The natural sugars have the extra beneficial action of stimulating tissue growth and feeding new cells. Dressings are changed three times a day. To draw out boils and carbuncles, a poultice is made by mixing equal parts of manuka honey and cod liver oil. This is applied on a gauze dressing and renewed every eight hours.

As some honeys contain spores from Clostridium bacteria, it may be wise to use a honey treated with gamma irradiation to prevent a theoretical risk of infection.

Bilberry
(Vaccinium myrtillus)

Bilberry is a small deciduous shrub native to central and northern Europe, northern Asia, and North America. It is related to the blueberry, blackcurrant and grape. While the American blueberry has creamy or white coloured flesh, that of the bilberry is purple so its content of antioxidant pigments is considerably higher.

Benefits
Its sweet, blue-black berries are used for culinary as well as medicinal purposes. They are a rich source of tannins, anthocyanins, and flavonoid glycosides that have powerful antioxidant and anti-inflammatory properties.

Bilberry has been used as a medicinal treatment for over a thousand years.

The dried berries were traditionally used for their astringent qualities in the treatment of diarrhoea, and have also been used to treat scurvy, cystitis, kidney stones and inflammation of the mucous membranes of mouth and throat.

Extracts are also used to strengthen blood vessels and the collagen-containing connective tissue that supports them, as well as improving circulation. These actions are used to treat easy-bruising syndrome, thread veins (telangiectasis), phlebitis, varicose veins and haemorrhoids for which it is particularly suited for use in pregnancy. In one study of almost 50 people with varicose veins, taking 480 mg bilberry extracts per day increased local circulation to reduce fluid retention, feelings of heaviness, pins and needles and pain, as well as improving the appearance of overlying skin. In addition, bilberry reduces the risk of stroke and inhibits unwanted clot formation.

Because of their beneficial effects on the circulation, bilberry extracts are prescribed in some parts of Europe for patients due to undergo surgery as it has been shown to reduce excessive bleeding by over 70 per cent.

Bilberry extracts are also established as a treatment for many eye disorders including macular degeneration, cataracts, night-blindness, glaucoma, retinitis pigmentosa and diabetic retinopathy. Its effectiveness in treating visual problems results from a number of actions. Its antioxidant blue-red pigments protect the membranes of light-sensitive and other cells in the eyes, reduce hardening and furring up of blood vessels, stabilize tear production, increase blood flow to the retina, regenerate the light-sensitive pigment rhodopsin, as well as increasing the strength of collagen fibres in capillaries and supportive connective tissues. Visual acuity improves by over 80 per cent within just 15 days.

Sufferers of diabetic retinopathy, in which haemorrhages form within the retina of the eye, especially benefit from these actions. The antioxidant effects also help to prevent the development and progression of cataracts, especially when combined with vitamin E. In one study of 50 patients with age-related cataracts, bilberry extract plus vitamin E stopped cataracts from progressing in 97 per cent of cases. Some researchers have also suggested that taking bilberry extracts can reduce short-sightedness after five months of regular use, perhaps by improving the reactivity and focusing ability of the eye lens.

The antioxidant anthocyanidins found in bilberries and other dark, blue-red pigmented fruits can lower uric acid levels and prevent gout attacks when around 250 g are eaten daily. They have also been found to help one in three women with breast pain due to benign fibrocystic disease and also to reduce painful periods through their muscle-relaxing action.

Bilberry contains a unique anthocyanoside called myrtillin which helps to lower a raised blood sugar level with a similar action to insulin. In the digestive tract, bilberry extracts have been shown to increase the secretion of protective mucus in the stomach to improve protection against peptic ulceration. One study found that bilberry extracts prevented ulcer development in over 60 per cent of people at risk versus just 12 per cent in those taking an inactive placebo.

Dose

20–60 g dried ripe fruit a day.

Dry extract (25 per cent anthocyanosides): 80–160 mg, three times a day. Diabetics may be advised to take more than this.

Excess

No toxicity has been found even at high doses, as bilberry extract is water soluble and excess is quickly excreted through the urine and bile.

Biotin

Biotin is a water-soluble member of the vitamin B group.

Benefits

It is important for the synthesis and metabolism of fatty acids, amino acids, genetic material, stress hormones and energy storage molecules. It is also essential for making and using glucose in the body, and for keeping skin, hair, nails, sweat glands and nerve cells healthy.

The EC RDA for biotin is only 0.15 mg (150 mcg) and biotin is widespread in the diet (e.g. in whole grains, rice, nuts, cauliflower, egg yolk, oily fish, liver and yeast extract). It is also produced by bacteria in the bowel although it may not be readily useable from this source.

Deficiency

Dietary deficiency of biotin is unusual, except in those following very low-calorie weight loss diets and in those eating large amounts of raw egg white over a long period (e.g. body builders who eat a dozen raw eggs a day): raw egg white contains a protein, called avidin, that acts as an anti-vitamin by binding to biotin in the gut and preventing its absorption. Cooked egg white does not have this effect.

People on long-term antibiotic treatment (e.g. for acne) may also be at risk of deficiency as this destroys normal bowel bacteria. When taking antibiotics, a good probiotic supplement containing plenty of friendly bacteria, such as *Lactobacillus acidophilus*, will help to overcome this effect.

It is estimated that one in every 123 people has an inherited inborn error of biotin metabolism. This is believed to affect their immunity against yeast infections and may be linked with recurrent vaginal thrush infections. In such cases high-dose biotin supplements will solve the problem if biotin deficiency is to blame.

There is some evidence that high-dose biotin might also improve the function of insulin to improve blood glucose levels in diabetics as well as improving nerve function.

Biotin deficiency might cause dry, flaky skin, a rash around the nose and mouth, brittle hair, patches of hair loss (alopecia), reversible baldness, tiredness, loss of appetite, nausea, depression, muscle pains and wasting.

Dose

For maintaining healthy skin, hair and nails, intakes of around 1 mg a day are taken. Two out of three people respond, with nails growing significantly thicker.

The upper safe intake is no more than 2.5 mg (2500 mcg) a day.

Black cohosh
(Cimicifuga racemosa)

Black cohosh – also known as squaw root or black snakeroot – is native to Canada and eastern parts of the USA.

Benefits

It is an adaptogen, known for its ability to help the body to adapt to changing situations, and valued for its hormone and mood-balancing properties.

The dried root of black cohosh is mainly used as a relaxant and a uterine stimulant to treat many gynaecological symptoms associated with raised levels of progesterone such as painful or irregular periods, labour pains, sex hormone imbalances and pre-menstrual syndrome, in which it can reduce feelings of depression, anxiety, tension, and mood swings. It contains a number of oestrogen-like plant hormones (phytoestrogens) of which formononetin is thought to be the most important, although it does not have an overt oestrogen action (see below).

The female menopause is associated with decreased levels of natural oestrogen which leads to increased levels of follicle-stimulating hormone (FSH) and luteinizing hormone (LH) as the brain tries to kick-start the ovaries. After the menopause, FSH and LH are secreted in large and continuous quantities. Many of the symptoms of menopause are suspected to be a result of the increased levels of LH.

Black cohosh is thought to work through the hypothalamus in the brain, and lowers levels of LH produced by the pituitary gland by as much as 20 per cent. This in turn decreases ovarian output of progesterone hormone to normalize oestrogen-progesterone balance. It also has a direct action on centres of the brain that help to control dilation of blood vessels, so reducing menopausal symptoms of hot flushes and sweating. Interestingly, it seems to enhance blood circulation in the genitals, and some evidence suggests that it causes a significant increase in weight of the uterus and ovaries as a result.

Black cohosh is the most widely used and thoroughly studied natural alternative to hormone replacement therapy (HRT). Several comparison studies have shown standardized extracts of black cohosh to produce better results in relieving hot flushes, vaginal thinning and dryness, depression and anxiety than those achieved by standard HRT (conjugated oestrogens). Trials suggest that four out of five women taking it describe its effects as either good or very good.

A German trial has shown that black cohosh plus St John's Wort was effective in treating 78 per cent of women with hot flushes and other menopausal problems. Most women experience significant improvement in symptoms within two to four weeks. In another study, black cohosh out-performed diazepam and oestrogen HRT in relieving depressive moods and anxiety. It will not protect against coronary heart disease or osteoporosis however.

Because its unique oestrogen action does not stimulate oestrogen-sensitive tumours (and may, in fact, inhibit them) black cohosh extracts have even been used in women with a history of breast cancer although this should only be done under the supervision of a qualified medical herbalist.

As black cohosh has a normalizing effect on female sex hormones, it may be used to improve low sex drive where this is linked with hormonal imbalances, such as after childbirth, irregular menstruation and around the time of the menopause. It is also used to help relieve symptoms of endometriosis.

Dose
Usually 80–160 mg standardized extracts daily.

Side effects
Some people experience headaches behind the eyes, nausea, or indigestion if they have taken too much black cohosh.

Although the German Commission E monograph recommends that treatment should be limited to six months, new toxicology studies suggest that black cohosh may be used long-term.

Contraindications
Black cohosh should not be taken during pregnancy or when breast-feeding.

Blue-green algae

Blue-green algae evolved over 3.5 billion years ago as the first successful life form on earth. A number of blue-green algae are widely available in supplement form, such as chlorella, spirulina and aphanizomenon.

Benefits

Blue-green algae are a rich whole-food source of over 100 synergistic and easily assimilated nutrients including antioxidants, vitamins, minerals, enzymes, essential fatty acids, essential (and non-essential) amino acids, iron, chlorophyll, protein and other protective substances. As the basis for the development of life on earth, algae are one of the most easily assimilable foods for the human body. The proteins found in algae, for example, are in the form of glyco-proteins – the necessary form for us to absorb and utilize – rather than as lipoproteins found in most other protein food sources.

Gram for gram, blue-green algae are the richest natural source of betacarotene, which protects against cell damage and ageing. Chlorella also contain a unique Chlorella Growth Factor (CGF) that has been found to act as an energy concentrate, immune enhancer, and tissue repair enhancer. Diabetic mice fed on chlorella live significantly longer than those not receiving chlorella supplements. Japanese research also suggests that a substance found in chlorella (chlon A) can increase immune reactions against tumour cells.

Substances extracted from blue-green algae have effects on laboratory cells that suggest they may help to prevent cancer, diabetes, coronary heart disease, degenerative disease and absorb toxic chemicals such as heavy metals and radiation. In one trial involving 44 people with pre-cancerous lesions of the mouth (oral leukoplakia), over half the lesions either vanished or significantly reduced in size in those who took 1 gram spirulina per day for one year, compared with no change in the lesions of those receiving a blue-green placebo supplement.

Blue-green algae are widely taken to improve bad breath (halitosis), aid digestion and to detox. Algae have a chelating action in the body which means they can bind to harmful toxins in the digestive tract (e.g. heavy metals) and help to remove them from the body. The blue phytochemical, phycocyanin, found in spirulina for example, has a powerful detoxifying action helping to reduce kidney damage due to heavy metals such as mercury. When toxins such as PCB, mercury copper, lead and cadmium are added to yeast cultures, cells start to die. If chlorella is added too, the yeast cells survive. Algae have an ability to absorb and neutralize toxins – they can even bind uranium.

The purest and most potent wild blue-green algae will only thrive in clean, unpolluted fresh water. Blue-green algae found in supplements are either derived from natural, unpolluted lakes, or are farmed in huge, alkaline, man-made lakes in places such as the Californian desert.

Dose

Varies from product to product, but typically 3 g a day. Large amounts may be consumed as a food without apparent harm. Some products have been contaminated with toxic algae, so ensure that you take a recognized, mainstream brand – preferably one that is certified organic, meaning it has grown in unpolluted waters.

Best taken with food.

Boron

Boron is a trace element obtained from fruit and vegetables, especially apples, grapes, pears, plums, prunes, strawberries, avocado and broccoli.

Benefits

Boron has several complex actions that depend on its ability to inhibit or stimulate a variety of enzymes. It is thought to be involved in normal brain function by affecting the movement of chemicals across the membrane of brain cells. It is also important for bone health through its ability to boost production of active vitamin D (needed for absorption of calcium from the intestines) and to reduce excretion of calcium and magnesium.

A group of post-menopausal women followed a normal, low-boron diet for 17 weeks and then took boron supplements (3 mg a day) for seven weeks. After just eight days on boron, they excreted 44 per cent less calcium and 33 per cent less magnesium than before. Their production of both oestrogen and testosterone hormones also doubled.

It can also improve oestrogen production in older women and a higher than average intake of boron in vegetarians (around 10 mg a day compared with 0.5–1 mg in non-vegetarians) may account for their lower risk of osteoporosis. Boron supplements were also found to increase both oestrogen and testosterone levels in athletes. Because of the way it raises steroid hormones, it is currently being investigated as a possible way to improve athletic performance.

Dose

A daily intake of 3 mg is suggested as optimum for bone health and some researchers have suggested that osteoporosis is a boron-deficiency disease.

Excess

Toxicity can occur at intakes of 100 mg a day or more, causing symptoms such as headache, muscle pain, nausea, vomiting, red eyes, rash and peeling skin plus reduced fertility.

Boswellia

Boswellia – known since biblical times as frankincense – is a gum resin that has recently been shown to have anti-inflammatory properties. It contains a number of fatty acids, including the anti-inflammatory boswellic acid.

Benefits

Boswellia products are used to treat chronic inflammatory conditions such as rheumatoid arthritis, asthma, ulcerative colitis, eczema and psoriasis, as well as tendonitis, ringworm and indigestion.

Sufferers of rheumatoid arthritis show significant reductions in pain, duration of morning stiffness and disability when treated with boswellia resin as compared with those taking a placebo.

In ulcerative colitis sufferers, 82 per cent of those taking boswellia went into remission compared with 75 per cent taking the usual anti-inflammatory or steroidal drug treatments, suggesting it to be at least as effective as standard medical treatment and without the side effects, as boswellia does not irritate the stomach.

Dose

200–400 mg, two or three times per day standardized to contain at least 37.5 per cent boswellic acids.

Brahmi

See **Gotu kola**

Brewer's yeast

Brewer's yeast is used medicinally to treat acute diarrhoea, acne, pre-menstrual symptoms and to prevent candida proliferation. Diarrhoea prevention has been shown in double-blind, placebo-controlled studies involving critically ill patients and in people taking penicillin. In one study, high-risk patients were given either brewer's yeast or placebo within 72 hours of starting a course of antibiotics. Yeast supplements were continued for three days following treatment and shown to halve the incidence of antibiotic-induced diarrhoea with no accompanying adverse side effects. In Germany, brewer's yeast strain Hansen CBS 5926 is approved for use in treating acute diarrhoea, and for preventing and treating traveller's diarrhoea. Oral intake of fermentable yeast can cause flatulence however, so although it may be helpful in reducing diarrhoea in some people with IBS, in others it may make symptoms such as bloating worse.

Brewer's yeast is a rich source of chromium. It is sometimes used to help repel mosquitoes.

Dose
250–750 mg a day.

Bromelain

Bromelain is a digestive enzyme derived from pineapples. It helps to clot milk and digest protein but, as it is absorbed intact into the circulation from the intestines, it is mainly used for its systemic effects.

Benefits
Bromelain has powerful anti-inflammatory actions, and is taken to reduce pain, swelling and inflammation associated with bruising, sprains, wounds, minor operations, burns and arthritis.

It is sometimes recommended before minor surgery and liposuction, to reduce post-operative swelling and bruising, and as a supplement to take after childbirth to boost healing. Bromelain is also sometimes taken to help reduce inflammation associated with urinary tract infections.

Bromelain has a useful blood-thinning action, and can reduce the risk of coronary heart disease, abnormal blood clotting and angina. In one study, people with angina who took 1000–1400 mg bromelain found that their symptoms either improved or disappeared within three months.

It has a useful mucus-thinning action and can help to reduce phlegm in respiratory conditions such as sinusitis, bronchitis and asthma.

Dose

250–500 mg three times a day. Select supplements containing at least 2000 milk clotting units.

Note: before undergoing liposuction, or any other surgery, it is best to consult a surgeon about taking bromelain.

Butcher's broom
(Cytisus scoparius)

Butcher's broom is an evergreen shrub found in most parts of Europe, whose leaves contain saponin glyosides such as ruscogenin.

Benefits

It is used to regulate abnormal heart rhythms associated with low blood pressure and heart pump failure.

Dose

150 mg, three times a day (standardized to 9–11 per cent ruscogenin).

Contraindications

Butcher's broom should not be taken by hypertension sufferers, as it constricts blood vessels, which puts blood pressure up.

C

Vitamin C is a water-soluble vitamin which cannot be stored in the body in appreciable amounts. It is the main antioxidant found in body fluids, protecting cells from damage due to exposure to excess free radicals – chemicals produced during normal metabolism. It is such an important antioxidant that many animals are able to make vitamin C themselves. The goat, for example, which weighs around the same as a man, produces between 2 and 13 g of vitamin C per day depending on its levels of stress and illness. Quite why we have either lost or never acquired the ability to synthesize our vitamin C requirements remains one of the greatest mysteries of human biochemistry. It is thought to have resulted from a genetic accident millions of years ago which, some scientists believe, essentially means that we all suffer from a genetic disease, named hypoascorbaemia – the final and potentially fatal result of which is scurvy. This genetic defect also increases our risk of a number of other common illnesses such as viral infections, raised cholesterol levels, coronary heart disease and cancer as well as reducing our ability to cope with the effects of stress.

Because our primitive ancestors ate a vegetarian diet full of vitamin C-rich plants such as purslane (just 100 g of which contained 12 mg vitamin E, 27 mg vitamin C and 2 mg betacarotene), their vitamin C intake was much higher than ours and has been estimated at 392 mg a day. Some researchers believe it may even have been as high as 10 g daily. This high dietary intake meant that humans were able to survive since the vitamin C they failed to make was adequately replaced by their food (It is found naturally in many fruits and vegetables including citrus fruits, blackcurrants, capsicum peppers, kiwi fruit and green leafy vegetables). Today, however, we eat a very different diet containing much lower levels of vitamin C, and supplementation seems to be an increasingly good idea.

Benefits

Vitamin C – ascorbic acid – is essential for the synthesis of collagen, a major structural protein in the body. It is necessary for proper growth and repair and for healthy skin, bones, teeth and reproduction. It is also involved in the metabolism of stress hormones. Some evidence suggests that vitamin C acts as a natural antihistamine and may help to damp down allergic reactions. It also has anti-viral and antibacterial actions and is used to treat or prevent common colds and influenza.

Perhaps the most important role of vitamin C is as an antioxidant. It is also vital for regenerating another antioxidant, vitamin E, which protects body fats such as those found in all cell membranes.

Studies have shown that men and women with the highest intakes of vitamin C have a lower risk of developing coronary heart disease and stroke. It also protects genetic material from oxidation and mutation and is therefore thought to protect against cancer.

Another useful role for vitamin C is its ability to increase absorption of iron – those taking iron supplements for anaemia should ideally wash down their tablets with a glass of orange juice.

Vitamin C as an immune booster

Vitamin C is one of the most powerful dietary immune-boosting nutrients. It is needed for immune cells to develop properly, has anti-viral and antibacterial actions and optimizes the actions of antibodies and immune cells. As an antioxidant, it also helps to neutralize the toxins, free radicals and inflammatory reactions associated with infections to reduce the severity and duration of symptoms. It only seems to have a beneficial effect on immunity in doses of 1 g per day or more, however.

Vitamin C and viral infections

Vitamin C is now one of the most popular supplements in winter as many people appreciate its benefits in relieving symptoms of the common cold. It has been shown to have an anti-viral action which works by suppressing the activation of viral genes. In order to produce symptoms, a cold virus – of which there are over 200 different types – must first infect cells in the respiratory tract and reprogramme them to make more cold viruses to escalate their attack. It seems the virus cannot survive in cells containing high-dose vitamin C so symptoms are less likely to develop. Studies involving school children and students found that taking vitamin C reduced the risk of catching a cold by as much as 30 per cent. Supplements have also been shown to provide protection for men doing heavy physical exercise, and who are more likely to develop respiratory infections. Military troops under training and participants in a 90 km running race were found to have half the risk of developing cold symptoms when taking vitamin C supplements of 600 mg–1 g per day. Researchers also believe that the powerful antioxidant action of vitamin C mops up inflammatory chemicals produced during a viral infection, so that supplements can improve symptoms and hasten healing even after a cold develops. Some researchers found that vitamin C at a dose of 1–6 g daily reduced the duration of a cold by over 20 per cent.

Vitamin C plus bioflavonoids (1800 mg complex) has also been shown to reduce the duration of recurrent *Herpes simplex* (cold sore) attacks by over half. The sores of those taking the vitamin C/bioflavonoids healed within 4.5 days as compared with 10 days in those taking an inactive placebo.

Interestingly, when you are ill your vitamin C needs seem to increase to such an extent that you become much more tolerant of high doses so you can take much higher amounts before developing loose bowel motions.

Heart attack and stroke

A study involving over 6600 men and women in the USA found that vitamin C levels were independently associated with risk of coronary heart disease and stroke to such an extent that just a small (0.5 mg a day) increase in blood vitamin C produced an 11 per cent fall in the risk of both coronary heart disease and stroke. Those with the highest vitamin C levels enjoyed a 27 per cent lower risk of coronary heart disease and a 26 per cent lower risk of stroke than those with low levels. Researchers concluded that these results are consistent with the hypothesis that increased vitamin C intakes may decrease the risk of coronary heart disease and stroke.

According to another study of 1605 middle-aged men, those who had vitamin C deficiency were 3.5 times more at risk of a heart attack than men with vitamin C levels above the deficiency level. Vitamin C may also play a role in preventing symptoms in those with existing coronary artery disease. Low levels of vitamin C are significantly linked with an increased risk of developing angina.

Dilation of arteries: recent research found that doses of 2 g a day could reverse the inability of diseased arteries to dilate within two hours of being taken, so blood flow improved through the artery by as much as 50 per cent. It is believed that vitamin C acts as an antioxidant to protect nitric oxide – the chemical needed for blood vessels to dilate (interestingly, nitric oxide is the same chemical needed for arterial dilation during a penile erection, and is the mediator through which Viagra, the anti-impotence drug, works).

Reduced dilation of arteries is also seen in diabetes and in people with congestive heart failure – two relatively common conditions in which vitamin C has now also been shown to have a beneficial effect. This suggests that breakdown of nitric oxide by free radicals contributes to abnormal blood vessel constriction in patients with insulin-dependent diabetes mellitus and in those with congestive heart failure and that high-dose antioxidant supplements may be helpful in these cases.

Vitamin C has also been found to reduce the sluggish action of arterial dilation seen after eating a high-fat meal – another factor linked with increased risk of a heart attack. In those undergoing surgery to open up narrowed coronary arteries, those taking vitamin C were less likely to experience re-narrowing of the arteries (40 per cent versus 24 per cent) and were 60 per cent less likely to need further surgery than those not taking vitamin C.

Blood fat levels: vitamin C has a beneficial effect on circulating blood fats, which independently reduces the risk of a heart attack. Researchers found that high levels of vitamin C are linked with increased levels of high-density lipoprotein – a protective transport protein that carries cholesterol around in the circulation so it is less likely to cause hardening and furring up of the arteries. In the laboratory, vitamin C has also been shown to reduce the uptake of harmful (LDL-) cholesterol by macrophages (the scavenger cells which deposit cholesterol in artery walls and contribute to atherosclerosis) by a massive 93 per cent.

Cancer

Those with the highest intakes of vitamin C seem least likely to develop certain cancers, including breast, cervical, colorectal, oesophageal, lung, pancreatic, prostate, salivary gland, and stomach cancers, and leukaemia and non-Hodgkin's lymphoma. If already diagnosed their prognosis may improve − especially when vitamin C supplements are taken together with vitamin E and mineral selenium.

Eye disease

The level of vitamin C found in the eye lens is 60 times that found in the circulation. This is because vitamin C is the main antioxidant that protects the lens of the eye from free radical attack leading to clouding from cataracts. In one study, it was found that those taking 300 mg vitamin C daily were 70 per cent less likely to develop cataracts than similar patients not taking supplements.

The Nurses' Health Study in 1993, involving over 87,000 nurses, found that 60 per cent of early cataracts occurred in women who had not taken vitamin C supplements. Those who had taken vitamin C for at least 10 years had a 45 per cent lower risk of developing cataracts than those who had not. Interestingly, the latter still had a naturally high dietary intake of vitamin C averaging 130 mg − twice as high as the EC RDA − but only those taking additional vitamin C seemed to benefit.

These findings were confirmed more recently when women who took vitamin C supplements for at least 10 years were found to have a 77 per cent lower risk of early lens opacities, and an 83 per cent lower risk of moderate lens opacities compared with women who did not use vitamin C. These studies suggest that long-term consumption of vitamin C supplements may substantially reduce the development of age-related cataracts.

Gallstones

Vitamin C affects the breakdown of cholesterol to bile acids, and it seems that in women, a good vitamin C intake may reduce the risk of symptomatic gallstones. A similar relationship was not found for men, however.

Lung disease

At least seven studies have shown that people with asthma have reduced symptoms and improved breathing when taking 1–2 g vitamin C per day. Increased vitamin C intakes are associated with improved lung function, and conversely, low intakes seem to be as harmful for lung function as smoking cigarettes for five years.

Osteoporosis

Since vitamin C is essential for the synthesis of collagen which makes up 30 per cent of bone volume, it is vital for healthy growth and repair of all tissues, including bone. It has been found to stimulate bone-building cells (osteoblasts), enhance vitamin D activity and boost calcium absorption from the gut. Not surprisingly therefore, researchers have found evidence of a positive association between dietary vitamin C intake and bone density at the hip. This link seems to be strongest in women aged 55–64 years who have used vitamin C supplements for at least 10 years and among women who have never used oestrogen hormone replacement therapy.

Osteoarthritis

Vitamin C may reduce the risk of cartilage loss and disease progression in people with osteoarthritis. Those with medium to high intakes of vitamin C had a 70 per cent lower risk of cartilage loss and of developing knee pain. For those who already had knee disease there was a three-fold reduction in knee osteoarthritis progression.

Helicobacter pylori

Helicobacter pylori is a motile bacterium that lives in the stomach of at least 20 per cent of the younger population and 50 per cent of those aged over 50. *H. pylori* increases the risk of indigestion and peptic ulcers by burrowing into the mucous lining of the stomach and exposing the stomach wall to acid attack. It survives exposure to gastric acid by producing an enzyme, urease, which converts urea into a bubble of ammonia gas. This alkaline bubble coats the bacterium and protects it. At the same time, the ammonia acts as another irritant to inflame the stomach wall. *H. pylori* is now known to be the main cause of gastritis, peptic ulcer disease and stomach cancer.

Researchers have found that vitamin C levels are significantly lower in the gastric juices of people with *H. pylori* infection compared with those who are *H. pylori* negative, and this finding is reversed when infection is eradicated with antibiotics. This suggests that vitamin C is consumed locally by the *H. pylori* bacteria and/or the inflammatory process/free radicals associated with the infection. High doses of vitamin C have now been shown to inhibit the growth of *H. pylori*.

Hay fever

Vitamin C has an antihistamine action that can help to damp down symptoms linked with pollen allergy.

Sperm health

Vitamin C is actively secreted into semen and is present at concentrations eight times higher than those found in the blood. It plays two roles in protecting sperm health – it stops sperm from clumping together and it also acts as a powerful antioxidant. Both of these actions are important in maintaining sperm quality and the power to fertilize an egg.

Semen contains a substance called non-specific sperm agglutinin. This is made up of a protein, a sugar, vitamin E plus several sulphur-containing groups. This substance exists in either an oxidized or a non-oxidized (reduced) form. In the reduced form, it binds to sperm heads and prevents sperm from clumping together. This increases sperm motility. In its oxidized form, it can't bind sperm and the sperm therefore stick to each other, causing them to become immobile. If 20 per cent or more of sperm are clumped together, infertility usually occurs. By acting as an antioxidant, vitamin C, keeps the agglutinin in its reduced form.

In one study, 35 infertile men were given 500 mg of vitamin C every 12 hours (i.e. twice a day) for one month. After only one week, the average percentage of sperm agglutination had dropped from 37 per cent to 14 per cent. After two weeks it had dropped to 13 per cent and at four weeks it was down to 11 per cent. As this study proceeded, the researchers confirmed a significant improvement in overall quality of the men's sperm, including the percentage of normal sperm present, sperm viability and sperm motility. Latest research also shows that vitamin C protects the genetic material (DNA) of sperm against the oxidizing reactions of free radicals. This reduces the risk of siring offspring with an inherited genetic disease.

In another interesting trial, a chemical resulting from damaged DNA was measured in the sperm of men on a relatively high-vitamin C diet – 250 mg per day. The vitamin C in their diet was then drastically reduced to only 5 mg per day, and the level of the chemical resulting from DNA damage promptly doubled. Researchers believe that this proves that vitamin C protects against sperm damage. They then raised the level to 10 and then 20 mg per day – with no effect. It wasn't until the daily intake of vitamin C rose to 250 mg per day that the protective effect returned.

While preparing for conception, a high vitamin C intake of at least 250 mg per day is ideal for optimum sperm health. Smokers need at least twice as much vitamin C as non-smokers as their blood levels are up to 40 per cent lower and their risk of sperm abnormalities are significantly greater.

Skin care
Exposure of skin to solar ultra-violet radiation causes long-term changes responsible for skin ageing and skin cancer. When ultraviolet light strikes the skin, it generates free radicals which set up an inflammatory reaction known as heliodermatitis. This damages skin structures and interferes with normal cell division. Enzymes released during the inflammatory process are also thought to dissolve elastin and collagen fibres. As a result of this 'photo-ageing', skin cells are unable to regenerate normally and collagen fibres – which make up 70 per cent of skin structure – become

matted, branched and twisted. As a result, skin that has been exposed to the sun over a long period of time eventually becomes dry, inelastic, thickened, yellow, scaly, mottled and wrinkled with a coarse, pebbly, leathery, rough texture. Vitamin C has been shown to protect against skin damage on UV exposure and to reduce the sunburn effect when taken at a dose of 2 g per day (plus 1000 IU vitamin E). This is not a sunscreen effect as vitamin C does not absorb light in the wavelength. Vitamin C is thought to help to neutralize free radicals as well as being needed for the production of new collagen. It is therefore now being added to many cosmetic creams designed to slow the visible signs of skin ageing. It is not easy to maintain it in a stable form in creams, however, and products need to be used quickly for maximum effect.

Reduced risk of premature death

A recent study involving 19,196 adults aged 45–79 showed that the risk of death from any cause during the four-year study period was greatly reduced in those whose vitamin C levels were in the top 20 per cent of the group compared with those whose vitamin C levels were in the bottom 20 per cent. An increase in circulating vitamin C levels equivalent to a daily 50 g increase in fruit or vegetable intake was associated with a 20 per cent decrease in risk of all causes of death, regardless of age, blood pressure, cholesterol levels cigarette smoking habit, diabetes or supplement use.

So, if you do nothing else after reading this book – consider increasing your intake of vitamin-C rich fruit and vegetables such as oranges or kiwi fruit!

Vitamin C deficiency

Mild deficiency of vitamin C is associated with non-specific symptoms (sometimes known as pre-scurvy syndrome) such as frequent colds and other infections, lack of energy, weakness and muscle and joint pain.

More severe lack of vitamin C leads to scurvy. A minimum daily intake of 10 mg vitamin C is needed to prevent this, although 20 mg per day is needed for normal wound healing. In scurvy, reduced conversion of the amino acid proline to hydroxyproline (an important component of collagen) results in:

- poor wound healing
- dry, rough, scaly skin
- broken thread veins in skin around hair follicles
- easy bruising
- scalp dryness
- misshapen, tangled, corkscrew, brittle hair
- hair loss
- dry, fissured lips
- inflamed, spongy, bleeding gums and loose teeth
- bleeding skin, eyes and nose
- weakness.

Dose

Vitamin C is now the most popular single nutritional supplement available. The EC RDA is 60 mg, but research suggests that high doses of vitamin C act in the body in a different way from smaller, nutritional doses, and increasing numbers of experts feel that a higher intake is preferable for optimum health. A general consensus is that 100–250 mg vitamin C is a good basic intake. Some researchers feel that the optimum intake is 1000–3000 mg a day.

Smokers and those with diabetes mellitus need twice as much vitamin C as other people as their metabolisms generate many more free radicals and harmful antioxidant reactions.

Intakes of at least 250 mg vitamin C a day are also advisable for those undergoing major surgery – both in its capacity as an antioxidant and because of the body's need for increased collagen production during the healing process.

To achieve a high vitamin C intake, it is best taken spread over several doses per day, as around 75 per cent of a 500 mg dose is absorbed from the gut in one go, while only around 50 per cent of a 1500 mg dose taken in one go is absorbed into the bloodstream.

The safety of vitamin C supplementation has been researched and established over a long period of time. The body's housekeeping mechanisms ensure that there is a consistent body pool size of around 20 mg/kg body weight (e.g. 1500 mg for someone weighing 75 kg) irrespective of intake, so that overloading does not occur even when dietary intakes are high.

Claims that large doses could trigger kidney stones have proved unfounded. A safety review in which vitamin C was taken in doses of 5 g or 10 g per day found only a marginal effect on urinary oxalate and these variations were within the normal range experienced with individuals who did not take vitamin C supplements.

In the large-scale Harvard Prospective Health Professional Follow-Up Study in 1997, those groups in the highest 20 per cent of vitamin C intake (higher than 1500 mg per day) were found to have a lower risk of kidney stones than those in the lowest 20 per cent of vitamin C intake. It is now therefore accepted that high doses of vitamin C do not increase the risk of calcium oxalate kidney stones in normal individuals. Those known to be recurrent stone formers, however, and people with renal failure who have a defect in ascorbic acid or oxalate metabolism, should restrict daily vitamin C intakes to approximately 100 mg.

Suggestions that high intakes of vitamin C interfere with the metabolism of vitamin B12 were due to faulty procedures in which vitamin B12 was lost during the analysis technique.

Recent alarmist headlines suggested that high doses of vitamin C might cause cancer. In fact, one of the authors of the recent paper in *Science*, published in 2001, was so worried that his results would be misreported that, in a phone interview with Reuters, he was quoted as saying 'Absolutely, for God's sake, don't say vitamin C causes cancer'. Unfortunately, many papers went on to do just that.

The study in question used vitamin C to induce conversion of lipid hydroperoxides (which are formed in the body during the oxidation of unsaturated fats) into compounds that can damage DNA. This effect demonstrated artificially in a test tube cannot occur in living cells where a number of enzyme systems exist to remove the damaging substances formed. In addition, fat-soluble Vitamin E protects lipid cell membranes in living systems from oxidative reactions and, as vitamin C is essential for the regeneration of vitamin E, it actually plays an important role in preventing the formation of lipid hydroperoxides in the first place. This seems ironic, given the adverse publicity.

Other factors that make this a non-story include the fact that researchers used lipid hydroperoxide concentrations 10,000 times greater than those found in the body, and that the methods used by the researchers to measure DNA could themselves have caused the damage noted. There is ample evidence that vitamin C is beneficial in doses of up to 2g daily. In fact, research into the antioxidant effects of vitamin C have raised the exciting possibility that vitamin C may have a specific and beneficial effect on the expression of certain enzymes involved in DNA repair which may account for its anti-cancer actions.

Excess

The only adverse effects of taking very high doses (e.g. as much as 10,000 mg per day) seem to be indigestion and a laxative effect. These are largely due to the acidity of vitamin C itself and are not a sign of toxicity. When vitamin C enters the alkaline environment of the lower digestive tract, so-called Acid Rejection Syndrome occurs which triggers inflammation, flatulence, diarrhoea and discomfort as well as reduced vitamin C absorption. Some people are more sensitive to the acidity of vitamin C than others. If indigestion occurs, it can usually be overcome by taking buffered vitamin C, or the non-acidic form, ester-C (see below). Timed-release supplements may also help.

Note:

● If you are taking high doses of vitamin C and you need to have a urine test, inform your doctor that you are taking a high-dose supplement as it can affect laboratory results.

● Some urine test kits used by diabetics are also affected by high dose vitamin C – use a kit that is not affected.

● High-dose vitamin C may mask the presence of blood in stool tests – inform your doctor if you are advised to have one of these.

- Do not take vitamin C and ginseng together in the same dose as this may reduce the effectiveness of the herbal remedy. Leave at least four hours between them.

- Sufferers of iron-storage disease (e.g. haemochromatosis) should only take vitamin C supplements under medical advice.

- Recurrent stone formers and sufferers of renal failure who have a defect in ascorbic acid or oxalate metabolism, should restrict daily vitamin C intakes to approximately 100 mg.

- Anyone who is taking a very high-dose supplement and needs to reduce their vitamin C intake should do this slowly over a few weeks rather than stopping suddenly, in order to avoid a so-called 'rebound scurvy' effect. Suddenly falling blood levels of vitamin C mean that enzymes activated by high levels of vitamin C are suddenly deprived of the extra vitamin C they need to work properly, and this can produce temporary symptoms of vitamin C deficiency.

Slow-release Vitamin C

Slow-release vitamin C (also known as timed release or prolonged release) provides a constant delivery of vitamin C over a six- to eight-hour period so that blood levels stay consistently higher for longer. This allows you to take a higher dose in one go and achieve the same effect as taking a lower dose two or three times a day. It is a useful way to take vitamin C for people with busy lifestyles.

Effervescent vitamin C

Effervescent vitamin C is designed to be dissolved in water to make a pleasant-flavoured drink for rapid absorption.

Buffered vitamin C

Vitamin C buffered with minerals such as calcium ascorbate or magnesium ascorbate has less acidity than standard vitamin C and is less likely to trigger indigestion.

Ester-C

Ester-C contains the active breakdown products of vitamin C produced by the body when standard vitamin C is metabolized. These naturally occurring metabolites (e.g. threonate) produce a vitamin C mixture which has a neutral pH and is therefore non-acidic. It does not trigger indigestion and, as it is 'body-ready', has the additional benefits of entering the bloodstream more quickly than normal vitamin C. This means that it produces higher vitamin C levels inside cells, and stays in the body for longer as less is excreted in the urine. Non-acidic ester-C zinc ascorbate has also been shown to strengthen gum tissues and inhibit bacteria associated with tooth decay and plaque formation, in contrast to normal vitamin C which can start to erode tooth enamel within minutes of prolonged contact. Ester-C is included in several mainstream brands of multinutrient supplements.

Vitamin C with bioflavonoids

Bioflavonoids are substances that are found together with vitamin C in fruits such as oranges, rosehips and acerola cherries. They help to increase absorption of vitamin C from the gut and also work together with vitamin C to strengthen body tissues and reduce inflammation. Many of the best supplements therefore contain these.

Vitamin C with antioxidants

Vitamin C is a powerful antioxidant that works within body fluids. Some supplements provide additional antioxidants, such as vitamin C, betacarotene and selenium, that also help to protect body fats or which work together with vitamin C for an overall improved antioxidant profile.

Calcium

Calcium is an important structural mineral and 90 per cent of that absorbed from the diet goes straight into the bones and teeth. The other 1 per cent (around 10 g) plays a crucial role in blood clotting, muscle contraction, nerve conduction, the smooth functioning of the immune system and the production of energy.

We each contain around 1.2 kg calcium – more than any other mineral. Most of this is stored in the skeleton as hydroxyapatite.

Calcium is absorbed in the small intestine, a process that is dependent upon the presence of vitamin D. Lack of calcium at any stage in life means that bone stores are raided, greatly increasing the risk of osteoporosis in the future. Good intakes of calcium are therefore vital throughout life, especially during childhood and adolescence when bones are still developing, and in later years when bones are naturally starting to thin down.

An adult needs a daily calcium intake of between 700 and 1000 mg, although those at risk of osteoporosis (e.g. women over the age of 45) will need as much as 1500 mg daily.

Calcium in the diet

Dietary sources of calcium include milk and dairy products, eggs, green leafy vegetables especially broccoli (but not spinach, whose oxalate content reduces its bioavailability), tinned salmon (including the bones), nuts and seeds, pulses and bread made from fortified flour. It is relatively easy to increase calcium intake by drinking an extra pint of skimmed or semi-skimmed milk per day. This provides as much calcium as whole milk but without the additional fat. The calcium found in milk is also in one of the most absorbable forms (calcium lactate).

Usually, only 30–40 per cent of the calcium present in food and drinks is absorbed. Some types of dietary fibre (phytates from wheat in unleavened bread e.g. chapatti) also bind calcium in the bowel to form an insoluble, non-absorbable salt. High-fibre diets, which speed the passage of food through the bowels, will also reduce the amount of calcium absorbed.

Benefits

Taking daily calcium supplements of 1000 mg helps to prevent bone loss in older women during the winter months when vitamin D levels are naturally lower.

Similarly, adding calcium supplements to the diet of elderly people reduces their risk of a vertebral fracture by 20 per cent, while giving them both calcium and vitamin D supplements may reduce their risk of non-vertebral and hip fracture by 30–40 per cent.

Calcium supplements seem to protect against the development of high blood pressure in pregnancy (pre-eclampsia) in those at risk, especially where calcium intakes are generally low. When calcium supplements are combined with linoleic acid (e.g. from evening primrose oil) the benefits are even greater.

Good intakes of calcium may also protect against cancer of the colon – possibly by buffering the effects of bile acids.

Calcium tablets are best taken with meals. Some evidence suggests that they are better taken with an evening meal rather than breakfast as calcium flux is greatest in the body at night, when growth hormone is secreted.

Calcium salts that seem to be most easily absorbed, other than calcium lactate (in milk) include calcium gluconate, calcium malate and calcium citrate (which is less likely to cause constipation than calcium carbonate and is also better for those with less stomach acid production, e.g. older people). The amount of elemental calcium supplied per gram of supplement will affect the recommended dose. Test your supplement by adding it to vinegar at room temperature and stirring every five minutes. If it hasn't dissolved after 30 minutes, it is unlikely to do so in your stomach either and you should switch to another brand. Effervescent tablets or calcium-enriched drinks usually help to improve absorption.

Deficiency

Low intakes of calcium have also been linked with high blood pressure and stroke. In fact, drugs that affect calcium channels in the body are highly successful in treating hypertension, angina, some irregular heart rhythms and poor circulation. Other symptoms that may be due to lack of calcium include muscle problems (aches, pains, twitching, spasm, cramps), palpitations, receding and infected gums and loose teeth.

Dose

Taking up to 2500 mg calcium supplements daily appears to be safe, although high doses should usually be taken together with other minerals such as zinc, iron and magnesium whose absorption it also affects. It is usually best to divide a large daily dose into two or even three doses spread throughout the day to improve absorption. People with a tendency to kidney stones should ideally take calcium supplements together with essential fatty acids but always seek medical advice first.

Those taking certain tetracycline antibiotics will need to ensure they do not eat or drink calcium-containing foods for at least an hour either side of taking their medication. This is because calcium binds with some tetracyclines to reduce their absorption.

Carnitine

L-carnitine is a non-essential amino acid that is made in the liver. Vitamins B3, B6, C and mineral iron are essential for its conversion.

Dietary sources include red meat, especially lamb and beef, offal and dairy products.

The only vegetable sources of L-carnitine appear to be avocado and the fermented soybean product, tempeh.

Benefits

The most important role of L-carnitine is in regulating fat metabolism. It is needed to transport long chain fatty acids into the energy-producing mitochondria found in all body cells where they are burned to produce energy. The more L-carnitine available, the more fat can be utilized – especially in heart muscle cells. L-carnitine is also needed to break down the branched-chain amino acids (leucine, isoleucine and valine) so they can be used as an energy source by muscle cells when other sources of energy are in short supply. By helping to mobilize fat stores and boost energy production, it may play a useful role in weight loss and in improving the appearance of cellulite.

L-carnitine aids digestion by stimulating the secretion of gastric and pancreatic juices and it has beneficial effects on blood fat levels by raising beneficial HDL (high-density lipoprotein) cholesterol while lowering total cholesterol and triglyceride levels overall. It may therefore be useful for treating hardening and furring up of the arteries (atherosclerosis), poor circulation and coronary heart disease.

When heart muscle cells do not receive enough oxygen, metabolism is impaired and free fatty acids build up and may damage heart cells. Research suggests that L-carnitine helps to neutralize these and may quickly become used up. Providing additional supplies may help to minimize heart damage in those at risk of a heart attack. Among a group of 44 men with angina, almost 23 per cent who took L-carnitine supplements for four weeks became free of exercise-induced angina compared with only 9 per cent taking inactive placebo.

L-carnitine has been shown to improve the distance walked without pain in patients with calf pain (intermittent claudication) due to hardening and furring up of the arteries (atherosclerosis). In one study 2 g carnitine taken twice daily allowed pain-free walking distance to increase by

75 per cent after three weeks of supplementation due to improved energy metabolism within muscle cells.

Taking 2 g carnitine before exercise has been shown to increase maximum oxygen uptake as well as the efficiency of muscle contraction at high exercise intensity. In another study, a group of marathon runners who took supplements of 2 g of L-carnitine daily for six weeks showed a 5.7 per cent improvement in peak treadmill running speed. Some other studies have not found a benefit for athletes taking L-carnitine supplements however.

As L-carnitine is needed for production of energy in muscle cells, it may play a role in chronic fatigue syndrome (CFS). When 18 patients with CFS were given 1 g carnitine three times a day, 12 significantly improved within four to eight weeks. L-carnitine can reduce feelings of fatigue and muscle weakness and it has been suggested as a possible treatment for people with muscle diseases such as muscular dystrophy, as these are associated with increased loss of carnitine in the urine.

L-carnitine is needed for energy production within sperm cells for optimum sperm motility. It may therefore be helpful for some men with infertility due to reduced sperm movements. When 100 men with low fertility were treated with 3 g L-carnitine per day, there was a statistically significant increase in total sperm count and in the proportion of sperm that could swim vigorously.

Dose
250 mg–1 g a day.

Excess

Diarrhoea may occur at doses in excess of 4 g a day. Increased body odour can occur when taking high doses. L-carnitine and co-enzyme Q10 seem to work synergistically.

Carotenoids

Over 600 carotenoids are present in fruit and vegetables, but only a few such as alpha-carotene, betacarotene, lycopene, lutein and zeaxanthin are currently recognized as being important for human health. They have an important antioxidant action in the body, especially in protecting cell membranes from free radical attack, but are generally less efficient antioxidants compared with vitamin E.

Carotenoids are found in yellow, orange, red and dark-green fruits and vegetables, including sweetcorn, carrots, pumpkins, spinach, mangoes, oranges, peaches, guavas, watermelons, spinach and other dark-green leafy vegetables. Some carotenoids, such as alphacarotene and betacarotene can be converted to vitamin A in the body.

By reducing oxidation of circulating fats, carotenoids help to reduce the risk of coronary heart disease. Among elderly people, those with the highest intakes of carotenoids were shown to be 50 per cent less likely to develop coronary heart disease, and 75 per cent less likely to experience a heart attack than those with the lowest intakes. Studies also show that an increased intake of a number of carotenoids is associated with a lower incidence of cataracts.

Betacarotene

Betacarotene is made up of two molecules of vitamin A joined together which can be split in the body to produce vitamin A when needed. It is estimated that 6 mcg betacarotene is equivalent to around 1 mcg of pre-formed retinol but this conversion is not always efficient, especially where intakes of other micro-nutrients such as zinc are low. It is estimated that only around half of ingested betacarotene is converted into vitamin A in the liver and in the cells lining the small intestine.

Benefits

Several studies suggest that natural dietary intakes of betacarotene and vitamin A are important in reducing the risk of coronary heart disease and a number of cancers, including breast, lung, skin cancer (melanoma) and possibly leukaemia. When synthetic, supplementary forms are taken however the same effect does not occur.

For example, a large study looking into whether taking high-dose supplements containing 30 mg betacarotene and 25,000 IU (7500 mcg) vitamin A could protect against lung cancer found no benefit in non-smokers and an apparent 46 per cent increased risk in those who smoked. The most likely explanation is that antioxidants do not work effectively on their own as they may temporarily be converted into free radicals themselves during their antioxidant reactions. They therefore need to be taken in balance with other antioxidants, including other carotenoids, vitamins C and E.

This balance is naturally obtained when consuming high intakes of betacarotene/vitamin A from dietary sources, and red-yellow-orange-green fruit and vegetables in particular contain a number of additional, beneficial plant substances known as phytochemicals. At present, the best way to ensure a good intake of natural betacarotene is to eat at least five servings of fruit and vegetables daily. Supplements containing natural betacarotene along with other fruit and vegetable extracts are also available.

Lutein

Those who eat the most carotenoids have at least a 60 per cent lower risk of developing age-related macular degeneration (AMD) of the eye than those with low intakes. Regular consumption of spinach, in particular, can reduce the risk by as much as 86 per cent. Poor dietary intake is thought to be the main cause of this condition and those who develop AMD have, on average, 70 per cent less lutein and zeaxanthin in their eyes than those with healthy vision. This is because carotenoids increase the thickness of the pigment layer in the macula and therefore protect against degeneration. This is partly because the antioxidant activity of carotenoids neutralizes harmful chemical reactions involved in light detection, and partly because their yellow colour filters out potentially harmful, visible blue light. In one study, in which two people took 30 mg lutein supplements per day, their macular density increased by 21 per cent and 39 per cent after 20 weeks. Even after lutein was discontinued, their maculae continued to improve for about six weeks.

High intakes of lutein and zeaxanthin may decrease the risk of coronary heart disease and lung cancer.

Lycopene

Lycopene is an important dietary carotenoid, that makes up at least 50 per cent of all carotenoids found in the body. It is best known as the red pigment in tomatoes. Cooking tomatoes releases five times more lycopene than is available from raw tomatoes. Tomato ketchup and tomato purée (which are concentrated) are therefore the richest dietary sources of lycopene. Pizza is also an excellent source as lycopene is fat-soluble and olive oil increases dietary absorption of lycopene as much as threefold.

Benefits

Like some other carotenoids, lycopene also protects against macular degeneration, and those with the lowest intakes have more than double the risk of developing AMD.

Increased dietary intakes of lycopene may lower the risk of certain cancers, with many studies showing a correlation between tomato intake or blood lycopene levels and reduced risk of cancers of the mouth, oesophagus, stomach, lung, colon, rectum, cervix or prostate gland. Women with the highest lycopene levels also appear to have five times less chance of developing pre-cancerous changes on their cervical smear than women with the lowest lycopene levels.

In one six-year study, men who ate two or more servings of tomato products a week reduced their risk of prostate cancer by up to 50 per cent. Interestingly, a family history of prostate cancer did not seem to reduce the protective effect of lycopene.

In another study 26 men with prostate cancer who were scheduled for surgical removal of the gland, were randomly assigned to receive 15 mg lycopene twice a day (as a pure tomato extract) for three weeks before their operation. Following removal of the prostates, those who had taken tomato extracts were found to have smaller tumours, which were more likely to be confined to the prostate, and to show signs of regression and decreased malignancy, than those not taking tomato extracts. Their levels of serum PSA (prostate specific antigen), a common marker used to detect prostate cancer) were also found to be lower.

No definite cause and effect relationship should be drawn from these observations, however, as lycopene may act as a marker for other potentially beneficial compounds found in tomatoes, and their synergistic effects, which must also be considered.

Similarly, after accounting for smoking, people with the lowest levels of lycopene are three times more likely to develop lung cancer than those with the highest intakes.

Lycopene may also play an important protective role against coronary heart disease. In one study, 19 young men followed a diet based on tomato products and experienced a significant increase in blood lycopene levels together with a reduction in circulating levels of LDL-cholesterol. Other studies show that those who consume the most lycopene from foods are half as likely to suffer a heart attack as those who consume the least.

Lycopene is depleted in skin exposed to ultraviolet light, suggesting that it also plays a role in protecting the skin from sun damage.

Some experts now believe that some of the benefits previously attributed to betacarotene may actually have been due to the presence of lycopene.

Ideally, at least five servings of lycopene-rich foods per day (e.g. tomato sauce, tomato juice, pizza), should be consumed, especially by those who smoke, drink or have a family history of cancer. A tomato-based lycopene supplement is also a good idea.

Supplements

It is usually best to take carotenoids as a mixed supplement. Studies suggest that intakes of carotenoids equivalent to those found in individuals who consume a carotenoid-rich diet reduce the incidence of coronary heart disease and some cancers, but this effect seems to be lost in high dose, and in smokers, although the reasons are not well understood.

The best advice is to avoid high-dose carotenoid supplements, and to combine a sensible dose (say 6–15 mg mixed carotenoids) with vitamin C, E, and selenium as a combination of antioxidants appears to be superior to high levels of any single antioxidant group.

Carotenodermia, in which the skin acquires an orange-colour due to a high intake of carotenoids, is harmless and will quickly resolve once intakes are reduced. In fact, this effect is deliberately sought to protect the skin in certain photosensitivity disorders where high-dose carotenoids have not shown any significant toxicity.

The usual recommended dose of mixed carotenoid supplements is the equivalent of at least 2500 IU (750 mg) vitamin A activity daily.

Contraindications
High doses of carotenoids should be avoided during pregnancy.

Cat's claw
(Uncaria tomentosa)

Cat's claw (also known as *uña de gato*) is derived from a South American vine.

Benefits

Its root and bark contain potent alkaloids, some of which have been found in the laboratory to possess anti-cancer and anti-viral activity. Cat's claw extracts also contain potent antioxidants and help to protect against environmental toxins including the genetic damage caused by ultra-violet light and smoking cigarettes.

Cat's claw is used to balance and support immune function by encouraging white blood cells to absorb and destroy (phagocytose) micro-organisms, abnormal cells and foreign particles. It can help to treat recurrent infections, including sinusitis, and conditions associated with long-term pain including gout. In some countries, it is only available on prescription.

Recent studies suggest that cat's claw may help to prevent the deposition of beta-amyloid plaques in brain tissues that occurs in Alzheimer's disease and this is under further investigation. It has also been shown to have anti-inflammatory actions, especially towards gastrointestinal inflammatory conditions such as gastritis.

Dose

It is generally advisable to start with a low dose (e.g. two 150 mg standardized capsules) and slowly build up to a therapeutic dose (five 150 mg standardized capsules).

Side effects

High doses of cat's claw may cause diarrhoea.

Contraindications

Cat's claw increases the immune rejection of foreign cells, and should not be used:
● during pregnancy or breast-feeding

- by anyone who has recently had – or is scheduled to receive – an organ/bone marrow transplant or skin-graft
- by those taking immunosuppressive drugs.

Some researchers also recommend that cat's claw is stopped two days before and after receiving chemotherapy.

Catuaba
(Erythroxylon catuaba)

Catuaba – known as the 'tree of love' – is native to Brazil. It is one of the most successful prosexual herbs available. The bark of the catuaba tree contains aromatic resins and non-addictive alkaloids – catuabins – that are distantly related to cocaine.

Benefits

Catuaba bark acts as a sexual stimulant and natural aphrodisiac, promoting erotic dreams and increased sexual energy in both men and women. Erotic dreams usually start between five and 21 days of taking extracts regularly, and these are followed by increased sexual desire. It also improves peripheral blood flow which may be another mechanism for boosting sexual performance, and it has been used to combat extreme exhaustion.

Interestingly, catuaba also has antibacterial and anti-viral properties. Research suggests that it may protect against infection with *Escherichia coli* and *Staphylococcus aureus*, and in cell cultures it has been shown to inhibit the cell-killing effect of HIV and the expression HIV markers on infected cells.

Dose

1 g on waking, and 1 g on going to bed.

Cayenne
(Capsicum frutescens)

Cayenne, or chilli pepper, is a perennial shrub native to Mexico, whose scarlet fruits filled with white seed are a popular 'hot' culinary spice.

Cayenne seeds contain steroidal saponins known as capsicidins, and weight for weight contain up to 1.5 per cent capsaicin (sometimes known as capsicum).

Benefits

Cayenne is widely known as a hot, spicy supplement that stimulates circulation to the hands, feet and genitals, and which promotes sweating. It is said to have aphrodisiac properties and to help maintain an erection. It aids digestion, relieves flatulence and reduces the risk of peptic ulcers by stimulating production of protective stomach mucus, and by improving blood flow in the stomach wall.

Chilli oil ointment may be helpful for reducing skin itching, pain due to fibromyalgia, and for stimulating poor circulation to the digits as occurs in Raynaud's syndrome.

Capsaicin is an effective topical painkiller when applied to the skin. It works by sinking down to nerve endings and reducing their content of a chemical, known as substance P, that is needed to transmit pain impulses to the brain.

Capsaicin is now available in a cream prescribed as a topical painkiller to relieve post-herpetic neuralgia (shooting pains that occur after shingles) and pain linked with diabetes (peripheral neuropathy).

It is also used to stimulate digestion, prevent infection and to treat some types of diarrhoea.

Dose
Usually around 500–1000 mg a day.

Note: chilli ointment or cream should not be applied to raw skin or to the eyes as this will be excruciatingly painful.

Chamomile
(Matricaria chamomilla or *M. recutita)*

German chamomile is one of the most important of all medicinal herbs. It was an important remedy used by the ancient Egyptians, Greeks and Romans to help soothe and relax, and also to reduce fevers, and it is still in widespread popular use today.

Benefits
It has anti-inflammatory, antacid, anti-parasitic, anti-spasmodic and sedative actions. It helps to relieve intestinal spasm associated with wind, colic and irritable bowel syndrome, and can also relieve menstrual cramps.

Chamomile is used externally to help reduce skin and mucous membrane inflammation, including eczema and inflammation of the genital region (baths and irrigation). It is also approved for inflammations and irritations of the respiratory tract (inhalations).

It is often applied to help cleanse and soothe bacterial infections of the skin, mouth, gums and eyes. Chamomile infusions may be used to soak a compress for application to burns, wounds and eyes.

It has a mild sedative action, helping to reduce anxiety, stress and to promote sleep.

Chamomile tea may be given to children and taken during pregnancy.

Dose
1–3 cups chamomile tea a day.

Chicken egg extracts

Chicken egg extracts (CEE) are used to help increase a low sex drive in both men and women. Egg consumption has long been associated with libido, and Casanova was reported to consume large quantities of raw egg to boost his testosterone levels.

Clinical trials involving male volunteers with low sex drive found that CEE significantly increased libido within three weeks compared with inactive placebo. Overall, 84 per cent of men experienced a good response with an overall increase in their desire for sexual activity. Almost half (45.2 per cent) experienced a major or very pronounced increase in sex drive. Only 16.1 per cent of men noticed no increase in libido. No participants reported any side effects.

CEE has also been shown to improve the frequency of desire, intensity of orgasm, general well-being, feelings of happiness and self-esteem, as well as energy levels.

When CEE were given to both men and women with low sex drive due to depression and the side effects of anti-depressant medication, 88 per cent reported a definite to very pronounced increase in sexual activity within two to three weeks.

Dose

First week: 6 capsules twice a day, morning and evening. Thereafter: 2 capsules twice a day. (Each 450 mg capsule contains 434 mg active ingredients.)

CEE is 90 per cent cholesterol-free.

Contraindications

Avoid CEE if you are sensitive to hens' eggs.

Chinese Milkvetch

See **Astragalus**

Chitosan

Chitosan is a fibre supplement derived from shellfish.

Benefits

Chitosan is believed to work as an aid to weight loss by absorbing dietary fat in the intestines so that less is absorbed and more is excreted. This helps to maintain a low fat intake and can also reduce circulating blood fat levels.

A number of randomized clinical trials have shown that when volunteers follow a low-calorie diet, those taking chitosan experience significantly more weight loss than those taking placebo over a four-week period. In one trial of 100 overweight or obese volunteers who followed a low-calorie diet, those taking chitosan supplements for four weeks lost 7.3 kg in that period compared with 3 kg in those taking placebo. A similar trial involving 90 adults showed weight reductions of 7.19 kg in the chitosan group versus 3.36 kg in the placebo group. Significant improvements in blood pressure and blood fat levels can also occur.

Dose
3–6 g a day.

Chloride

Chloride is a negatively charged electrolyte of chlorine.

Benefits
Chloride, together with sodium (outside the cells) and potassium (inside the cells), regulates the body's fluid, electrolyte and acid/alkaline balance. It also aids digestion through the production of hydrochloric acid in the stomach, and through cleansing body wastes in the liver. Foods containing chloride include fruits, vegetables, kelp, seafood, table salt and processed foods. As chloride is widespread in foods, deficiency is unlikely except in excessive vomiting.

The body contains around 115 g of chloride ions, kept constant by the excretion of excess salts in sweat, urine and faeces.

Dose

There is currently no EC RDA for chloride and dietary supplements are rarely needed.

Choline and phosphatidyl choline (Lecithin)

Choline is an essential, vitamin-like substance that must be obtained from the diet. Until recently it was thought that the body could make enough to meet its needs from other nutrients, including folic acid and vitamin B12. Since 1998, however, this has been thought to no longer be the case, especially in later life. Conditions that may be due to lack of choline include fatty liver degeneration, hardening of the arteries, Alzheimer's disease, high blood pressure, nervousness, learning difficulties, depression and stomach ulcers.

Choline in the diet

Most dietary choline is derived from the closely related substance, phosphatidyl-choline (also known as lecithin).

Choline is obtained from many food sources, including liver, meat, fish, egg yolk, wheatgerm, nuts and green leafy vegetables. Commercial lecithin found in most supplements is extracted from soybeans.

Benefits

Choline is vital for the structural integrity of cell membranes and, if it is in short supply, cells cannot function properly and are programmed to die (apoptosis). Choline and lecithin also act as emulsifiers to help break down dietary fats into smaller particles that can be absorbed and used in the body. It helps to boost concentration and alertness by acting as a building block to stimulate production of certain neurotransmitters in the brain, including acetylcholine, noradrenaline and dopamine.

Oral supplements of choline can increase brain levels of acetylcholine and improve memory storage and retrieval. In one study, 61 healthy adults aged 50–80 took either 2 tablespoons of lecithin or an inactive placebo for five weeks. By the end of the study, memory test scores of the lecithin group improved significantly and a 48 per cent decrease in memory lapses was reported. People with depression, who failed to respond to prescribed drugs have also benefited from taking choline supplements.

Choline and lecithin appear to reduce the risk of coronary heart disease (CHD) by lowering abnormal cholesterol levels by inhibiting intestinal absorption of cholesterol and increasing excretion of cholesterol in bile. In one study involving 32 people with high blood lipids who took 10.5 g lecithin for 30 days, average total cholesterol and triglycerides decreased by one-third, harmful LDL-cholesterol decreased by 38 per cent and beneficial HDL-cholesterol increased by 46 per cent. The researchers concluded that lecithin should be administered for the prevention and treatment of atherosclerosis. Choline may also reduce the risk of CHD by boosting metabolism of homocysteine, an amino acid strongly linked with increased risk of circulatory problems.

Lecithin can restore normal movement to abnormal sperm cells in the laboratory, and nearly double the ability of sperm to enter and fertilize an egg. It is also essential for implantation of a fertilized egg into the womb lining.

As choline is essential for optimal development of the brain and nervous system, its concentration in blood reaching the foetus is 14 times greater, and that found in breast milk is 100 times higher, than levels found in the mother's bloodstream. Studies suggest that high intakes of choline during pregnancy may enhance memory and learning capacity in the foetus and have long-lasting effects on the memory of offspring – especially if taken during the last three months of pregnancy.

Research suggests that lack of choline is linked with an increased risk of developing liver cancer. If choline is in short supply, liver cells are unable to process and export dietary fats, which build up inside them to produce fatty liver degeneration and liver cell death. Abnormal regeneration of liver tissues then results in a build up of collagen (fibrosis), cirrhosis and can trigger cancerous changes. Choline also helps to eliminate toxins from the liver and gall bladder and may be recommended for people with gallstones.

Lecithin and choline supplements have been shown to improve athletic performance – possibly due to improved communication between nerve and muscle fibres. Blood choline levels have been found to fall by 40 per cent in marathon runners during the course of a race, with similar falls found in swimmers and triathletes. When choline supplements were given before the race, the fall in choline levels was less drastic and, in some cases, performance improved. In one double-blind crossover study, long-distance runners in a 20-mile race improved their time by an average of five minutes, after taking 2.8 g of choline chloride. Less intense activities of short duration do not seem to benefit, however.

Dose
Choline
As choline is not stored in the body, recommended daily intakes are:

- 550 mg a day for men
- 425 mg a day for non-pregnant women, rising to 450 mg during pregnancy and 550 mg when breast-feeding.
- Choline can be taken in doses as high as 1 g three times a day for improving mental function.

Phosphatidylcholine
Capsules: 1–2 g a day, usually divided into three doses.

Lecithin
2–10 g. One tablespoon of lecithin granules provides 1725 mg phosphatidylcholine and 250 mg choline – a little less than that found in a hen's egg. They are best taken with meals to boost absorption.

Choline and lecithin supplements should ideally be taken with vitamin B5 to improve their effect in the body.

Contraindications
Choline and lecithin supplements should not be taken by those with manic depression except under medical supervision in case it worsens the condition.

High doses of choline (e.g. 10 g daily) can cause indigestion, anorexia, sweating and, over time, nerve and cardiovascular distress as well as a strong, fishy body odour. Lecithin supplements are therefore generally preferred.

Chromium

Chromium exists in several forms in nature. The hexavalent form of chromium (used in industry) is toxic and can cause skin and mucous membrane ulceration, gastro-enteritis, liver and kidney problems. Contact leads to dermatitis while inhalation can trigger asthma, perforation of the nasal septum and even cancer.

The trivalent form of chromium is the only one that can be used in the body, and which is non-toxic at recommended doses. Supplements usually contain either chromium picolinate or chromium polynicotinate.

Trivalent chromium is an essential trace element that is needed in minute amounts to form an organic complex known as the Glucose Tolerance Factor (GTF). This complex also contains vitamin B3 (niacin) plus amino acids, and is also known as chromium dinicotinic acid glutathione.

GTF interacts with the pancreatic hormone, insulin, to regulate the uptake of glucose by cells. It also encourages the production of energy from glucose, especially in muscles, increases protein synthesis and lowers blood fat levels, including harmful LDL-cholesterol. It may also suppress hunger pangs through a direct effect on the satiety centre in the brain. Most refined carbohydrates have little chromium content and people eating processed foods will have low intakes. In general, the more carbohydrate you eat, the more chromium you need.

When supplements providing 200 mcg chromium per day were given to diabetics, almost half needed less insulin or blood sugar-lowering tablets. The effects were twice as good in those with non-insulin dependent than in those with insulin-dependent diabetes. Some trials have found little improvement in glucose tolerance when chromium was given to elderly people with stable insulin-independent diabetes, however.

Chromium may help to reduce the risk of coronary heart disease by lowering blood levels of harmful low-density lipoprotein (LDL) cholesterol and raising levels of beneficial high-density (HDL) cholesterol.

Because chromium has an effect on appetite, hunger pangs and fat metabolism, it is widely recommended as a slimming aid, and when combined with a sensible diet and regular exercise, chromium supplements may help some people to lose weight (especially if they are deficient in chromium). While some studies have shown it to be beneficial in weight loss, others have shown little benefit however, and more research is needed.

Chromium in the diet

Foods containing chromium include egg yolk, red meat, cheese, fruit and fruit juice, whole grains, honey, vegetables and condiments such as black pepper and thyme.

Brewer's yeast is a particularly good source of chromium as it is already in the form of GTF, making it at least ten times more effective than that obtained from other food sources. Special chromium-enriched yeast strains have now been developed.

Deficiency

Chromium deficiency is thought to be common. One estimate suggested that 90 per cent of adults are deficient as most people get less than 50 mcg from their diet, and only around 2 per cent of this is in an absorbable (trivalent) form. Intestinal absorption is low (0.5–2 per cent) except where chromium is present in the form of GTF.

Interestingly, chromium levels are highest just after birth. They then rapidly decrease especially after the age of ten. Low levels of chromium have been linked with poor glucose tolerance and diabetes, and it is now widely believed that dietary lack of chromium is a risk factor of maturity-onset (insulin-independent) diabetes as well as cardiovascular disease. Other symptoms that may be due to chromium deficiency include poor tolerance of alcohol, abnormal blood fat levels, muscle weakness, hunger pangs and weight gain, nervousness, irritability, confusion, depression, thirst, decreased sperm count and impaired fertility.

Dose

There is currently no EC RDA set for chromium. Intakes of 50–200 mcg per day are considered both safe and adequate. Supplements are best absorbed when taken with vitamin C, while calcium-containing supplements will reduce absorption.

Excess

Do not exceed the stated dose as this may affect zinc and iron absorption.

CMO (cis-9-cetyl myristoleate)

CMO is a waxy oil which is highly lubricant and also has a natural anti-inflammatory action. It helps to lubricate joints and is mainly taken to improve symptoms of rheumatoid arthritis. It is often taken together with fish or flaxseed oil, vitamin E and glucosamine sulphate and sometimes with an enzyme, lipase, to aid its digestion. A double-blind, randomized trial provided results from 382 people with inflammatory arthritis (e.g. rheumatoid, psoriatic) who had failed to respond to non-steroidal anti-inflammatory drugs. Some took CMO alone for 30 days, some took it combined with another agent (glucosamine hydrochloride, sea cucumber extracts or hydrolyzed cartilage) and one group took only placebo. Treatment response rates were 63 per cent in the CMO group, 87 per cent in the CMO plus additional agent group, and 15 per cent in the placebo group.

Dose

600 mg daily was administered in the above trial.

Tobacco and caffeine use are reported to reduce the effectiveness of CMO.

Despite these results, CMO is expensive – the cost of one month's supply varies from £50 to over £70. Although some practitioners claim that only one course may be needed, other supplements such as omega-3 fish oils and glucosamine sulphate used alone may be more cost-effective.

Cobalamin

See **Vitamin B12**

Co-enzyme Q10

Co-enzyme Q10 (CoQ10) – also known as ubiquinone – is a vitamin-like substance that improves oxygen utilization and energy production. It is present in all body cells, with the heart, liver cells and sperm cells containing the greatest amounts.

CoQ10 is needed to process oxygen in cells, and to generate energy-rich molecules. Without CoQ10, the energy hidden in food molecules could not be converted into a form of energy in muscle cells, including those of the heart. After the age of 20, levels of CoQ10 start to decrease as dietary CoQ10 is absorbed less efficiently from the intestines and its production in body cells starts to fall. Dietary sources include meat, fish, whole grains, nuts and green vegetables. Average adult dietary intakes of CoQ10 are estimated at 3–5 mg daily among meat eaters and 1 mg daily among vegetarians.

Benefits

CoQ10 acts together with vitamin E to form a powerful antioxidant defence against oxidation damage to body fats – including those in the circulation. Like other antioxidants, CoQ10 seems to protect against hardening and furring up of the arteries (atherosclerosis), reduce heart disease and is often helpful for those with Raynaud's syndrome.

Low levels of CoQ10 mean that cells do not receive all the energy they need so they function at a sub-optimal level and are more likely to become diseased, age and even die. Research suggests that falling CoQ10 levels play a significant role in age-related medical conditions such as coronary heart disease. CoQ10 is now also being added to skin-care preparations to reduce skin damage that leads to premature wrinkles, especially following exposure to UVA in sunlight.

Biopsies of heart muscle from patients with various forms of heart disease have shown that up to 75 per cent are deficient in CoQ10. At least one study has found that the more severe the heart disease, the lower the levels of CoQ10. It has therefore been used by some doctors in the USA and Japan to treat coronary heart disease and heart failure with excellent results.

Supplements have been used to normalize high blood pressure and, in a trial involving 18 patients with essential hypertension, a daily dose of 100 mg CoQ10 was found to significantly reduce blood pressure compared with a placebo. CoQ10 is thought to lower hypertension by improving the elasticity and reactivity of the blood vessel wall. In another trial involving 109 people with essential hypertension, an average daily dose of 225 mg CoQ10 was added to their existing drug regime. A significant, gradual improvement in BP occurred and, overall, 51 per cent of participants were able to stop between one and three antihypertensive drugs within 4.4 months of starting CoQ10.

CoQ10 is vital for production of the energy sperm need for motility. Men with reduced sperm motility showed significant improvements in sperm function when taking CoQ10 supplements, and in fertility treatments their sperm were over twice as likely to fertilize an egg compared with those not taking CoQ10.

CoQ10 supplements – both given alone and with vitamin B6 – increase the number of antibodies made after vaccination, and also increase the number of certain immune cells to boost immunity. It may also be useful in weight loss by stimulating lipid metabolism in mitochondria. Two groups of obese individuals were placed on a controlled reducing diet and one group also took CoQ10. Within nine weeks, the group on CoQ10 lost an average of 30 pounds, compared with an average of 13 pounds for the other group.

CoQ10 can help to protect against gum disease. Diseased gum tissue has been shown to have significantly reduced levels of CoQ10 compared with healthy gum tissue from the same patients. When CoQ10 supplements are combined with periodontal treatments, periodontal disease can be improved enough to save some teeth scheduled for removal.

In a study involving 25 Finnish top-level cross-country skiers, those taking CoQ10 supplements showed significant improvement in all measured indexes of physical performance. Ninety-four per cent of the athletes felt CoQ10 had improved their performance and recovery time compared with only 33 per cent of those taking an inactive placebo.

Some researchers believe that CoQ10 helps to improve survival rates in people with breast, prostate and possibly other cancers, although this is still under investigation.

Dose

The optimal dietary intake of CoQ10 is unknown. Commercially available dietary supplements recommend 10–100 mg CoQ10 daily – often taken as two separate doses. Intakes of up to 180 mg daily are recommended for general use by some researchers. Higher doses of 300–600 mg daily are used to treat illnesses such as heart disease and high blood pressure.

CoQ10 is best taken with food to improve absorption as it is fat soluble. It usually takes at least three weeks and occasionally up to three months before the full beneficial effect and extra energy levels are noticed. To utilize CoQ10 to the full, you also need to ensure a good intake of B and C vitamins.

Side effects

Only occasional and transient, mild nausea have been reported at high doses.

Conjugated linoleic acid

Conjugated linoleic acids (CLA) are fatty acids mainly found in meat and dairy products. They are formed in animals with more than one stomach by the action of an enzyme (linoleic acid isomerase) produced by an intestinal bacteria (*Butyrivibrio fibrisolvens*) which acts on dietary linoleic acid before it is absorbed into body tissues. CLA can also be produced commercially from sunflower, safflower and other oils.

Because it is a fatty acid, CLA is laid down in cell membranes, where it is involved in cell growth. It differs from linoleic acid only in the placement of two double bonds within its fatty acid chain, which changes its biological actions.

Benefits

CLA alters the type of chemicals produced by cells when they react to stimulants such as foreign proteins, injury or even exercise. It can reduce the inflammatory response, artery constriction and abnormal blood clotting by reducing synthesis of prostaglandin PGE-2 into which it is incorporated.

Research shows that CLA helps to promote a healthy body fat composition by increasing the breakdown of fatty tissue (lipolysis) and increasing lean body mass (LBM). It is thought to work by regulating the action of enzymes in fat cells so that less fat is laid down in these fat cells, and more is broken down and discharged from the cell, although the exact mechanism is not yet known. Once released the fatty acids are then transported to muscle cells to act as an energy source – building muscle at the expense of fat. Research has confirmed that CLA reduces the size of fat cells.

CLA cannot be synthesized in the human body, and changes in farming practices, food processing and reduced consumption of milk and high fat foods mean that CLA intakes have fallen by 80 per cent compared with the amounts eaten by our stone age ancestors. As a result, it is often referred to as the 'missing link' in weight-loss management. Some researchers have even claimed that obesity is a CLA deficiency disease, as it is essential for the mobilization and transport of dietary fats away from fatty tissues to muscle cells where it is burned for fuel.

CLA was originally patented for improving growth, and for use in preventing the changes in body composition that can accompany the use of steroids, and infection. It is now also believed to help reduce risk factors associated with heart disease, increase bone density, reduce chronic inflammation and possibly normalize a raised blood glucose level by increasing sensitivity to the effects of insulin.

In one study, 64 per cent of a group of 22 people with diabetes showed improvements in insulin levels after eight weeks (compared with improvement in 40 per cent taking a placebo), with a moderately reduced blood fasting glucose level. They also had reduced triglyceride levels after 8 weeks (reduction of 50 mg/dl compared with 10 mg/dl in those not taking supplements). Further large-scale studies are still needed.

When 71 obese volunteers followed a calorie-restricted diet and took moderate exercise, 35 were also given 3 g daily of CLA supplements (one gram with each meal) while the other 36 were given a sunflower oil placebo. Both groups lost around 5 pounds in weight over six months, and CLA did not seem to contribute to weight loss. However, when the dieters went back to eating 'normally' and regained weight, those taking CLA were more likely to gain lean tissue (muscle) rather than fat. Usually, weight gain would be expected to consist of at least three times more fat than muscle, but those taking CLA gained fat and lean tissue in nearly equal proportions. Those taking CLA experienced no side effects, but experienced less depression, negative feelings and upset stomach than those not taking it – it helped them stick to their diet. These findings suggest that CLA would be most helpful as a weight-management aid rather than a weight-loss aid.

In another study, ten subjects (including both genders) each took 3 g CLA daily, and another group of ten took a placebo. After three months, those taking CLA had only lost around 2 lbs in weight but their body fat percentage changed significantly from 21.3 to 17 per cent. Those taking a placebo gained half a pound in weight and their body fat percentage increased slightly from 22 per cent to 22.4 per cent.

In another study, 19 healthy volunteers took 3 g CLA daily and were instructed not to carry out any other changes in their diet or lifestyle during the three-month trial period. Although the changes experienced were small, 74 per cent of volunteers lost weight even though they did not make any other changes to their normal diet or lifestyle. Interestingly, several of the participants – including those who had maintained or gained weight, reported that their waists had reduced in size, clothes were looser fitting and some dropped a clothing size due to changes in distribution of weight between fat and muscle.

CLA research is currently looking into possible protective actions against coronary heart disease by reducing blood triglyceride and cholesterol levels, and reducing formation of atherosclerotic plaques involved in hardening and furring up of the arteries. It is also under investigation for anti-cancer activity, especially against breast cancer. Laboratory research suggests that it may be 100 times more effective in reducing growth of tumour cells than fish oils.

Researchers estimated that the average diet supplies 100–300 mg CLA daily, while the most beneficial effects occur at intakes of around 3000 mg daily.

Dose

1 g capsules (equivalent to 0.6 g CLA) three times a day with food. Swallow with 200 ml water.

Products with a strength of at least 75 per cent CLA are most beneficial. Consider taking antioxidants with them to help protect them from oxidation.

Contraindications

CLA should not be taken during pregnancy as its effects are unknown.

Copper

Copper is the third most abundant essential trace element in the body after zinc and iron. It is obtained from a number of dietary sources, including crustaceans and shellfish (prawns, oysters, lobster, crab), nuts, pulses, whole-grain cereals, avocado, artichokes, radishes, garlic, mushrooms and green vegetables grown in copper-rich soil. Brewer's yeast supplements are also an excellent source.

Benefits

Copper balance in the body is now known to be controlled by two genes, and is needed for healthy growth, liver, brain and muscle function, immunity, white and red blood cell development, iron absorption from the gut, and for cholesterol and glucose metabolism. It is essential for the function of a number of enzymes involved in antioxidant protection, and others needed to synthesize brain chemicals, and the two pigments melanin and haemoglobin. It is also involved in regulating blood cholesterol levels and may help to protect against hardening and furring up of the arteries (atherosclerosis).

Copper is involved in vitamin C metabolism and the synthesis of collagen – a major structural protein. It is therefore needed to maintain healthy bones, cartilage, hair and skin – especially their elasticity. In fact, if vitamin C intakes are optimal, copper deficiency can quickly occur if dietary intakes are limited.

In one trial involving menopausal women, those taking 3 mg copper supplements did not lose significant bone density compared with those taking a placebo, who experienced a significant fall in bone mineral density, suggesting that supplements may help to prevent osteoporosis.

Up to 70 per cent of dietary intake remains unabsorbed because it is bound to other bowel contents such as sugars, sweeteners, refined flour, raw meat, vitamin C, zinc and calcium. Supplementation is therefore important, especially if the diet is deficient.

The risk of copper deficiency is greater when zinc intakes are high. The ideal dietary ratio of copper to zinc is 1:10.

Deficiency

Lack of copper can occur in conditions such as Crohn's or coeliac disease or in people with a hereditary inability to process copper properly. This can lead to heart muscle problems (cardiac myopathy). Other problems that may be linked with lack of copper include anaemia, low white cell count, increased susceptibility to infection, fluid retention, loss of taste sensation, raised blood cholesterol levels, abnormal structure and pigmentation of body hair, abnormal pigmentation and loss of elasticity in skin, irritability, impaired fertility and osteoporosis.

Copper-deficient diets have been shown to reduce bone mineralization and strength. Many people with arthritis have low blood levels of copper, and are helped by wearing a copper bracelet so that trace amounts are absorbed through the skin.

Excess copper (e.g. from drinking water supplied through copper pipes) is toxic at levels just twice as high as the norm, and can lead to restlessness, nausea, vomiting, colic, diarrhoea and, in long-term cases, to copper-induced cirrhosis of the liver.

Dose

There is currently no EC RDA for copper. Intakes of between 0.8 and 3 mg are suggested as both safe and adequate for adults. Generally intakes are low, however, with an average of around 1.6 mg a day (and 50 per cent of people get less than this) and copper deficiency is common as the dietary sources are not always eaten frequently. In supplement form it is best taken as copper citrate or copper picolinate.

Cranberry
(Vaccinium macrocarpon)

Cranberries are native to North America, and are widely used to make sauces and jelly, and are also juiced to make a popular and refreshing fruit drink.

Benefits

Traditionally, cranberries were used as a poultice to dress wounds, and to prevent or treat scurvy as they have a high content of vitamin C. More recently it was recognized that cranberry juice has a beneficial effect on the urinary tract to reduce the incidence of urinary infections.

Research shows that drinking 300 ml cranberry juice daily can almost halve the risk of developing cystitis. A double-blind, placebo-controlled trial randomized 153 elderly women to drink either 300 ml cranberry juice per day for six months, or a synthetic placebo that was indistinguishable in taste, appearance, and vitamin C content but lacked cranberry. Those drinking cranberry juice were 42 per cent less likely to develop pus cells in their urine (pyuria) than people not drinking it.

Cranberry fruit solids also have beneficial anti-adhesin (preventing bacteria) properties, and standardized cranberry supplements prepared from these can also help to reduce the symptoms of urinary tract infections. In one clinical trial, 24 women with a history of recurring urinary tract infections where given prophylactic antibiotics for six months. Then, they were divided into two groups, and half took cranberry extracts for the next six months, while the second group continued with antibiotics. Those taking cranberry supplements (Cran-Max) had only one urinary tract infection within the group compared with 25 relapses (average of 2.3 per patient) in those continuing with prophylactic antibiotics. They also did not have side effects, while those on antibiotics experienced diarrhoea, Candida, vomiting and skin reactions.

Cranberry is also helpful for reducing the unpleasant odours associated with urinary incontinence.

Research is currently looking into other beneficial actions of cranberry anti-adhesins, including their ability to reduce dental plaque in the mouth. Recent research from Tel Aviv University also provides preliminary evidence suggesting that cranberry juice can help to stop *Helicobacter pylori* sticking to cells in the stomach lining. This may help to flush *Helicobacter* from the stomach so they are expelled more easily to help reduce the risk of gastritis and peptic ulcers.

Dose

Cranberry juice: 300 ml daily
Cranberry supplements: 500 mg daily

Note: if a urinary tract infection is suspected medical advice should always be sought – especially during pregnancy.

D

Vitamin D is a water-soluble vitamin, whose natural form is known as cholecalciferol. This can be synthesized in the body by the action of sunlight (UVB rays) on a cholesterol-like molecule (7–dehydrocholesterol) in the skin. Blood levels of vitamin D are therefore naturally higher in the summer and lower in winter. Cholecalciferol and synthetic versions (in the form of ergocalciferol) are broken down in the body to form a hormone called calcitriol.

Foods containing vitamin D include oily fish, fish liver oils, fortified margarine and breakfast cereals, liver, eggs, fortified milk and butter.

Benefits

Vitamin D is essential for the absorption of dietary calcium and phosphate in the small intestine and for their deposition in bone, and for bone modeling. If vitamin D is lacking during childhood, deformed bones (rickets) result, while in adulthood, vitamin D deficiency leads to weakened, softened bones known as osteomalacia.

Bone thinning (osteoporosis) in menopausal women is partly regulated by the amount of vitamin D obtained in the diet or from supplements. When vitamin D is in short supply, less calcium is absorbed from the diet and blood levels therefore have to be maintained by leaching calcium from bones. Four out of five people with hip fracture have evidence of vitamin D deficiency.

In a study of post-menopausal women with low vitamin D levels, increasing intakes to 12.5 mcg for one year significantly reduced bone loss in late winter and increased bone density in the spine. Adding calcium supplements to the diet of elderly people reduces their risk of a vertebral fracture by 20 per cent, while giving both calcium and vitamin D supplements reduces the risk of hip fracture by up to 40 per cent.

Vitamin D also has an important action on skin health and may be effective in treating some forms of psoriasis. Vitamin D was also found to reduce growth and division of cancer cells in the laboratory, and may play a role in reducing the risk of certain cancers, especially those affecting the prostate, colon and breast. These findings are currently under investigation.

Excess intake of fluoride causes mottling of teeth known as fluorosis. This was thought to be irreversible, but a study in which children with fluorosis were given vitamin C (500 mg), calcium (250 mg) and vitamin D (20 mcg or 800 IU) daily showed marked reversal of dental mottling.

Deficiency

Most people get enough vitamin D from their diet and from exposure to sunlight. People living in high altitudes, in northern latitudes (including Scotland), and those who cover up their skin in sunlight, use high-factor sunscreens, or who stay indoors all day may not be exposed to enough sunlight to meet their vitamin D needs. Older people are also at risk of deficiency as they synthesize less vitamin D.

Symptoms that may be due to lack of vitamin D include constipation, muscle weakness, lowered immunity with increased susceptibility to infections, poor growth, irritability, bone pain, bone deformities (in rickets) and deafness (in osteomalacia).

Dose

The EC RDA for vitamin D is 5 mcg (200 IU). People over the age of 50 usually need at least double this amount.

Note: doses of vitamin D are sometimes expressed in International Units (IU) rather than micrograms: 1 mcg vitamin D = 40 IU.

Excess

Excess vitamin D is toxic and can lead to headache, loss of appetite, nausea, vomiting, diarrhoea or constipation, palpitations and fatigue.

Damiana
(Turnera diffusa aphrodisiaca)

Damiana is a small shrub with aromatic leaves (smelling similar to chamomile) whose long tradition of use as an aphrodisiac can be traced back to the ancient Mayans of Central America. Its reputation is so well established that it is even reflected in the botanical name, *Turnera aphrodisiaca*.

Benefits

The volatile, aromatic oils of damiana have a stimulant and gently irritating effect on the genitals to produce localized tingling and throbbing sensations. Its alkaloids may also boost circulation to the genital area and increase sensitivity of nerve endings in the clitoris and penis. Blood flow to the penis also increases so that erections are firmer and more long lasting.

These combined effects are said to increase sexual desire, enhance sexual pleasure and stimulate performance. Some herbalists have suggested that the alkaloids in damiana could have a testosterone-like action but there seems to be no research to support this.

When drunk as a tea damiana produces a mild euphoria and some people use it almost as a recreational drug. It is also used as a tonic for the nervous system, mild laxative, urinary antiseptic and for headaches and bed-wetting. It is specifically used in cases of anxiety and depression where there is a sexual problem such as low sex drive, impotence, premature ejaculation and recurrent genital herpes infections.

Dose
Capsules/tablets: 200–800 mg a day, usually taken on an occasional basis when needed rather than regularly, often combined with other prosexual herbs.

Side effects
Some evidence suggests that damiana may reduce iron absorption from the gut and therefore it should not be used long term.

Dandelion
(Taraxacum officinalis)

Dandelion is a well-known perennial weed found throughout most parts of the world. The leaves were traditionally eaten in spring as a cleansing herbal tonic.

Benefits

Dandelion is widely used for liver and digestive problems. The root (usually obtained from two-year-old plants) is also used in an effective detoxifying supplement that works on the liver, increasing detoxification functions and stimulating the flow of bile so more toxins are eliminated through the bowels. It also has a gentle laxative action that helps to improve constipation.

Dandelion leaf is used for its diuretic action on the kidneys, helping to increase the elimination of water-soluble toxins from the body. Dandelion also has a useful mineral content, including potassium which helps to flush excess sodium through the kidneys. This makes it an excellent treatment for water retention and bloating – in fact, the medieval name for dandelion was 'piss-a-bed'.

Dandelion may be taken to help treat liver problems, including gallstones, jaundice and hepatitis but is best used under medical supervision. It should not be taken during an acute attack of gallstones, or if obstructive jaundice is present, for example.

As dandelion improves bile flow, it is useful for relieving symptoms caused by hormone imbalances, especially oestrogen excess, such as endometriosis and cyclical breast pain. It also promotes absorption of dietary iron and is sometimes used, therefore, to treat anaemia.

Dose

5–10 g fresh root daily divided between two or three doses or 500 mg extracts twice a day.

Side effects

Large doses can cause nausea and diarrhoea.

Contraindications

Should not be taken by anyone who has active gallstones or obstructive jaundice.

Devil's claw
(Harpagophytum procumbens)

Devil's claw is named after the sharp hooks that develop on its fruit. It is a South African desert plant whose tap root produces potato-like tubers to store water.

Benefits

Devil's claw tubers contain compounds known as iridoid glycosides such as harpagoside and harpagide that have a natural anti-inflammatory and painkilling actions similar to those of aspirin.

Devil's claw is taken to treat low back pain, and painful, inflamed joints due to osteoarthritis, rheumatoid arthritis, gout or sports injuries.

It is also traditionally used as a tonic to help digestive problems, headaches and to reduce fevers. Some practitioners use it in an ointment to be applied to sores, boils and ulcers. Devil's claw has also been found to encourage excretion of uric acid, reducing the risk of recurrent gout.

Research in Germany has found improvement with devil's claw in conditions of the upper duodenum related to the pancreas and clinical evaluation has indicated a marked reduction in raised cholesterol levels.

In one study 105 patients with chronic back pain were given either Devil's claw (800 mg, three times a day) or an inactive placebo, and were allowed to take additional painkillers if necessary. After four weeks, 9 out of the 51 people receiving Devil's claw were pain-free compared with only 1 of the 54 receiving placebo. The investigators suggest that further trials with devil's claw investigating pain reduction would be worthwhile.

Another double-blind, placebo-controlled trial showed significant reductions in muscle pain, pain sensitivity and muscle tension in those suffering from shoulder neck and back pain with benefits appearing after around two weeks of treatment.

Against this, however, a trial involving 197 patients aged 18–75 with chronic back pain found that devil's claw had only a mild beneficial effect in which only one in ten people seemed to respond well. It was found to be beneficial for those who would also be helped by painkillers, manipulation or attendance at back school.

Dose

1–10 g daily depending on concentration of extract, to provide around 50 mg harpagoside daily.

Contraindications

Devil's claw should not be taken by:

- sufferers of peptic ulcers or indigestion as it promotes secretion of digestive juices
- pregnant or breast-feeding women.

Dong quai
(Angelica sinensis)

Dong quai, or Chinese angelica, is native to China and Japan where it is widely used as a female tonic and sometimes referred to as 'female ginseng'.

Benefits
Its aromatic rhizome is harvested after two years' growth and is a good source of vitamins E and B12, iron and oestrogen-like substances that interact with oestrogen receptors in the body. This helps to damp down the effects of excess oestrogen production (as in some cases of pre-menstrual syndrome, cyclical breast pain, endometriosis, fibroids) and also provides additional oestrogen activity where natural oestrogen levels are low (e.g. at the menopause).

In Asia, dong quai is valued as an adaptogen with hormone and mood-balancing properties. It is second only to Korean ginseng in popularity and is frequently combined with other herbs (e.g. chasteberry, liquorice, Siberian ginseng).

Chinese angelica is traditionally combined with other herbs as a natural form of hormone replacement therapy for women experiencing menopausal symptoms such as hot flushes and night sweats. However, a 12-week placebo controlled study involving 71 women was widely reported to find no significant difference in menopausal symptoms between those taking dong quai as a single agent, and those taking an inactive placebo. This does not prove lack of efficacy, however, as Chinese angelica is usually prescribed in combination with other herbs with which it may act in synergy.

Dong quai is also used to ease menstrual cramps and, in one study, was found to be 1.7 times more effective as an analgesic than aspirin for relieving muscle spasms. In addition it is taken as a nourishing tonic for anaemia, to stimulate the circulation, as a laxative and to improve cyclical mood swings and headaches. It is said to increase blood circulation to the pelvis, supports normal ovarian function and helps to regulate an irregular menstrual cycle.

Dose
Capsules standardized to 9000 ppm ligustilide: 200 mg three times daily.

Contraindications
Dong quai should not be taken by:
- anyone who has peptic ulcers
- pregnant or breast-feeding women
- women who experience heavy menstruation, abnormal bleeding or who take anticoagulants such as coumarin or aspirin regularly.

Note: Chinese angelica contains anticoagulants and should not be taken in large quantities. It also contains psoralene, a compound that increases skin sensitivity to sunlight and may cause a skin rash on exposure to sun in some people, especially those with fair skin; they should only, therefore, take small quantities.

E

Vitamin E consists of two groups of fat-soluble compounds, the tocopherols and tocotrienols. The most active of these is alpha-tocopherol, and the vitamin E content of foods and supplements is usually expressed in terms of alpha-tocopherol equivalents. Synthetic alpha-tocopherol (dl-alpha tocopherol) has less biological strength than natural source vitamin E (d-alpha tocopherol) due to the different symmetries of the molecules present.

Vitamin E in the diet
Foods containing vitamin E include wheatgerm oil, avocado, margarine, eggs, butter, whole grains, nuts, seeds, oily fish and broccoli. Vitamin E is unstable when frozen – up to 80 per cent of the vitamin E content is destroyed. Heating also destroys around 30 per cent vitamin E content. Fresh raw foods and supplements are therefore the best sources.

Benefits
Vitamin E is a powerful antioxidant which acts as a preservative to protect body fats from the harmful effects of excess free radicals. Vitamin E protects cell membranes, nerve sheaths, circulating cholesterol molecules, dietary fats and body fat stores from oxidative damage and rancidity. In general, the more polyunsaturated fatty acids you eat, the more vitamin E is obtained.

Vitamin E also has a strengthening effect on muscle fibres to relieve muscle cramps, it boosts immunity (by working together with selenium to increase antibody production), improves skin suppleness and healing and also seems to improve glucose use in the body. It therefore helps people with diabetes to develop a better response to insulin hormone and improved glucose balance.

Vitamin E has a powerful protective effect in the circulation by reducing hardening and furring up of the arteries, helping blood vessels to dilate and reducing abnormal blood clotting. In a study involving over 125,000 people, the risk of coronary heart disease was reduced by up to 50 per cent in women and 25 per cent in men who had taken vitamin E supplements for two years or more.

In the Cambridge Heart Antioxidant Study (CHAOS), over 2000 patients with coronary heart disease were divided into two groups. Half took vitamin E for 18 months, while half received a placebo. Taking high-dose vitamin E (400 or 800 IU daily = 268 mg or 536 mg) was found to reduce the risk of a heart attack by 77 per cent. Not only was the difference highly statistically significant, it seemed that the group treated with vitamin E were at no greater risk of a heart attack than people without coronary heart disease. The results need further investigation however as not all trials have shown such a beneficial result.

Smokers generate a large number of free radicals which are linked with a number of diseases including coronary heart disease, high blood pressure, stroke, osteoporosis and cancer. Low dietary intakes of antioxidant vitamins (e.g. vitamins C and E) increase the risk of these illnesses, whereas high dietary intakes seem to be protective.

An interesting study of over 11,000 people aged 67 years and over found that those taking vitamin E had a reduced risk of premature death at any age by around a third compared with those not taking vitamin E supplements. Risk of death from coronary heart disease was reduced by 63 per cent, and risk of death from cancer reduced by 59 per cent. These results took into account other factors such as alcohol use, smoking history, aspirin use and known medical conditions. A protective effect against some cancers was also found in a study of over 35,000 women in which a strong reduction in colon cancer risk occurred in those with high intakes of vitamin E supplements among women under the age of 65.

Laboratory experiments suggest that when lycopene and vitamin E act together, prostate cancer cells are stopped from growing and multiplying by as much as 90 per cent. A diet high in vitamin E seems to provide some protection against cataracts and age-related macular degeneration – both conditions that can cause loss of sight in later life. In one study involving 1380 people, those with high levels of vitamin E had less than half the risk of lens opacities (cataracts) compared to those with the lowest levels.

Other studies have shown that vitamin E is beneficial in the treatment of peripheral vascular disease and neurological problems such as Parkinson's Disease, tardive dyskinesia and epilepsy.

Some studies have found that vitamin E intake is linked with lung function in older people. For example, for every 1mg increase in vitamin E in the daily diet, the amount of air that can be blown out in one second increases by 42 ml.

Vitamin E creams or oil are often used to improve the quality of skin healing after surgery; however, as many as one in three people develop sensitivity to topical vitamin E.

Deficiency

Lack of vitamin E has a harmful effect on the nervous system and can produce symptoms such as lack of energy, lethargy, poor concentration, irritability, muscle weakness and poor co-ordination. In severe, long-term lack (such as that due to malabsorption) serious effects such as blindness, dementia and abnormal heart rhythms can occur. The EC RDA for vitamin E is 10 mg.

Dose

10–1000 mg or more under supervision. High intakes of vitamin E can be toxic, but this only usually occurs at doses above 3000 mg daily. Select supplements containing a natural source (d-alpha tocopherol) for their greater bioactivity.

Note: sometimes the amount of vitamin E is expressed in International Units (IU) rather than milligrams:
1 IU=0.67 mg alpha-tocopherol equivalents or, conversely, 1mg = 1.5 IU.
  Vitamin C is needed to regenerate vitamin E after it has acted as an antioxidant, therefore adequate supplies of both vitamins are essential.

See also **Carotenoids – Lycopene**

Echinacea
(Echinacea purpurea)

Echinacea, or purple coneflower, is a traditional remedy first used by native American Indians such as the Sioux to treat blood poisoning, snake bites, boils, fever, eczema and to relieve allergic reactions.

Benefits

Echinacea contains several unique polysaccharides known as echinacins that help to stimulate the immune system by increasing the number and activity of white blood cells responsible for attacking viral, fungal and bacterial infections. It stimulates phagocytosis – the process in which white blood cells ingest bacteria and viruses before destroying them – and also boosts production of a natural anti-viral substance called interferon. It also contains flavonoids that have an antioxidant action.

Echinacea boosts immunity, promotes healing and is now mainly used to help prevent and treat recurrent upper respiratory tract infections such as the common cold, laryngitis, tonsillitis, otitis media or sinusitis, viral infections such as herpes cold sores, and skin complaints. A tincture of echinacea can be used as a mouthwash to treat and help to prevent recurrent oral thrush.

In people who take it, echinacea has been shown to almost double the length of time between infections compared with those who do not, and when infections do occur, they tend to be less severe.

In one study involving 180 people with influenza, those taking echinacea extracts daily had a significant reduction in symptoms compared with those taking a placebo. Most studies show that it reduces susceptibility to colds by around a third. In a second study of just over 100 people with a common cold, some were given echinacea and others a placebo. After eight weeks, those taking echinacea had longer times between recurrent infections, less severe symptoms and recovered faster when infection did occur than those taking the placebo.

Echinacea also has detoxifying effects and encourages elimination by promoting sweating. Its benefits to the immune system mean that it is often helpful in auto-immune conditions such as eczema, psoriasis, lupus, multiple sclerosis and rheumatoid arthritis. It is sometimes also helpful in chronic fatigue syndrome – especially where this has followed on from a viral illness. It may help to improve survival in those with cancer, but this is still under investigation.

Dose

300 mg, three times daily to treat colds and influenza, or 200 mg, three or four times a day for lesser infections. Select products standardized to contain at least 3.5 per cent echinicosides.

Opinions on how to take echinacea vary. It seems to work by stimulating the activity of white blood cells that absorb viruses and bacteria before destroying them. This activity remains above normal for several days after a dose, so taking it only on week days, and not at weekends, for example, or for two weeks out of four, should not reduce its effectiveness.

The manufacturers of one of the leading echinacea tinctures (Echinaforce) do not place any restriction on its long-term use, and say it may be taken in low dose, long term to reduce infections, or in a higher dose just when you feel an infection coming on.

There is no evidence of any harm done by taking it long term.

Other manufacturers prefer their products to be used intermittently, e.g. for no more than two weeks without a break. Always follow manufacturer's guidelines on how to use their products, as they do contain different balances of ingredients which means they should be used in a different way.

When taking them intermittently, goldenseal can be taken during the time that echinacea is not being taken to maintain immune vigour.

Echinacea is also applied to the skin as dilute solutions to treat a variety of inflammatory and infective skin conditions.

Echinacea seems to be safe during pregnancy and breast-feeding, although as with all supplements it should only be taken during pregnancy under supervision from a qualified practitioner.

Elderberry
(Sambucus nigra)

Elder trees are native to northern Europe, and elderberries are a familiar autumn fruit widely used in home-made country wines and jams.

Benefits

Elderberry juice contains an anti-viral compound termed 'antivirin' and has been shown in double-blind, placebo-controlled trials to reduce the severity and duration of common cold and influenza infections. It is active against influenza types A and B, including the most virulent strains. In one trial involving 40 people (children and adults) with respiratory viral infections, including influenza, 93 per cent receiving elderberry extracts showed significant clinical improvement within two days, whereas it took six days to achieve similar improvement in those receiving placebo.

In another randomized, placebo-controlled trial involving 27 people with Panama flu type B, 15 took elderberry extracts, and 12 took a placebo. Within two days, 93 per cent taking elderberry extracts showed significant clinical reduction in symptoms and fever, while 92 per cent of those taking placebo took up to six days to improve.

A similar trial involving 60 people aged 18–54 years with flu-like symptoms for 48 hours or less found that those taking elderberry syrup were relieved of influenza symptoms on average four days earlier than those taking the placebo. Levels of antibodies were found to be significantly higher in those taking elderberry extracts than in those on placebo.

Elderberry extracts also seem to be active against *Herpes simplex* viruses and HIV.

Dose
Standardized elderberry syrup: 15 ml twice a day.

Essential Fatty Acids

Essential fatty acids (EFAs) belong to a group of oils known as long-chain polyunsaturated fatty acids (LCPs). While your body can make small amounts of EFAs from other dietary fats, they are often in short supply and must come from the diet. There are two main EFAs:

- linoleic acid – an omega-6 PUFA
- linolenic acid – an omega-3 PUFA.

In addition, arachidonic acid – an omega-6 PUFA – may be essential if supplies of other EFAs (from which it can be synthesized) are low.

Once in your body, these two EFAs act as building blocks to make cell membranes, sex hormones, and hormone-like chemicals (prostaglandins) found in all your body tissues. EFAs can also be converted into two other types of LCPs:

- arachidonic acid (AA) which you make from linoleic acid
- docosahexaenoic acid (DHA) which you make from linolenic acid.

Dietary Sources of Essential Fatty Acids

- Linoleic acid alone is found in sunflower seeds, almonds, corn, sesame seeds, safflower oil and extra virgin olive oil.
- Linolenic acid alone is found in evening primrose oil, starflower (borage) seed oil and blackcurrant seed oil.
- Both linoleic and linolenic acid are found in rich quantities in walnuts, pumpkin seeds, soybeans, linseed oil, rapeseed oil and flax oil.
- Arachidonic acid is found in many foods (e.g. seafood, meat, dairy products) and can also be made from linoleic or linolenic acids.
- Gamma-linolenic acid is found in evening primrose oil, starflower (borage) seed oil and blackcurrant seed among others.

EFAs are found in nuts, seeds, green leafy vegetables, oily fish, whole grains or in supplements such as evening primrose oil. It is estimated that as many as eight out of ten people do not get enough EFAs from their diet.

Once in the body, EFAs are fed into a series of metabolic reactions (the EFA pathway) that convert them into hormone-like substances called prostaglandins:

Linoleic → Gamma-linolenic → dihomo-gamma → arachidonic → prostaglandins
acid   acid   linolenic acid   acid
        (evening primrose oil)

Prostaglandins are involved in a variety of balancing metabolic reactions. As you can see from the EFA pathway, some gamma-linolenic acid can be synthesized from dietary linoleic acid, but this reaction needs an enzyme (delta-6–desaturase) that is easily blocked by a number of factors associated with an unhealthy diet, lifestyle and toxicity, including:

- excess intakes of saturated (animal) fat
- excess intakes of trans-fatty acids (e.g. found in hydrogenated margarines)
- excess intakes of sugar
- drinking too much alcohol
- dietary lack of vitamins and minerals, especially vitamin B6, zinc and magnesium
- crash dieting
- smoking cigarettes
- exposure to pollution.

Taking an essential fatty acid supplement (such as evening primrose oil, flaxseed oil) overcomes any enzyme blocks by feeding into the middle of the EFA pathway.

Deficiency

When you do not get enough EFAs from your diet, the metabolism can make do with the next best fatty acids available (e.g. those derived from saturated fats) but as a result prostaglandin imbalances are common. Prostaglandins made from other sorts of fat cannot be converted into prostaglandins made from the EFAs. This increases the risk of imbalances, especially of sex hormones, and is linked with dry, itchy skin, chronic inflammatory diseases (e.g. rheumatoid arthritis, psoriasis and eczema) and gynaecological problems such as cyclical breast pain. Other symptoms due to lack of essential fatty acids include thirst, urinary frequency, pimply skin and acne, dry hair and dandruff, brittle nails, lowered immunity with frequent infections, prostate problems and low sex drive. Lack of EFAs during early childhood has also been linked with an increased risk of allergies such as eczema, asthma and hay fever in later life, and may also be linked with cradle cap – a scaly scalp condition – in newborn infants.

EFAs are especially important in pregnancy, yet as many as eight out of ten pregnant women have poor dietary intakes. Essential fatty acids are important for the structure and development of a developing baby's eyes and brain. Also, prostaglandins help to reduce the risk of premature delivery, protect against high blood pressure during pregnancy and soften the cervix to trigger childbirth when the time is right. Studies suggest that male babies have a higher need for EFAs than females.

Research in many countries, including the UK, USA and Netherlands, shows that even in normal pregnancy, a mother's EFA status is marginal, with low EFA levels that tend to fall lower with each successive pregnancy. EFA deficiency is especially likely with multiple pregnancies when the needs of two or more babies must be met.

As pregnancy requires such high levels of EFAs, and as intakes are generally low, maternal essential fatty acid status declines throughout successive pregnancies: stores are not readily replenished and, with each subsequent pregnancy, essential fatty acid deficiency becomes increasingly marked.

Some researchers have observed that first babies are often more intelligent than their younger siblings and have speculated that lack of EFAs – especially DHA – may be involved. Research in the Netherlands involving 244 women who were pregnant for up to the seventh time showed that maternal blood levels of DHA were significantly lower in those women who had previously given birth compared to those pregnant with their first child. Blood samples from the umbilical artery and vein also showed significantly higher DHA levels in first children compared with those born afterwards. Birth order was found to play a significant role in determining how much DHA was available to the developing baby. Further research is needed to see what effect this has on the intellectual potential for children born second or later in a family. Certainly women planning a second or subsequent pregnancy are well advised to take essential fatty acid supplements to protect themselves and their baby from the potential effects of deficiency.

During pregnancy, women lay down over 5 kg fat. The composition of fats in these stores will depend on their dietary intake. By eating the right sorts of fats – especially essential fatty acids – EFA reserves will be stored to help top up the amount present in their breast milk. In other words, any excess eaten over and above the baby's immediate needs during pregnancy will not be wasted. A significant proportion can be stored and mobilized later, while breast-feeding, to continue the supply needed for eye and brain development during the first four to six months of the baby's life after birth. After this time, a baby's metabolism is mature enough to start making small amounts of DHA from other dietary essential fatty acids, assuming these are available.

Dose

A healthy adult woman needs around 6–10 g EFAs a day. During pregnancy and while breast-feeding, these needs are increased to an average of 14g a day (equivalent to about 4000 g per pregnancy).

Eucalyptus
(Eucalyptus globulus)

There are over 700 different types of eucalyptus of which over 500 produce essential oils. The blue gum (*Eucalyptus globulus*) is most widely used medicinally.

Benefits

Eucalyptus, sometimes known as the fever tree, is a traditional Aboriginal medicine used as an antiseptic, fumigant, to reduce fever, and as a decongestant to treat catarrh and the common cold. In addition to its antiseptic, antibacterial, anti-inflammatory and expectorant properties, it also stimulates blood flow, is mildly anti-spasmodic and helps to dilate the small airways (bronchioles) of the lungs. It is also used to deter mosquitoes.

Eucalyptus leaf medicinal tea is taken for bronchitis and sore throat. It is sometimes included in herbal cough mixtures.

Dose
Infusion: 2–3 g in 150 ml water, twice a day.
Tincture 1:5 (g/ml): 10–15 ml, twice a day.
Extract 5:1 (w/w): 500 mg, twice a day.

Evening primrose oil

Evening primrose is native to North America. Its seed oil is a rich source of gamma-linolenic (also known as gamolenic) acid (GLA) which helps to overcome lack of dietary EFAs.

GLA (gamma-linolenic acid) is metabolized in the body to form hormone-like substances known as prostaglandins which are found in all body tissues and play a major role in mediating inflammation, blood clotting, hormonal balance and are involved in the immune response against infections and cancer.

Benefits
Evening primrose oil (EPO) is one of the most popular and useful food supplements available as up to 10 per cent of its essential fatty acid content is GLA. It can be used to help a wide range of problems from dry itchy skin, eczema, psoriasis, rosacea and acne to pre-menstrual syndrome, menopausal problems, endometriosis and cyclical breast pain. It has also proved useful in the treatment of diabetic

neuropathy, irritable bowel syndrome, rheumatoid arthritis, high cholesterol levels and high blood pressure.

When taken for eczema, EPO helps to reduce itching, scaliness and fluid weeping as well as reducing the amount of topical corticosteroid creams needed. It is also helpful for people trying to give up alcohol by reducing cravings.

When taken in combination with fish oils, the beneficial effects of EPO are multiplied. Research into the effects of evening primrose oil and fish oil (taken in a ratio of 4:1) on drug usage in rheumatoid arthritis found that, after six months, nearly all of those taking it were able to reduce their dose of painkillers (non-steroidal anti-inflammatory drugs) and felt much better in themselves.

The fact that evening primrose oil (EPO) could help prostate problems was first noted when a 69-year-old man was given a dose of 3 g daily to treat a raised cholesterol level. The cholesterol level reduced and the man also reported that his prostatic symptoms of urinary retention, urgency, frequency and nocturia improved progressively until he was symptom-free. Three other men with prostate problems were then also given EPO and their symptoms duly improved around three months after starting the treatment.

Dose

500–1000 mg EPO daily for general health (equivalent to 40–80 mg GLA).

Up to 3 g daily (equivalent to 240 mg GLA) may be taken to treat hormone imbalances (such as those associated with cyclical breast pain, pre-menstrual syndrome or menopausal symptoms). It can take up to three months to notice a beneficial effect, however.

As an oil, it is best taken with food to boost absorption. The action of GLA is boosted by vitamin E which also helps to preserve it. Certain vitamins and minerals are also needed during the metabolism of essential fatty acids. These are vitamins C, B6, B3 (niacin), zinc and magnesium. If you are taking evening primrose oil, you should therefore ensure that your intake of these is adequate.

Contraindications

Only people who are allergic to it and those with a particular nervous disorder known as temporal lobe epilepsy should not take evening primrose oil.

See also **Essential Fatty Acids**

Feverfew
(Tanacetum parthenium)

Feverfew is a common European plant belonging to the daisy family.

Benefits

Feverfew leaves contain a substance called parthenolide that inhibits release of a neurotransmitter, serotonin, in the brain circulation. This blocks the sudden widening or constriction of blood vessels involved in the development of migraine, and is effective in reducing the severity and frequency of attacks.

In clinical trials, 70 per cent of people taking feverfew leaf extract found it either prevented headaches or lessened their severity, as well as related symptoms of nausea and vomiting. In one trial involving 60 migraine sufferers, those taking feverfew had 25 per cent fewer attacks and also less nausea and vomiting.

Feverfew is also used to help painful periods and is thought to reduce synthesis of the hormone-like chemicals (prostaglandins) that trigger menstrual cramps.

Dose

125-250mg daily depending on strength of extract. Select a product containing at least 0.2 per cent parthenolide for every 125 mg feverfew extract. Non-standardized supplements may contain very little parthenolide.

It may take four to six weeks before benefits are noticed, and feverfew usually needs to be taken long-term to prevent a recurrence of migraine attacks.

Contraindications

● Feverfew should not be taken during pregnancy or breast-feeding as it may affect contraction of the uterus.

● Feverfew should not be taken by anyone who is on anticoagulant drugs as it may inhibit blood clotting.

Fibre

Dietary fibre – or roughage – is the fibrous plant substances that pass through the small intestines undigested. We lack the enzymes necessary to break down these substances, such as cellulose, hemicellulose, lignin, pectins and gums. Once fibre reaches the large bowel however, enzymes released by bacteria start to ferment soluble fibre to release gases, while insoluble fibre is excreted largely unchanged.

Fibre in the diet

Dietary sources of fibre include whole-grain cereals, nuts, seeds, root vegetables and fruits. Fibre supplements include bran, psyllium seed, linseed and ispaghula husks.

A healthy diet ideally provides at least 18 g fibre per day – around 40 per cent higher than the current average intake. Increasing fibre intake to 30 g per day can relieve both diarrhoea and constipation by helping to normalize bowel function. Some people experience feelings of bloating and distension on increasing their fibre intake; this effect normally disappears after two or three weeks and can be avoided altogether if fibre intake is increased very gradually. When increasing fibre intake it is also important to drink at least 2–3 litres of fluids per day to help bulk up the fibre for optimum effect.

Foods containing 3 g of fibre or more per 100 g are considered high-fibre choices. These include:

- bran (40 g fibre per 100 g portion)
- dried apricots (18 g)
- prunes (13 g)
- brown bread (6 g)
- walnuts (6 g)
- peas (5 g)
- white bread (4 g)
- cooked wholemeal spaghetti (4 g)

New research suggests that bowel bacteria quickly adapt to the types of roughage in your diet, so it is important to eat as many different sources of fibre as possible. If you mainly eat fibre of one type (e.g. bran) bowel bacteria will respond within a week or two by increasing their output of enzymes to ferment this. The fibre reaching your colon will then be broken down more quickly so that you lose much of the benefit gained.

Benefits

Although it provides little in the way of energy or nutrients, fibre aids in the digestion and absorption of other foods. Soluble fibre is important for the function of the stomach and upper intestines, where it absorbs fats and sugars to slow the rate at which they pass into the circulation. It also encourages the muscular contractions that propel digested food forwards.

Insoluble fibre is more important in the large bowel, where it absorbs water, bacteria and toxins, bulks up the faeces and hastens stool excretion.

Experiments show that for every gram of fibre eaten, bowel motions increase by around 5 g in weight. This is because dietary fibre provides nutrients for bacterial growth, and much of the increased bowel motion bulk due to a high-fibre diet is due to increased bacterial multiplication in the gut. Fibre also absorbs water, which increases stool bulk, and toxins (e.g. harmful chemicals found in a non-organic diet) so they are more likely to be excreted rather than absorbed.

If the diet is lacking in fibre, very little bulk will reach the lower bowel. Instead of the small muscular contractions needed to move bulky stools downwards, the intestinal walls have to squeeze tightly to propel the smaller pellets on their way. This may trigger prolonged muscle spasm and pain in some people with irritable bowel syndrome (IBS). There is no consistent link between symptoms of IBS and fibre intake however, and it is unlikely that lack of fibre is the sole cause.

Overall, following a high-fibre diet helps around one third of people with IBS. In up to a quarter of sufferers, changing to a high-fibre diet initially makes the bloating and distension of IBS worse. However, this effect disappears after two or three weeks so it's worth persevering gradually so that the bowel has time to get used to the higher intake. In one study of 100 patients, 55 per cent said that bran made their symptoms worse with only 10 per cent finding bran helpful. Of those whose symptoms worsened, 67 per cent rated their deterioration as substantial, while 33 per cent said it was moderate. If you cannot tolerate bran – as at least half of IBS sufferers can't – taking supplements containing other forms of fibre such as ispaghula, psyllium or sterculia is often effective. Psyllium seed/powder is an excellent and popular fibre source as it quickly swells in the bowel to produce a gentle scouring action.

Fibre also binds cholesterol and other fats in the bowel to reduce their absorption and can have a significant effect on cholesterol levels. Just 10 g psyllium seed taken daily for at least six weeks can reduce LDL-cholesterol levels by between 5 and 20 per cent.

A group of people with ulcerative colitis who were given psyllium husk fibre supplements during remission were found to have significantly greater improvement than those not taking them.

Other benefits attributed to a high-fibre diet include improved sex hormone balance.

Researchers have found that a low-fibre (which is also usually high-fat) diet is associated with relatively high levels of circulating oestrogen. As a result, people following this type of eating pattern are more likely to develop hormone-dependent cancers such as those of the breast or prostate gland. This is because sex hormones pass from the bile into the gut from which they are absorbed back into the circulation. This so-called 'enterohepatic circulation' helps to maintain relatively high sex hormone levels. If the gut contains dietary fibre residues, however, these mop up a significant amount of sex hormones so that more are excreted and less reabsorbed. As a result, oestrogen levels tend to be lower and a high-fibre diet helps to protect against both breast and prostate cancer.

Women who have followed a lifelong low-fibre diet are also more likely to have menopausal symptoms of oestrogen withdrawal – their tissues are used to a relatively high level of circulating hormones, and they seem to tolerate the menopausal drop less well. However, switching to a healthier, low-fat, high-fibre diet around the time of the menopause can also make symptoms of oestrogen withdrawal worse (by lowering oestrogen levels further), unless the amount of plant hormones (e.g. isoflavones obtained from soy) eaten is also increased.

Research involving a group of 665 patients with a previous history of colorectal adenomas – benign growths in the large bowel which can develop into malignant tumours if left untreated – compared how they fared when randomly assigned to receive either calcium supplements, fibre (3.5 g ispaghula husk) or a placebo. After three years, 552 participants who completed the study had a colonoscopy to look for recurrence of the benign adenomas. The participants found recurrences in 16 per cent of those taking calcium, 29 per cent receiving fibre and 20 per cent in the placebo group. The authors concluded that a low-fat, high-fibre diet plus supplementation with wheat-bran fibre or ispaghula husk may not be effective strategies for the prevention of colorectal adenoma recurrence. This should not be extrapolated to mean that fibre supplements might increase the risk of colon cancer in the general population, however, although it was widely misreported as such.

Dose

Start with a small increase in fibre intake, e.g. 2 g with each meal, and slowly increase to obtain the desired effect. An intake of between 18 and 30 g a day (*including* that obtained from your diet) is considered optimum for health.

Note:
● Fibre in the bowel absorbs large quantities of water and can dry the gut out. Fluid intake must also be increased to avoid problems.

● It is possible that a high-fibre diet may reduce absorption of calcium and iron in the bowel.

● Fibre supplements – especially psyllium – should not be taken within two hours of any prescribed medication as it may interfere with its absorption.

Fish oils

Omega-3 fish oils are a rich source of essential fatty acids (EFAs) such as docosahexaenoic acid (DHA) and eicosapentaenoic acid (EPA). Levels of EFAs such as DHA and EPA are typically three times greater in oils from the flesh of oily fish such as salmon, herrings, sardines, pilchards and mackerel than they are in oils extracted from cod liver. New techniques have now been developed that can concentrate these EFAs when making fish oil supplements, however.

Ideally, everyone should aim to eat at least 100 g oily fish two or three times per week, which for most people means increasing our average fish intake by a factor of ten! Healthy staple foods such as margarines, bread and even milk containing refined fish oil are now also available in a number of countries to help boost intakes in those who do not each much fish. Omega-3 essential fatty acids supplements (oils, capsules) are also available. Emulsified oils help to prevent the fish aftertaste that some people find off-putting.

Benefits

Omega-3 polyunsaturated fatty acids (n3–PUFAs) help to balance the action of omega-6–polyunsaturated fatty acids (n6–PUFAs mostly derived from vegetables oils) in the body, and have a protective action against long-term inflammatory diseases such as asthma, rheumatoid arthritis and psoriasis. In one study of 80 people with psoriasis, omega-3 fish oils significantly reduced psoriasis patches within four to eight weeks. This is because they are processed to form hormone-like chemicals, known as prostaglandins, that help to damp down rather than trigger inflammation. This anti-inflammatory action is also beneficial against rheumatoid arthritis.

In ulcerative colitis, another chronic inflammatory disease, a four-month study confirmed that taking fish oil supplements resulted in weight gain and decreased colonic inflammation so that those who required oral steroids could halve their intake of these drugs. Similar benefits are experienced by Crohn's disease sufferers, with around 70 per cent of those taking fish oil supplements experiencing remission.

Omega-3 fish oils also have a thinning effect on the blood, reduce blood stickiness and decrease the risk of hardening and furring up of the arteries. Even a modest increase in dietary intakes of oily fish can help to prevent death due to coronary thrombosis (heart attack). In those who have already had a heart attack, eating more fish significantly reduces the chance of a second heart attack. If one does occur, the chances of dying from this second heart attack is significantly decreased. Studies have also found that people who eat oily fish once or twice a week are less likely to die from stroke. The blood-thinning action is also beneficial in Raynaud's syndrome and for peripheral arterial disease such as intermittent claudication (calf pain due to poor circulation during minimal exercise).

Painful periods seem to be worse in women who do not eat much fish, and taking omega-3 fish oil supplements has been shown to significantly improve painful periods in teenage girls. This is because omega-3 essential fatty acids have a beneficial effect on the types of prostaglandins produced in the womb lining (endometrium) to reduce muscle spasm.

Fish oils may have a role in reducing the risk of cancer, by interfering with the growth of tumour cells and reversing the weight loss that can occur in people with cancer. In one study, pre-cancerous polyps of the colon also responded dramatically to treatment with fish oils and reduced in frequency by 50 per cent.

Dose

Usually 1–4 g a day. For severe inflammatory diseases such as inflammatory bowel disease and rheumatoid arthritis, doses of 6 g daily may be recommended. Added vitamin E stops rancidity.

Side effects

Belching and mild nausea are possible side effects of taking fish oil supplements. They may also exacerbate asthma in patients sensitive to aspirin. There are no serious side effects, however, and fish oil has many widely accepted nutritional benefits on cardiovascular health.

Contraindications

● Cod liver oil products should not be taken during pregnancy as they contain vitamin A, an excess of which can be harmful to a developing baby.

● Some research suggests that fish oils increase blood sugar levels in diabetics. However, omega-3 fish oils protect against the increased risk of coronary heart disease that occurs in diabetes. Monitor sugar levels carefully.

● Seek medical advice before taking fish oil supplements if you have a blood-clotting disorder or if you are taking a blood-thinning drug such as warfarin (may increase tendency to bleed).

Fish oils and pregnancy

Two LCPs (*see* **Essential Fatty Acids**), arachidonic acid (AA) and docosahexaenoic acid (DHA), are vital for development of normal brain and eye function, especially during the last three months of pregnancy. The placenta extracts them from the maternal circulation and concentrates them in your baby's circulation, so that foetal levels of AA and DHA are twice as high as in the mother.

AA is important for making strong, flexible, elastic blood vessel walls that reduce the risk of bleeding into the brain, especially in premature infants. DHA is transported to the baby's central nervous system and incorporated into brain cell membranes to make up 10–15 per cent of the weight of the baby's cerebral cortex. It is found mainly in the areas of membrane occurring in synaptic connections between brain cells. DHA is also concentrated in the light-sensitive cells at the back of a developing baby's eyes where it makes up 50 per cent of the weight of each retina.

It is now believed that a low-fat diet providing too few EFAs during pregnancy may be linked with an increased risk of the offspring developing dyslexia, attention deficit hyperactivity disorder, autism and schizophrenia. One in three people with schizophrenia, for example, have abnormally low levels of AA and DHA. This occurs in those with a form of the disease known as neural development schizophrenia in which symptoms come on at a young age, and which is associated with a decline in reasoning and ordered thought.

Lack of dietary EFAs may not be the root cause of these conditions, but could trigger it in those predisposed to them through other genetic or environmental factors. It is also possible that the conditions are linked with poor ability to absorb EFAs from the gut, or problems with the way in which EFAs are handled once they reach the brain. Most evidence suggests that the problem is a dietary one, however, with higher rates of schizophrenia in children conceived during times of starvation, and in those with a poor diet, as well as in babies who are not breast-fed.

If a pregnant woman is lacking in EFAs, her baby will obtain some of the AA and DHA he needs from her body's richest store – her own brain. This may account for the slight shrinkage (2–3 per cent) in maternal brain size seen in some pregnant women, causing the poor concentration, poor memory, forgetfulness and vagueness that many women experience during the last few months of pregnancy.

Boosting dietary intake of EFAs, AA and DHA throughout pregnancy can help to:

- improve the development of the baby's eyes and brain
- improve the baby's visual acuity
- reduce the risk of pregnancy-associated high blood pressure (pre-eclampsia)
- reduce the risk of a preterm delivery
- reduce the risk of a low-birthweight baby
- reduce fluid retention during pregnancy (oedema)
- reduce the risk of poor concentration and 'scattiness' towards the end of pregnancy
- reduce the risk of dry, itchy skin problems
- possibly reduce the risk of stretch marks
- possibly increase the baby's intelligence through improved brain development.

Interestingly, studies suggest that women carrying a male baby need higher intakes of EFAs than those carrying a female baby.

Note:
Many EFA supplements especially designed for pregnancy are now available, and tend to contain DHA, DHA plus AA, or DHA, AA plus GLA.

Fish oil supplements containing other EFAs (e.g. eicosa-pentaenoic acid) are best avoided as their blend of EFAs may have an excessive blood-thinning effect which may not be desirable during pregnancy. Cod liver oil supplements should also be avoided, as they contain potentially harmful high levels of vitamin A (retinol).

See also **Essential Fatty Acids**

Flaxseed oil
(Linum usitatissimum)

The medicinal properties of flaxseed (also known as linseed) oil have been recognized for over 5000 years. Flaxseed is the richest known plant source of an omega-3 essential fatty acid (alpha-linolenic acid) similar to the essential fatty acids (EFAs) found in fish oil, but less potent. For those who are allergic to fish, or who don't like fishy burps, flaxseed oil is a good alternative. Flaxseed oils also contains a beneficial omega-6 essential fatty acid, linolenic acid.

Benefits

The EFAs in flaxseed oil are incorporated into cell membranes to make them more fluid and supple, to alter the way in which they interact with hormones (which seems to protect against some cancers) and to improve immune function to increase cell resistance to infection. By improving nerve transmission, flaxseed oil is helpful for those with nervous system disorders, numbness and pins and needles. The omega-3 oils also have a powerful anti-inflammatory effect in conditions such as arthritis, psoriasis and colitis.

Flaxseed oil has beneficial effects on circulating blood fats, including LDL-cholesterol, and is widely recommended for people with coronary heart disease and high blood pressure. Some evidence suggests that, as with fish oils, if taken by those who have had a heart attack it may reduce the chance of a second heart attack occurring.

Flaxseed oil is also one of the richest sources of oestrogen-like plant hormones known as lignans. It is therefore recommended for menstrual problems, including pre-menstrual syndrome, painful periods and for cyclical breast pain. It is also helpful for certain male hormone imbalances including prostate problems.

Flax seeds are a good fibre source and are useful for improving constipation, diverticular disease and irritable bowel syndrome.

Note:

- It is important not to confuse the medicinal cold-pressed linseed oil extracted from ripe seed with the toxic raw linseed oil (from immature seed) used by artists and furniture makers. The latter contains warnings that it should not be taken internally.

- Medicinal flaxseed oil degrades on exposure to light and if not processed and stored properly quickly turns rancid.

- Liquid flaxseed oil must be stored carefully (e.g. in the fridge in opaque bottles).

- Avoid oil that is past its use by date, or which has a strong odour.

Dose

Oil: 1 teaspoon–1 tablespoon once or twice a day.

Flax seeds: 1–2 tablespoons with water twice a day.

Best taken with food to enhance absorption.

Taking it in the form of seeds or as capsules is most convenient. Do not exceed stated doses.

Fluoride

Fluoride is a mineral that is important for healthy bones and teeth. It binds to tooth enamel and strengthens it to help prevent decay. In the same way, small amounts of fluoride can bind to bone to produce calcium fluoroapatite which is more resistant to reabsorption.

Dietary sources of fluoride include tea leaves (which provide 70 per cent of average intakes), fluorinated water supplies, seafood (especially oysters), milk, eggs, lettuce, cabbage, lentils and whole grains.

People who drink large amounts of tea may gain some benefit in the long-term prevention of osteoporosis.

Dose

There is currently no EC RDA for fluoride. Intakes of 1.5 mg–4 mg have been suggested as desirable. Fluorination of drinking water supplies 1–3 mg fluoride a day.

Excess

Excess fluoride can cause formation of abnormal, weakened bone and discoloured teeth (fluorosis). Fluorosis seems to triple the risk of osteoporotic fractures and may also increase the risk of bone cancer.

Folic acid

Folic acid is the synthetic, monoglutamate form of the naturally occurring folate (polyglutamate form) that is widely found in fruit, green leafy vegetables, nuts, pulses and yeast extracts. It is difficult to obtain optimum levels from these sources, but folic acid found in fortified foods and supplements is absorbed more efficiently than naturally occurring folate and has a greater bioavailability in the body.

Benefits

Folic acid is involved in a wide number of metabolic reactions and in protein and sugar metabolism. It works together with vitamin B12 in the synthesis of nucleic acids during cell division, to ensure that cell duplication is normal and it is especially needed by cells with a rapid turnover. When folate levels are low, newly replicated chromosomes are more likely to be abnormal and cells – especially red blood cells – become larger than normal.

Because of its effects on cell division, folic acid may help to protect against the development of certain cancers, including cancers of the cervix, oesophagus, mouth (especially in smokers), colon, rectum, smoking-related cancers of the lung and breast cancer in women with a high alcohol intake.

Folic acid is also essential during pregnancy, especially in the first few weeks of a baby's development, often before a mother is aware that she is pregnant. Its effects on cell division mean that deficiency is associated with a type of congenital abnormality in which the spinal cord and, occasionally, the brain do not develop properly. These abnormalities arise between the 24th and 28th day after conception and are known as neural tube defects. If folic acid is in short supply, the neural tube – which eventually develops into the brain and spinal cord – does not fuse fully along its length, so a gap is left at the top or bottom of the spine. The most common example of this is spina bifida. As a result, all women of reproductive age should consider taking a vitamin and mineral supplement containing folic acid, in case of unplanned pregnancy (it is estimated that at least one in three pregnancies is unplanned). Folic acid supplements of at least 400 mcg daily can reduce the risk of spina bifida by as much as 75 per cent if taken during the first 12 weeks of pregnancy. Because dietary folate is less readily absorbed, a threefold increase in existing dietary folate intakes would be needed to obtain 400 mcg per day through diet alone. Folic acid supplements are therefore essential for women who are planning to conceive.

A raised blood level of the amino acid homocysteine is now recognized as an important risk factor for developing coronary heart disease and stroke. Homocysteine is formed in the body from the breakdown of the dietary amino acid methionine. Homocysteine becomes highly reactive and toxic as it accumulates in the circulation, causing oxidation damage to the lining of artery walls so they become narrow and inelastic. Normally, its level is tightly controlled by three different enzymes that convert homocysteine to cysteine – a safe end product used by cells for growth.

Two of the three enzymes that control homocysteine levels depend on folic acid for their activity. Those who do not obtain enough folic acid for optimal enzyme function will have a raised homocysteine level and consequently an increased risk of circulatory problems. A study of 14,000 people in the USA found that those with higher than normal homocysteine levels had three times the risk of a heart attack.

Genetic mutations can also decrease the activity of any one of the three controlling enzymes to raise homocysteine levels and around one in ten people is affected, inheriting higher than normal blood levels of homocysteine to triple their risk of these diseases. One in 160,000 people has extremely high levels with 30 times the risk of premature heart disease and osteoporosis. After the menopause, some women are also less able to process homocysteine so levels build up to increase the risk of osteoporosis and coronary heart disease.

The risks associated with an elevated homocysteine level are comparable to those of an abnormally raised cholesterol level, only they are more easily corrected through dietary intervention.

Deficiency

Folic acid and folate are both water soluble and the body can therefore store very little at a time. As a result, dietary lack rapidly causes deficiency and it is believed to be the most widespread vitamin deficiency in developed countries. Lack of folic acid causes a variety of symptoms, including a red, sore tongue, anaemia, cracking at the corners of the mouth, diarrhoea, tiredness, insomnia, weakness and muscular cramps. Emotional symptoms of irritability, forgetfulness, confusion and depression can also occur.

Low blood levels of folic acid have recently been linked with an increased risk of Alzheimer's disease. This is thought to result from the increased risk of vascular disease that is now known to be associated with an elevated blood level of the amino acid, homocysteine.

People with the skin depigmentation condition vitiligo often have low blood levels of folic acid, and sometimes vitamin B12 and/or vitamin C. In some people with this condition, prolonged treatment with vitamin supplements, plus safe, sensible exposure to the sun, can result in repigmentation without side effects.

In one study of 60 people with chronic fatigue syndrome, 50 per cent had low levels of folic acid and there is preliminary evidence showing that taking B group vitamins (including folic acid) can help a significant number of people with chronic fatigue.

Dose

The EC RDA for folic acid is 200 mcg.

Taking a vitamin and mineral supplement providing as little as 200 g folic acid per day is effective in lowering plasma homocysteine levels. High levels of homocysteine can be reduced by taking folic acid supplements (400–650 mcg per day). People with a family or personal history of coronary heart disease may wish to consider taking supplements of at least 400 mcg folic acid daily.

Women who are pregnant or planning to be need a daily intake of at least 400 mcg per day, preferably in the more readily available form, folic acid. They should be started before trying to conceive and ideally continue for at least 12 weeks. Women who have previously conceived a child with a neural tube defect are advised to take supplements ten times larger, containing at least 4–5 mg folic acid daily to help reduce the risk of a recurrence.

The recommended upper safe limit for folic acid is to take no more than 1000mcg daily.

Note:

● Some anti-epilepsy drugs result in low levels of folic acid. People taking drugs to treat epilepsy should tell their doctor if they take folic acid supplements so blood levels of their medication can be monitored where appropriate.

● For women on anti-epileptic drugs, it is vitally important to obtain advice about taking extra folic acid supplements before trying to conceive a baby.

● Folic acid should usually be taken together with vitamin B12. This is because lack of vitamin B12 (which leads to damage of the nervous system, especially the spinal cord) is masked by taking folic acid supplements (as this prevents the occurrence of pernicious anaemia which usually allows lack of vitamin B12 do be detected).

● Interesting new research suggests that taking high dose folic acid supplements may increase the chance of conceiving twins.

Fo-ti
(Polygonum multiflorum)

Fo-ti – also known as *he shou wu* – is one of the oldest Chinese tonic herbs whose dried roots are harvested when they are three to four years old. Raw fo-ti roots are laxative and also toxic but curing the root – for example by boiling for hours in black soybean broth – converts it into a highly valued tonic that has mostly lost its laxative and toxic effects.

Benefits

Fo-ti is famous for its rejuvenating and revitalizing properties. It is widely used in the East as a general restorative, to promote fertility, sexual function and boost a low sex drive. Research shows that it can reduce abnormally raised cholesterol and may have some antibiotic effects against tuberculosis and malaria. It is also used to reduce premature greying of hair. It is often taken together with *Panax ginseng* (*see* **Ginseng**).

Dose

Tablets: 5 g daily.

Contraindications

Fo-ti is best avoided if suffering from diarrhoea.

Garlic
(Allium sativum)

Garlic is such a popular culinary herb that, worldwide, average consumption is equivalent to one clove per individual per day.

Benefits

Garlic has a number of medicinal uses and is antioxidant, antiseptic, antibacterial and anti-viral. It is used to treat viral warts, stomach and respiratory infections but its most important effect is its ability to maintain a healthy circulation and reduce the risk of coronary heart disease and stroke.

Clinical trials using standardized tablets have shown that taking garlic regularly can reduce high blood pressure, lower levels of harmful blood fats (LDL-cholesterol and triglycerides), reduce blood stickiness and improve circulation. Regular use reduces the risk of hardening and furring up of the arteries up to 25 per cent.

The main substance derived from garlic that protects against coronary heart disease is allicin, which gives a crushed clove its characteristic smell. Allicin is not present in whole garlic cloves, however, which contain an odourless precursor called alliin, which is an amino acid unique to the garlic family. Alliin is stored within garlic cells, separated from the enzyme (alliinase) designed to break it down. It is only when alliin and alliinase come together that beneficial allicin (diallyl thiosulphinate) is made. This natural reaction occurs as soon as a clove of garlic is cut or crushed, and releases its characteristic odour. Allicin prevents cells from taking up cholesterol, reduces cholesterol production in the liver and hastens excretion of fatty acids, thereby discouraging atherosclerosis. Sulphur compounds formed by the degradation of allicin are also beneficial and are incorporated into long-chain fatty acid molecules, to act as antioxidants. Antioxidants protect blood LDL-cholesterol molecules against oxidation and reduce their uptake by scavenger cells to protect against atherosclerosis.

Garlic powder extracts can lower blood pressure (BP) enough to reduce the risk of a stroke by up to 40 per cent. At daily doses of 600–900 mg, for periods of between 28 and 180 days, systolic BP was reduced by an average of 8 per cent (and up to 17 per cent) while diastolic BP was reduced by an average of 12 per cent (and up to 16 per cent). This reduction is a gradual process requiring a minimum of two to three months treatment.

Garlic powder tablets reduce diastolic BP by an average of 12 per cent, which lowers risk of coronary heart disease (CHD) by a massive 38 per cent just through its action on blood pressure. This effect is thought to be due to a combination of increasing the fluidity of blood (i.e. decreasing its stickiness), through a beneficial effect on the way sodium and potassium ions cross cell membranes, and dilation of blood vessels by relaxing smooth muscle cells. The blood vessel dilation effect can be seen within five hours of taking a single dose.

Garlic has such a powerful medicinal action that, in Germany, garlic powder tablets containing the equivalent of 4 g of fresh cloves are available on prescription to treat high blood cholesterol levels and high blood pressure.

Another benefit of garlic is that it helps to improve the circulation, especially through small arteries (arterioles) and small veins (venules). Garlic dilates the arterioles by an average of 4.2 per cent and the venules by 5.9 per cent. As a result, it can improve blood flow to the skin by almost 50 per cent (helpful for sufferers of Raynaud's syndrome and chilblains) and to the nail folds by as much as 55 per cent.

By inhibiting platelet clumping which is one of the first events to trigger atherosclerosis, garlic, if taken regularly can protect against both the first and later stages. Platelet clumping is significantly decreased after a dose equivalent to half a clove of garlic and lasts for three hours. Some of the ingredients in garlic (ajoene, methylallyl trisulphide and dimethyl trisulphide) seem to be as potent as aspirin in this respect.

Another interesting study found that garlic powder tablets can increase the elasticity of the aorta so that the heart has to work less hard to pump blood out into the body.

For people who experience calf pain on walking more than 100 yards due to reduced blood flow to the legs (intermittent claudication), taking garlic powder tablets for just three months has been shown to increase the distance that can be walked before calf pain starts by as much as 30 per cent.

As well as all the above benefits, most people also notice an improvement in their general well-being. One study assessed people's psychological state before and after four months' treatment with standardized garlic tablets. There was a marked improvement in positive mood characteristics (activity, elated mood, concentration, sensitivity) and a drop in negative mood characteristics (anxiety, irritation) in those taking garlic tablets, compared with no significant change in those taking an inactive placebo.

Taking garlic powder tablets during pregnancy can reduce the risk of pregnancy-associated high blood pressure (pre-eclampsia) and improve circulation through the placenta so that growth retardation associated with pre-eclampsia is less problematic. Garlic has also been shown to boost placental production of factors that stimulate foetal growth. Intriguingly, garlic in the bloodstream stimulates nasal smell receptors and babies in the womb have been shown to be sensitive to garlic.

There are no reports of interactions between garlic and other medications. The blood-thinning effects of garlic will add to those of aspirin and fish oils however. Garlic may increase bleeding tendency.

Dose

600–900 mg standardized garlic powder tablets a day.

Garlic powder tablets seem to be more effective than garlic oil capsules – in one randomized trial of 80 patients, garlic powder tablets reduced cholesterol levels by 11 per cent and garlic oil by only 3 per cent over four months.

Enteric coating of garlic powder tablets reduces garlic odour on breath and protects the active ingredients from degradation in the stomach.

Note: if applying raw garlic juice or oil to warts, protect surrounding skin with petroleum jelly. Some people are allergic to topical application of garlic.

Ginger
(Zingiber officinale)

Ginger is a perennial, tropical plant native to the jungles of south-east Asia. It is one of the oldest medicinal spices known and the rhizome contains a variety of unique chemicals such as gingerol, zingerone and essential oils.

Benefits

Ginger has analgesic, antihistamine, stimulating, anti-inflammatory and anti-nauseant properties. It also has a warming action that promotes sweating, and is popular for treating chilblains, Raynaud's syndrome, colds and fevers.

Ginger is frequently used to quell motion sickness, morning sickness during pregnancy, and to relieve post-operative nausea. It can also help to relieve indigestion, flatulence, diarrhoea, suppressed menstruation, poor circulation, dizziness and migrainous headaches.

Gingerol has a similar structure to aspirin, and was recently found to be at least as effective as garlic in reducing blood clotting, boosting the circulation and lowering blood pressure.

Its anti-inflammatory action is helpful in relieving muscle and joint aches and pains, including those of rheumatoid and osteoarthritis. In a recent trial involving 247 people with moderate osteoarthritis of the knee, those taking ginger extracts had significantly more pain relief on standing (as assessed using a visual analogue scale) than those taking a placebo.

Dose

Powdered ginger root standardized for 0.4 per cent volatile oils: 250 mg, two to four times a day.

Fresh powdered ginger: 1–2 g every four hours as necessary.

Note: recommended doses must not be exceeded during pregnancy.

Ginkgo
(Ginkgo biloba)

The *ginkgo biloba*, or maidenhair tree, is one of the oldest known plants on earth. It has remained virtually unchanged during the last 200 million years and is often described as a living fossil.

Benefits

Ginkgo's fan-shaped leaves contain a variety of powerful antioxidants, flavoglycosides, bioflavones and unique chemicals known as ginkgolides and bilobalides. These have been found to relax blood vessels in the body and boost blood circulation to the brain, hands, feet and genitals by stopping cell fragments in the blood (platelets) from clumping together.

Ginkgo is one of the most popular health supplements in Europe. Many people find it helps to improve memory and concentration, as well as easing dizziness and improving their peripheral circulation. It is also effective for improving depression linked with reduced blood flow to the brain. In one double-blind study, 40 depressed patients aged 51 to 78 years who had not benefited from standard anti-depressant drugs, were given either 80 mg of ginkgo extract three times daily or a placebo. After eight weeks, those taking ginkgo showed a threefold improvement in their Hamilton Rating Scale for Depression (average score 14 dropped to 4.5) compared with a drop from 14 to only 13 in those taking the placebo.

A recent randomized, double-blind, placebo-controlled trial showed that ginkgo can significantly improve memory in older people – probably by improving circulation in the brain. The most effective dose was 120 mg taken in the morning. Other trials have also shown good results in people with Alzheimer's and multi-infarct dementias.

Field trials suggest that over 70 per cent of those taking ginkgo for Raynaud's syndrome found it helpful. Studies show that within one hour of taking ginkgo the blood flow to nail fold capillaries is significantly increased.

Ginkgo extracts have also been shown to help migraine – perhaps by reducing abnormal platelet clumping and improving blood circulation in the brain. Ginkgo is also used to treat an irregular heartbeat, varicose veins, haemorrhoids, leg ulcers, chilblains, tinnitus and anxiety. It might also be helpful for reducing the risks of deep vein thrombosis on long-haul flights (so-called economy-class syndrome).

Ginkgo is a true prosexual supplement. Research shows that it can improve blood flow to the penis to strengthen and maintain an erection, even at a relatively low dose of 60 mg a day for 12–18 months. Research involving males with erectile dysfunction showed a beneficial effect after six to eight weeks of treatment, and after six months half of those studied had regained full potency. In a trial involving 50 males who took ginkgo for nine months, all those who had previously relied on injectable drugs to achieve an erection regained the ability to have unaided erections. Of the 30 men who were not helped by medical drugs, 19 regained their erections with ginkgo.

Dose

Extracts standardized for at least 24 per cent ginkgolides: 40–60 mg, twice or three times a day. One-a-day formulations are also available. Take a minimum of 120 mg daily. Effects may not be noticed until after ten days treatment and it may take up to 12 weeks for gingko to have a noticeable beneficial effect.

Note:

● A handful of cases have appeared in the medical literature in which bleeding within the skull (subarachnoid haemorrhage or subdural haematoma) has occurred in people taking ginkgo extracts in combination with warfarin (a powerful blood-thinning drug) or aspirin. Although ginkgolides found in *Ginkgo biloba* do inhibit platelet aggregation, these are present in small concentrations and at usual therapeutic doses no effects on platelet aggregation have been found. Certainly in people not taking blood-thinning agents, there appears to be no cause for concern. In a double-blind, placebo-controlled, randomized trial of ginkgo extracts in cases of dementia, out of 309 patients the one subdural hematoma that occurred was in the placebo group. For people taking warfarin or aspirin, however, it is best to err on the side of caution and to avoid using *Ginkgo biloba* until any possible interactions have been fully investigated.

- Do not use unprocessed *Ginkgo* leaves as these contain powerful chemicals that can cause allergic reactions.

Ginseng
(Panax ginseng; P. quinquefolium)

Ginseng – usually referred to as Chinese, Korean or Asian ginseng – is one of the oldest known herbal medicines, used in the Orient as a revitalizing and life-enhancing tonic for over 7000 years. High-quality ginseng roots are collected in the autumn from plants that are five to six years old. White ginseng is produced from air-drying the root, while red ginseng (which is more potent and stimulating) is produced by steaming and then drying the root. The closely related American ginseng (*P. quinquefolium* from the woodlands of east and central USA and Canada) has a similar action and is, in fact, generally preferred in Asia as it is sweeter tasting and thought to have more 'yin' (heat-reducing capacity) than Chinese ginseng. American ginseng is said to be best for fatigue caused by nervous conditions, anxiety and insomnia, while Korean ginseng is better for fatigue with general weakness and loss of energy.

Benefits

Ginseng contains at least 28 different ginsenosides that make up 3–6 per cent of the dry root weight. Research suggests that American ginseng contains more of the calming and relaxing Rb1 ginsenosides, while Korean ginseng contains more of the stimulating Rg1 ginsenosides.

Clinical trials have confirmed that ginseng helps the body to adapt to physical or emotional stress and fatigue. It is stimulating and restorative, improving physical and mental energy, stamina, strength, alertness and concentration. It has a normalizing effect on hormone imbalances and boosts metabolic rate. It also improves peripheral circulation, including blood flow to the genitals.

Ginseng lowers cholesterol levels, improves lung function, reduces a build up of lactic acid in exercising muscles and improves oxygen uptake in cells. Research shows that people taking ginseng have faster reaction times than those not taking it, and it improves stamina while reducing muscle cramps and fatigue. A group of hospital nurses who took ginseng were better able to stay awake and perform their night duties than those not taking it.

Ginseng is also prized as an aphrodisiac, sexual balancer and fertility enhancer. Many of the steroidal compounds it contains are similar in structure to human sex hormones and to adrenocorticotrophic hormone (ACTH). Ginseng seems to increase production of ACTH from the pituitary gland in the brain, which in turn stimulates the adrenal glands to increase their output of corticosteroids and sex hormones (usually around 5 per cent of circulating sex hormones such as testosterone are produced by the adrenal glands). Several studies suggest that ginseng increases levels of nitric oxide (NO) in the spongy tissue of the penis. NO is a nerve communication chemical (neurotransmitter) that is essential for a number of physiological processes, including increasing blood flow to the penis for normal erectile function and sexual arousal. This action is similar in effect to that of the new anti-impotence drug, sildenafil (Viagra). In a study in which men with impotence were given either Korean red ginseng or an inactive placebo for 60 days, frequency of sexual intercourse, morning erection, firmness of penis and size of tumescence were significantly increased in those taking the ginseng.

It is best to avoid taking other stimulants such as caffeine-containing products and drinks while taking ginseng.

Dose

Depends on grade of root. Choose a standardized product, preferably with a content of at least 5 per cent ginsenosides. This will generally be more expensive, but cheap versions may contain very little active ingredient. Start with a low dose and work up from 200 mg to 1000 mg a day. An optimum dose is usually around 600 mg daily. It should not be taken for more than six weeks without a break. In the East, ginseng is taken in a two weeks on, two weeks off cycle. Some practitioners recommend taking it in a six weeks on, eight weeks off cycle.

Side effects

Long-term use of ginseng has been reported to cause sudden high blood pressure, diarrhoea, painful breasts (mastalgia), difficulty in sleeping, nervousness, skin eruptions and euphoria. Together, these symptoms are known as ginseng abuse syndrome and have occurred in people taking 3 g crude root daily for two years. This mimics corticosteroid poisoning and is thought to be due to over-stimulation of the adrenal or pituitary glands. High doses of 15 g resulted in feelings of depersonalization and depression. Other hormonal effects, such as post-menopausal bleeding and painful breasts (mastalgia) in older women, have also been reported.

When taken in therapeutic doses in a two weeks on, two weeks off cycle, side effects should not be a problem. If Chinese ginseng is too stimulating, however, it could be worth trying American ginseng which seems to have a more gentle action.

Contraindications

Ginseng is not recommended for people with:

- high blood pressure (may make hypertension worse)
- a heart rhythm abnormality
- an oestrogen-dependent condition, such as pregnancy, cancer of the breast, ovaries or uterus (as it contains oestrogenic compounds).

Glucosamine

Glucosamine sulphate is a substance that is naturally made in the body from a sugar (glucose) and an amino acid (glutamine). It is needed in the body to produce molecules (glycosaminoglycans) for laying down new framework tissues in damaged joints. Glucosamine is essential for the production of new cartilage and synthesis of the joints' oil (synovial fluid). Larger quantities are needed when damaged joints are healing and, as production of glucosamine is normally a slow process, it is often in short supply.

Benefits

Glucosamine boosts regeneration of cartilage and improves production of synovial fluid – the joint's oil – to make it thicker, more cushioning and protective. As a result, inflammation is reduced. It also strengthens the jelly-like centre of intervertebral discs in danger of prolapse. Glucosamine sulphate is also needed for healthy formation of nails, tendons, skin, eyes, bone, ligaments and mucous membranes of the digestive, respiratory and urinary tracts.

Research suggests that a glucosamine sulphate supplement can help injuries such as torn cartilage, sprained ligaments, strained tendons and prolapsed intervertebral discs. Researchers have also reported a reversal of cartilage damage in those receiving active treatment.

Glucosamine sulphate also improves the pain and stiffness of rheumatism and arthritis. In one study in which 212 patients with osteoarthritis of the knee took glucosamine sulphate or an inactive placebo for three years, those taking the placebo developed worsening symptoms with increased narrowing of the knee joint. Those taking glucosamine supplements found that their symptoms improved, however, and there was no joint narrowing.

In many people, glucosamine supplements are at least as effective – and sometimes more so – at damping down joint symptoms than non-steroidal anti-inflammatory painkillers such as ibuprofen. They are especially helpful for men with back pain, arthritis or sports injuries. In a study involving 178 people with osteoarthritis of the knee, those randomized to receive glucosamine at 1500 mg a day for four weeks showed improvements similar to those seen with ibuprofen at 1200 mg daily, but with fewer side effects. Two weeks after stopping treatment, those who had taken glucosamine had a better residual therapeutic effect than those taking the non-steroidal anti-inflammatory drug.

Glucosamine sulphate is also available combined with extracts of New Zealand green-lipped mussels which have powerful anti-inflammatory effects. Other combination products are also available, containing other nutrients (e.g. vitamin C, manganese), herbs (e.g. curcumin and ginger) and oils (e.g. grapeseed and fish oils) for additional effects.

Dose
1000–2000 mg a day in divided doses.

Contraindications
It should not be used in pregnancy as its effects have not yet been investigated.

Glutamine

Glutamine is an amino acid that has several important roles in metabolism. Its synthesis (from glutamate) is the main pathway for removing toxic ammonia from the body. Glutamine plays a role in maintaining normal blood glucose and acid levels, and if glucose is in short supply, brain cells can burn glutamine for energy instead. Glutamine is also used by the brain to make chemical messengers (neurotransmitters) and helps to overcome mental fatigue, anxiety and improve mood.

Glutamine is the most abundant free amino acid in muscle, cerebrospinal fluid and in the circulation. It is used as a source of energy and for synthesis of genetic material in rapidly dividing cells, such as those lining the gut. If glutamine is in short supply, the intestinal lining becomes 'leaky' and when it was first discovered, glutamine was initially referred to as 'intestinal permeability factor'. Other rapidly dividing cells that need good supplies of glutamine include red blood cells, immune cells, and those in hair follicles.

Glutamine in the diet

Glutamine can be synthesized in the body but may become essential for adults under stress or for those who are recovering from injury, infection or surgery. The best dietary sources of glutamine are meat, chicken and eggs but only in the raw form – once heated, glutamine becomes inactive. Its precursor, glutamic acid is present in grains, grapes, nuts and chocolate.

Benefits

Glutamine is used to reduce sugar cravings, alcohol cravings, boost immunity and to help treat colitis, Crohn's disease, peptic ulcers, irritable bowel syndrome and diarrhoea. It is an important muscle-building amino acid and helps replenish muscle glycogen stores after exercise. Some researchers consider glutamine may have an anti-ageing effect by preserving muscle, encouraging fat metabolism and boosting growth hormone levels by up to fourfold.

One hour after a marathon run, blood glutamine levels are reduced and there is a marked change in blood immune cell balance (reduced T-helper to T-suppressor ratio) which lowers immunity (possibly one reason why athletes who over-train are more prone to colds etc). Seven athletes were shown to reduce their blood glutamine level by 45 per cent after a single short-distance sprint. After ten days of long-distance running, their blood glutamine level also dropped by 50 per cent and in some was still depressed after six days suggesting they needed more glutamine than they could make or their diets provided.

Glutamine is also used as a fuel by some immune cells and taking 5 g glutamine supplements was shown to reduce the rate of infections in athletes to less than 20 per cent compared with a greater than 50 per cent infection rate in those not receiving glutamine.

Eighty-four critically ill patients in an intensive care unit were randomly assigned to receive an intravenous feed containing glutamine or one without. After six months, significantly more patients receiving glutamine had survived (57 per cent) compared with those not receiving glutamine (33 per cent). The treatment costs for length of stay and treatment of complications such as infections were also reduced by 50 per cent.

In people with cancer, glutamine seems to enhance the effectiveness of chemotherapy and radiation treatments while reducing toxicity. Daily doses of around 0.5 g help to decrease infections, weight loss and improve healing of radiated intestines. In one study, 13 out of 14 patients receiving chemotherapy suffered less inflammation and ulceration of the mouth (stomatitis) than expected as a result of swishing and swallowing 4 g glutamine liquid twice a day.

Some researchers have found that the behaviour of children and adults with attention deficit hyperactivity disorder improved when taking glutamine.

In one study, nine healthy volunteers aged 32 to 64 were either given 2 g glutamine or a placebo. Those taking glutamine had accelerated fat burning (while preserving muscle tissue) compared to those taking the placebo and it may prove beneficial as part of a weight-loss regime.

Dose

0.5 g to 2 g a day. Glutamine is sometimes taken after an intense fitness workout at a dose of around 2–3 g along with plenty of water.

Contraindications

● Diabetics appear to have an abnormal glutamine metabolism, with more glutamine being broken down for the production of glucose. Diabetics should not take glutamine supplements except under medical advice.

● People with chronic renal failure should avoid glutamine supplementation.

Goldenseal
(Hydrastis canadensis)

Goldenseal is a plant native to North America, but which has been collected so extensively it is now cultivated commercially.

The dried root contains many unique substances, including alkaloids such as hydrastine and canadine, as well as containing berberine.

Benefits

Goldenseal has a natural antibacterial and anti-viral action, and boosts immunity by activating the body's scavenger cells known as macrophages. It also increases blood circulation to the spleen, where bacteria and other foreign substances are rapidly filtered from the blood. Goldenseal is widely used to overcome infections such as sinusitis, cold sores, common cold, influenza, urinary tract and eye infections. As an immune booster, it is often helpful against chronic fatigue syndrome, recurrent herpes attacks and shingles. It is also helpful against nausea and vomiting.

Freshly prepared goldenseal infusion (i.e. tea) may be strained and used as an eyewash to relieve infections such as conjunctivitis or styes, while goldenseal tincture (prepared using alcohol) may be applied topically to treat mouth ulcers and warts.

Dose

125 mg extract, twice to four times daily (standardized to at least 8 per cent alkaloids or 5 per cent hydrastine).

Goldenseal is only usually taken for up to two weeks at a time. It is often taken with echinacea (*see also* **Echinacea**). Goldenseal is usually only taken when symptoms are present, and stopped as soon as they have improved, except when it is being alternated with echinacea (e.g. two weeks on, two weeks off) to maintain immune vigour.

Side effects

Very high doses may cause mouth dryness.

Contraindications

Goldenseal should not be used during pregnancy, breast-feeding, or by sufferers of high blood pressure or glaucoma.

Gotu kola
(Centella asiatica)

Gotu kola is one of the most important Ayurvedic herbs, also known as brahmi. It is reputed to increase longevity and is also referred to as the Fountain of Youth. In Asia, many people regularly eat one leaf of gotu kola a day in the hope of prolonging their life though unfortunately, there is little evidence that it is effective in this respect.

Benefits

The dried leaves, stems and flowers contain glycosides and triterpenoids which are present in concentrations of 1–8 per cent. Gotu kola is not related to the kola nut (*Cola nitida* or *Cola acuminata*) and does not contain caffeine.

Research confirms that when used externally, gotu kola promotes healing of wounds, chronic ulcers, burns, psoriasis plaques and keloid scars. It also improves cellulite by acting directly on fibroblasts (fibre-producing cells) to improve connective tissue structure and reduce connective tissue hardening (sclerosis) which makes it especially helpful for symptoms associated with varicose veins. Several studies have shown that at least eight out of ten people with varicose veins show significant improvement.

Gotu kola is also taken by mouth to relieve anxiety and depression, improve memory and concentration (especially in those with learning difficulties), promote calm (in larger doses), relax muscle tension, boost adrenal function during times of stress and to relieve pain. It is also said to have blood-cleansing properties, to stop bleeding and increase physical and mental energy levels. It has also been used to treat diarrhoea, fever, absent or irregular periods and vaginal discharge. In people with liver cirrhosis, gotu kola has been shown to improve the microscopic appearance of liver tissue and to reduce inflammation.

Dose

● Standardized extracts, e.g. containing asiatic acid (30 per cent), madecassic acid (30 per cent), asiaticoside (40 per cent), or madecassoside (1–2 per cent): take 60–120 mg a day.

● Standardized to 10 per cent asiaticosides: take 200 mg, twice or three times daily.

● Extracts standardized to contain 25 mg triterpenes: two to four capsules a day.

Side effects

High doses may cause headache. Large doses are calming rather than energizing.

Grapefruit seed

Grapefruit seed extracts were first investigated when it was noted that they did not rot when thrown on a compost heap.

Benefits

Grapefruit seed extracts have a natural broad-spectrum antibacterial, anti-fungal, anti-viral and anti-parasitic action that may be used internally or externally. They have been proven effective against candida yeasts, herpes viral infections, the parasite *Giardia lamblia*, and the following bacteria: *E. coli*, *Staphylococci*, *Streptococci*, *Salmonella*, *Pseudomonas*, *Klebsiella*, *Shigella*, *Chlamydia*, *Helicobacter*. They are non-toxic and may be helpful for people with recurrent infections such as candida.

Dose

3–15 drops liquid extract, diluted into water or juice, daily.

Grapefruit seed extracts may be applied undiluted to warts and corns (one drop, twice daily).

Grapeseed

Extracts from the seeds of red grapes contain antioxidant substances known as proanthocyanidins which are more powerful than vitamins C or E, and more concentrated than those that give red wine its widely appreciated health properties.

Benefits

Antioxidants help to mop up free radicals – harmful molecular fragments that trigger oxidation reactions and damage all components of body cells – including genetic information. Free radicals are formed as by-products of our metabolism, and are produced in increased amounts in certain conditions.

Grapeseed extract has a beneficial effect on blood vessels, reducing hardening and furring up of the arteries, thinning the blood and reducing the risk of coronary heart disease and stroke. It strengthens fragile capillaries and protects cell structures from damaging oxidation reactions which has earned it a place in several cosmetic preparations. It is widely recommended to treat conditions associated with poor circulation, such as diabetes, impotence, varicose veins, thread veins, rosacea, macular degeneration, peripheral vascular disease, intermittent claudication and leg cramps.

One study suggested that taking grapeseed extracts for two months was helpful for people with eyestrain due to prolonged working with computer VDU screens.

As an antioxidant, it is likely to protect against cancer.

Dose

100–200 mg daily (standardized extracts containing at least 92 per cent proanthocyanidins).

Grapeseed oil also has beneficial properties and taking 30 ml daily can both increase levels of beneficial HDL cholesterol (which protects against coronary heart disease), and reduce triglyceride levels by around 15 per cent within one month.

Green-lipped mussel
(Perna canaliculus)

Raw extracts of New Zealand green-lipped mussels contain glycoproteins that damp down inflammation in arthritic joints. They seem to work by preventing white blood cells from moving into the joints, where they would have released powerful chemicals making pain and swelling worse.

Benefits

Extracts produce significant reductions in pain and stiffness and have been shown to outperform non-steroidal anti-inflammatory drugs (NSAIDs) such as ibuprofen and indomethacin.

In a trial of 86 patients, 67 per cent of those with rheumatoid arthritis and 35 per cent of those with osteoarthritis benefited.

Green-lipped mussel extracts do not produce gastric side effects and may even protect against NSAID induced ulceration.

Dose

200–1250 mg a day.

Green tea

Green and black tea are similar in that both are made from the young leaves and leaf buds of the same shrub, *Camellia sinensis*. Two main varieties are used, the small-leaved China tea plant (*C. sinensis sinensis*) and the large-leaved Assam tea plant (*C. sinensis assamica*).

Green tea is made by steaming and drying fresh tea leaves immediately after harvesting, while black tea is made by crushing and fermenting freshly cut tea leaves so they oxidize before drying. This allows natural enzymes in the tea leaves to produce the characteristic red-brown colour and reduced astringency.

Benefits

Tea is one of the most popular drinks in the world, and its origins date back to ancient China where legend claims tea was introduced as a beverage in 2737 BC when leaves from a camellia bush fell into the emperor's cup of hot water.

Over 30 per cent of the dry weight of green tea leaves consists of powerful flavonoid antioxidants such as catechins. These are converted into less active antioxidants (such as theaflavins and thearubigins) during fermentation but even so, drinking four to five cups of black tea per day still provides over 50 per cent of the total dietary intake of flavonoid antioxidants (other sources include fruit and vegetables especially apples and onions). Tea is a rich source of phytochemicals and the trace element, manganese. It is also one of the few natural sources of fluoride and may protect against tooth decay.

The antioxidants in green tea extracts appear to be at least 100 times more powerful than vitamin C, and 25 times more powerful than vitamin E.

Research suggests that drinking either type of tea has beneficial effects on blood lipids, blood pressure, blood stickiness and can decrease the risk of coronary heart disease and stroke. Research suggests that people who drink at least four cups of tea a day are 50 per cent less likely to have a heart attack than non-tea drinkers (its antioxidants reduce oxidation of LDL-cholesterol so less is deposited in artery walls) and are also less likely to suffer from high blood pressure. High intakes (around eight to ten cups a day) may also reduce the risk of some cancers, especially those of the stomach, colon, rectum, pancreas, breast, skin and bladder. This is believed to result from a catechin known as EGCG (epigallocatechin gallate) which is one of the most powerful anti-cancer compounds found. It seems to block the production and action of an enzyme (urokinase) needed by cancer cells, without which the abnormal cells undergo a natural process of programmed cell death known as apoptosis.

Antioxidants found in green tea extracts are also known to increase resistance to infection, and to protect against premature ageing – hence they are now added to a variety of skin-care preparations.

As green tea is an acquired taste, some people prefer to drink a blend of black and green teas, or to take green tea extracts.

Dose
Drink four cups of green tea daily, or take supplements of 500 mg daily (standardized to contain at least 50 per cent polyphenols).

Guarana
(Paullinia cupana)

Guarana is derived from a Brazilian bush and known locally as the 'food of the gods'. The dried seeds contain a complex of natural stimulants, including guaranine – a tetramethyl xanthene similar to caffeine (a trimethyl xanthene) – theobromine, theophylline plus saponins similar to those found in Korean and American ginseng.

Benefits

Guarana increases physical, mental and sexual energy levels and relieves fatigue. It is less likely to produce the irritability, poor sleep and tremor linked with excess caffeine intake as the guaranine is buffered by oily saponins that produce a natural timed-release effect. Although it acts as a stimulant, it also has a calming effect and does not usually interfere with sleep or worsen stress-related symptoms. Some people are sensitive to it however, and respond in the same way as they do to the caffeine found in coffee.

Research in Denmark has found that after taking guarana extracts for three months, volunteers had a significant increase in energy levels and reacted better to stress.

In Japan, doctors advise long-distance lorry drivers to chew guarana gum to stay awake and as a result the number of accidents due to drivers falling asleep at the wheel has dropped significantly. Guarana also seems to boost the immune system, thin the blood, reduce fluid retention, decrease appetite and raise metabolic rate. It relieves tension headache, pre-menstrual syndrome and period pains.

Guarana is useful for preventing jet lag, when taken before, during and after a long-distance flight. Research is looking into its potential to reduce the incidence of abnormal blood clotting associated with economy-class syndrome.

Dose

1 g a day.

Note: guarana is a restricted substance for some sports.

Gynostemma pentaphyllum

Gynostemma (also known as jiaogulan) is native to southern China, where it is referred to as the herb of immortality as those taking it regularly are said to live to over 100 years. In Japan, it is known as the sweet tea vine.

Gynostemma is newly recognized to contain triterpenoid saponins, four of which are identical to those found in Korean ginseng, and some are identical to those found in liquorice (*Glycyrrhiza glabra*). Whereas Korean ginseng contains 28 of these important saponins, however, over 80 have been identified in gynostemma and as most are unique to it, they are known as gypenosides.

Benefits

Gynostemma has similar antioxidant, tonic and adaptogenic effects to Korean ginseng and increases vigour, alertness and reflexes as well as reducing anxiety. It supports the function of the adrenal glands in times of stress, and has been shown to lower blood pressure, reduce abnormally raised cholesterol levels, improve circulation through the coronary arteries, brain and peripheral circulation. It is currently under investigation for its ability to protect the liver from toxins and to fight cancer by increasing the activation of natural killer immune cells.

It is widely used to treat bronchitis, due to its anti-inflammatory expectorant action, and is likely to become a popular supplement in the near future – perhaps as popular as Korean ginseng itself.

Dose

20 mg, two or three times a day (standardized to 85 per cent gypenosides).

Hawthorn
(Crategus oxycantha and C. monogyna)

The flowering tops and berries of the hawthorn provide one of the most beneficial herbal remedies available for treating the heart and circulation.

Benefits

Hawthorn extracts contain a substance, known as vitexin, that normalizes the cardiovascular system, either relaxing or stimulating it as necessary, and may therefore be recommended to treat opposing problems. It can lower high blood pressure, relieve angina, improve heart pump efficiency in heart failure, and help to correct an abnormal heart rhythm.

Hawthorn helps to reduce high blood pressure by relaxing peripheral blood vessels and dilating coronary arteries through its ability to block the action of an enzyme (ACE or angiotensin-converting enzyme), which improves blood circulation to heart muscle and the peripheries. It has a mild diuretic action that discourages fluid retention, and can also slow or possibly even reverse the build up of atheromatous plaques to reduce hardening and furring up of the arteries (atherosclerosis). Hawthorn extracts also increase the strength and efficiency of the heart's pumping action. These actions have been shown to reduce shortness of breath, ankle oedema and exercise tolerance in people with heart problems compared with those taking a placebo.

Hawthorn preparations are so effective in helping angina and hypertension that they are currently under research in the search for new drugs.

Other beneficial actions of hawthorn include promoting calm, reducing stress-related symptoms and overcoming insomnia.

Dose

100–450 mg a day (standardized to at least 1.8 per cent vitexin). Larger amounts are usually divided between three doses. It may take up to two months for hawthorn extracts to show an appreciable effect.

Side effects

Side effects are rare, although nausea, sweating and skin rashes have been reported.

Contraindications

Anyone who suffers from a heart condition should check with their doctor before taking hawthorn, especially if they are on prescribed medication.

Hemp seed oil
(Cannabis sativa)

Oil from the seed of the non-drug strain of Cannabis, known as the hemp plant, contains both omega-6 and omega-3 essential fatty acids in a ratio of 3 to 1, which includes gammalinolenic acid (GLA).

Benefits
Hemp seed oil has similar uses to evening primrose, flaxseed and omega-3 fish oils. It is used to correct hormone imbalances such as those occurring in pre-menstrual syndrome, help maintain a healthy circulation, and also for its anti-inflammatory action in conditions such as arthritis, psoriasis and colitis.

Hemp seed oil supplements do not contain the psycho-active chemical (tetrahydrocannabinol) found in other (marijuana) strains of the cannabis plant.

Dose
5–15 ml a day, best taken with food.

Histidine

L-Histidine is an amino acid that is converted into histamine in the body. Histamine acts as a neurotransmitter in the brain, and is the chemical that triggers orgasm when released from mast cells in the genitals.

Benefits
High levels of histidine promote orgasm in both males and females. Taking too much histidine has been linked with temporary premature ejaculation and may therefore be helpful for men with retarded ejaculation. It is sometimes taken as a prosexual supplement to enhance sexual activity.

Dose

50–500 mg, twice a day with meals. No more than 1.5 g should be taken daily except under medical supervision. (Histidine may be prescribed at doses of 4 g a day to relieve pain in rheumatoid arthritis, for example.) Some nutritionists recommend taking histidine together with B group vitamins for maximum effect.

Contraindications

Histidine should not be taken by:

- women who suffer with heavy menstrual bleeding
- anyone who has a history of depression
- anyone who is taking antihistamine medications for allergic conditions.

Horsechestnut
(Aesculus hippocastanum)

Horsechestnut seed extracts are derived from the common deciduous tree.

The main active ingredients are triterpene saponins together known as escin (aescin). This has been shown to tighten small blood vessels and reduce excessive permeability, to help stop fluid leakage from the circulation into the peripheral tissues. It may also reduce the activity of enzymes that lead to excessive breakdown of supporting tissues around capillary walls so that it has a strengthening effect on tissues supporting peripheral blood vessels. Clinical studies have shown that Horsechestnut extracts significantly reduce fluid exudation across capillaries compared with placebo, and double-blind placebo controlled trials have shown that extracts can reduce sensations of tiredness, heaviness, tension, itching, cramping, pain and swelling in the legs in those with varicose veins and chronic venous insufficiency. Extracts are also used to treat haemorrhoids and may help to reduce nosebleeds. They have also been used to reduce swelling following sprains and strains.

Dose
250–500 mg, daily, corresponding to 100 mg escin daily.

Select extracts standardised to contain 16% to 21% escin where possible.

Side effects
Occasional side effects of itching, nausea, and indigestion may occur.

5-hydroxy-tryptophan

Products containing 5-hydroxy-tryptophan (5-HTP) are derived from the seed pods of a West African plant, *Griffonia simplicifolia*.

5-HTP is derived from an amino acid, tryptophan, which in the diet is also found in chicken, meat and dairy products. 5-HTP is able to pass from the bloodstream into the brain where it is converted into a neurotransmitter (a chemical essential for brain communication), serotonin (5-hydroxy-tryptamine or 5-HT), which helps to lift mood and also influences appetite.

Benefits

When you eat carbohydrate, serotonin is released to lift your mood slightly and also helps to signal that you have eaten enough – that's why you tend to feel full up more quickly when eating a starchy meal than when eating a fatty meal. Serotonin also soothes, calms and gives rise to feelings of contentment. Some serotonin is converted by the pineal gland into melatonin, the hormone that helps determine our sleep/wake cycle.

In one study, overweight women taking 5-HTP supplements felt fuller, ate less calories and lost more weight than those taking an inactive placebo. In a study involving 20 obese people, those taking 5-HTP for 12 weeks while following a calorie-controlled diet lost five times more weight than those taking the placebo, as they felt less hungry and were less interested in food.

Lack of serotonin has been linked with depression, uncontrollable appetite, obsessive-compulsive disorder, autism, bulimia, social phobias, pre-menstrual syndrome, anxiety and panic, migraines, schizophrenia and violence. There seems to be an increased serotonin activity in people with anorexia and reduced serotonin activity in those with bulimia.

5-HTP is used to treat insomnia, depression, anxiety, panic attacks, obesity and attention deficit disorder. It may also be helpful in the treatment of migraine, fibromyalgia and eating disorder.

Researchers have found impurities in some 5-HTP supplements and the unknown contaminant, which has not yet been identified has been called 'Peak X'. This has previously been associated with a serious illness known as eosinophilia myalgia syndrome (EMS) and in the USA, doctors recommend that people only take a 5-HTP supplement that has been independently verified as 'Peak X free'. There is some suggestion that the contamination was spurious however, and may even have been deliberate, so it's difficult to know the exact story.

Dose
150–300 mg a day (divided into three doses) for up to three months, best taken on an empty stomach.

Side effects
Side effects are uncommon but can include headache, nasal congestion, nausea and constipation.

Contraindications
● Since 5-HTP may cause drowsiness, it should not be used while driving a car or operating heavy machinery.

● 5-HTP should not be taken with anti-depressant drugs as these affect chemical messengers in the brain including serotonin and can interact to cause a variety of symptoms such as anxiety, palpitations, sweating and diarrhoea.

● The effects of 5-HTP in pregnancy has not been studied, so it should not be taken by pregnant or breast-feeding women.

Indian ginseng
See **Ashwagandha**

Indian mustard
(Brassica juncea)

Indian mustard is a member of the cabbage family. Its roots have an unusual ability to absorb and concentrate minerals from the soil in which it is grown, and has been used to clear areas of toxic heavy metals such as lead and uranium. It is therefore known as a primary accumulator, or nature's magnet.

Indian mustard is taken as a mineral source depending on how it is grown. That grown hydroponically in a selenium-enriched environment, for example, will accumulate selenium and is taken as a natural selenium source. A zinc-rich supplement is soon to become available. Each is concentrated to produce a one-a-day supplement so that only one tablet/capsule need be taken a day.

Indian mustard is also a good source of phytochemicals, such as glucosinolates similar to those found in broccoli, which have a protective action against cancer.

Dose
One-a-day tablets enriched with particular minerals such as selenium.

See also **Selenium, Zinc**

Iodine

Iodine is an essential trace element that has only one known function in the body: it is vital for the production of the two thyroid hormones, thyroxine (T4) and tri-iodothyronine (T3). These hormones control the metabolic rate, the conversion of food and fat stores into energy and how much body heat is produced.

Dietary sources of iodine include marine fish, seaweed products, iodized salt and crops or cattle reared on soils exposed to sea spray. Lack of iodine is common in many parts of the world, however.

Benefits

Iodine plays a major role in preventing lethargy, tiredness, and excessive weight gain. The normal range for thyroxine hormone is wide, and sub-optimal intakes of iodine may account for feelings of lethargy and difficulty in losing weight in many whose T4 level is in the low normal range.

Deficiency

Symptoms that may be linked with iodine deficiency include underactive thyroid gland, swollen thyroid gland (goitre), tiredness, lack of energy, weight gain, muscle weakness, susceptibility to the cold, coarse skin, brittle hair and nails, breast tenderness and increased production of mucus.

Lack of iodine in pregnancy leads to an underactive thyroid which shows up after birth as a condition known as cretinism. As well as an underactive thyroid, the child's brain cannot develop properly leading to severe mental retardation. This is a serious problem in some parts of the world, including parts of Europe, New Zealand, Brazil and the Himalayas. In some areas, iodine deficiency affects nine out of ten of the population. In Indonesia, for example, there are currently an estimated 1.5 million severely mentally retarded children and 800,00 with cretinism. This is a devastating condition that is entirely preventable if expectant mothers are given injections of iodized oil – preferably during the preconceptual period. Treatment must be given before the sixth month of pregnancy to protect the brain against the effects of iodine deficiency. When treatment is not given until the last three months of pregnancy, it does not seem to improve brain function. In the Western world, newborn babies are screened for cretinism as part of the heel-prick test carried out soon after delivery.

Gross iodine deficiency leading to swelling of the thyroid gland (goitre) may occur in people who restrict their salt intake and who do not eat iodine-rich foods (e.g. seafood).

Supplements providing iodine act as a mild thyroid stimulant and may encourage a more efficient metabolism if your iodine intake has been sub-optimal. It is therefore included in many products designed to aid weight loss. It may also improve energy levels and quality of skin, hair and nails.

Selenium plays a role in the metabolism of thyroid hormones, and the effects of iodine deficiency are made worse by low selenium intakes.

Dose

The EC RDA for iodine is 150 mcg a day (adults). Those who are physically active may need more iodine than people who are inactive as iodine is lost in sweat – an athlete in heavy training can lose the full RDA of 150 mcg iodine in sweat alone.

Iodine is best obtained from natural extracts of kelp, bladderwrack (*Fucus*) or from an A to Z-style vitamin and mineral supplement.

Up to 3 per cent of people are allergic to iodine, and taking supplements long-term (especially those derived from kelp) can cause sensitivity reactions.

Excess
Excess iodine may lead to a metallic taste in the mouth, oral sores, headache, diarrhoea, vomiting, rash and – as with a deficiency – can also lead to thyroid swelling (goitre).

Iron

Iron is an essential mineral needed for the production of haemoglobin, the red blood pigment which transports oxygen and the waste gas, carbon dioxide, around the body. Many enzyme systems also rely on iron to function properly, including those involved in the production of energy from carbohydrate, fat and protein.

Iron is found in a protein, myoglobin, which binds oxygen in muscle cells for ready access during exercise, but two thirds of your body's iron stores are present in haemoglobin.

Deficiency
Lack of iron quickly leads to the production of red blood cells that are much smaller and paler (due to lack of haemoglobin) than normal. This results in iron-deficiency anaemia with symptoms of paleness, fast pulse, tiredness, exhaustion, dizziness, headache and even shortness of breath and angina if anaemia is severe.

Lack of iron also impairs concentration and learning ability especially for school children.

Other symptoms that can occur in iron deficiency include generalized skin itching, concave brittle nails, hair loss, sore tongue, cracking at the corners of the mouth, reduced appetite and difficulty in swallowing.

Worldwide, iron deficiency is the most common nutritional disease, with most cases going unrecognized. Women are more at risk of iron deficiency than men, because of blood loss during menstruation. This can result in a low-grade iron deficiency that is enough to impair immunity, without causing frank iron-deficiency anaemia.

If anaemia is suspected, it is important to seek medical advice before taking iron supplements, as the cause needs to be determined and iron supplements may mask iron deficiency.

Various studies have suggested that up to 20 per cent of the menstruating women in developed countries are iron deficient, but less than half of these have anaemia.

Iron plays an important role in immunity as white blood cells use powerful iron-containing chemicals to destroy invading micro-organisms (bacteria, yeasts, viruses) and one of the signs of iron deficiency is often increased susceptibility to infection, especially recurrent thrush and *Herpes simplex* virus attacks. As this can occur when levels of iron are not low enough to cause anaemia, it will not be picked up with a simple test to measure haemoglobin levels. Instead, it is necessary to measure the amount of iron-binding protein (ferritin) present in the circulation to detect low iron stores.

Iron requirements are thought to double during pregnancy as a woman's red blood cell and haemoglobin count goes up by 30 per cent although a lot of this will be obtained through the absence of normal losses associated with menstrual bleeding.

Although iron is important during pregnancy, many doctors no longer routinely recommend iron supplements to pregnant women. However, in a study in which 99 women were given regular iron supplements from the 28th week of pregnancy, the prevalence of anaemia and iron deficiency decreased markedly in comparison with that in women who were not given supplements. Three months after delivery, the iron status of infants born to mothers who had taken supplements was significantly higher compared with those born to mothers who had not.

Iron forms part of an antioxidant enzyme system (iron catalase) that helps to protect the brain from damage from free radicals during pregnancy. This enzyme may provide some protection against cerebral palsy during development in the womb. Taking iron supplements during pregnancy may also halve the risk of the offspring developing a type of brain tumour (astrocytoma) during childhood.

Lack of iron can trigger pica – a condition characterized by cravings for eating strange things such as soil, coal, paper. This is especially common during pregnancy, and iron deficiency should always be checked for.

Dietary sources of iron include shellfish, red meats, sardines, wheatgerm, wholemeal bread, egg yolk, green vegetables and dried fruit. Overboiling vegetables decreases their iron availability by up to 20 per cent. Vegetarians and those who eat little red meat are at increased risk of iron deficiency. Their intakes are dependent on absorbing inorganic non-haem iron, and food supplements play an important role.

Dose
The EC RDA for iron is 14 mg for adults.

Iron exists in two main forms: ferrous iron and ferric iron. Iron must be in the ferrous form to be absorbed properly, so avoid supplements supplying iron in the ferric form – especially as this also inactivates vitamin E. Iron-rich spa water is available as a liquid iron tonic, as are iron-rich solutions/tablets obtained from plant sources (herbal tonics) which are also well tolerated and may act more quickly.

Vitamin C increases the absorption of inorganic (non-haem) iron when taken at the same time, by keeping it in the ferrous form, so it is a good idea to wash down supplements with fresh fruit juice.

Phytate fibre, calcium and tannin-containing drinks decrease iron absorption. Coffee, for example, can reduce iron absorption by up to 39 per cent if drunk within an hour of eating. Iron is therefore best taken on an empty stomach unless it causes irritation.

Ferrous fumarate or ferrous gluconate is usually better tolerated than ferrous sulphate.

Iron supplements given alone can decrease absorption of zinc and other essential minerals (such as manganese, chromium and selenium) so it is usually advisable to only take iron in combination with these, e.g. in an A to Z-style vitamin and mineral supplement (unless prescribed individually by a doctor).

Excess

Avoid taking too much iron as this can cause constipation or indigestion and excess is toxic (especially for children). Some studies also suggest that excess intakes may increase the risk of heart disease and colon cancer, especially in males.

Most men and post-menopausal women do not need to take iron-containing supplements.

Note:
- Some people have an inherited tendency to absorb too much iron, leading to a potentially dangerous condition known as haemochromatosis which usually only occurs in males. Early signs of haemochromatosis include loss of sex drive, reduced size of testicles, fatigue and joint pains.

- Keep iron supplements well away from small children – eating just a few has been known to be fatal.

Isoflavones

There are three main types of dietary plant hormones that have a similar structure to human oestrogens: isoflavones, flavonoids and lignans. The isoflavones (genistein, daidzein, formononetin, biochanin A and glycitein) have been most extensively studied and are found in members of the pea and bean family such as chickpeas and soya. Flavonoids are present in high concentrations in many fruits and vegetables – especially apples and onions – and are also found in green and black tea leaves. Lignans are found mainly in linseed but also in sesame seeds, wholegrain cereals, fruit and vegetables.

Benefits

Isoflavones have an oestrogen-like action in the body which is 500–1000 times weaker than that of human oestrogens. Also known as phytoestrogens, they can damp down high oestrogen states by competing for the stronger natural oestrogens at oestrogen receptors. This reduces the amount of oestrogen stimulation a cell receives. As they have a weak oestrogen action, phytoestrogens also provide a useful additional hormone boost when oestrogen levels are low after the menopause. They therefore act as a natural form of hormone replacement therapy.

In cultures such as Japan where soy is a dietary staple, intakes of isoflavones are 50–100 mg a day as compared with a typical Western consumption of only 2–5 mg. As a result, less than 25 per cent of menopausal Japanese women complain of hot flushes, compared with 85 per cent of North American women.

In one study involving over a hundred post-menopausal women, isoflavones from soy extracts significantly reduced the number of hot flushes experienced per day. By the 12th week of treatment, women taking soy had a 45 per cent reduction in hot flushes versus 30 per cent with a placebo.

Isoflavones mimic some of the beneficial effects of oestrogen on the circulation, helping to dilate coronary arteries, increase heart function, reduce blood levels of harmful LDL-cholesterol (typically by 10 per cent) and reduce blood stickiness to prevent unwanted clotting. These findings may help to explain why the Japanese have one of the lowest rates of coronary heart disease in the world.

Based on evidence from over 50 independent studies, the US Food and Drug Administration (FDA) have authorized health claims on food labels saying that 'A diet low in saturated fat and cholesterol, and which includes 25 g soya protein per day, can significantly reduce the risk of coronary heart disease'.

Phytoestrogens also have a beneficial action on bone, boosting formation of new bone and reducing absorption of old bone. A daily intake of 2.25 mg isoflavones has been shown to significantly increase bone mineral content and density in the lumbar spine and to protect against spinal bone loss and osteoporosis.

Isoflavones may also play an important role in protecting against breast and prostate cancers. As well as reducing the total amount of oestrogen stimulation these glands receive (by blocking oestrogen receptors so that stronger human oestrogens cannot stimulate them) isoflavones reduce the activity of tumour growth factors in the laboratory, so that new blood vessels do not form in developing tumours and tumour cells fail to thrive. They also seem to protect genetic material from harmful mutations.

Some scientists believe that eating just one bowl of miso soup (made from fermented soya beans) per day may reduce the risk of stomach cancer by more than 30 per cent.

Dose
At least 2.25–50 mg isoflavones a day.
(NB: 60 g of soy protein provides 45 mg isoflavones.)

K

Vitamin K activity is found in three fat-soluble compounds: phylloquinone (K1), menaquinones (K2) and menadione (K3).

Vitamin K is essential for normal blood clotting. It acts as an essential co-factor for the production of clotting proteins II, VII, IX, X, protein C and protein S in the liver. High doses of vitamin K are used to counteract an overdose of the blood-thinning drug, warfarin.

Vitamin K in the diet

Most of our vitamin K requirements are met by beneficial bacteria in our gut that produce vitamin K2, which is then absorbed into our circulation and used. Dietary sources of vitamin K usually supply around a fifth of our needs; it is found in cauliflower (the richest source), broccoli, kelp and other dark green leafy vegetables, yoghurt (in which it is produced by the bacteria present), egg yolk, alfalfa, safflower, rapeseed, soya and olive oils, fish liver oils, liver, tomatoes, meat, potatoes and pulses.

Benefits

A single dose of vitamin K is offered to all newborn infants either by injection or orally, to prevent a condition known as haemorrhagic disease of the newborn. This arises during the first few days of life and causes haemorrhage into the brain due to vitamin K deficiency. Some research initially suggested an increased risk of childhood leukaemia associated with giving vitamin K by injection (rather than orally) at birth, but this has now been discounted.

Vitamin K is also needed for the synthesis of osteocalcin – a calcium-binding protein found in bone matrix – and it is now recognized as being as important for bone health as calcium. Lack of vitamin K has been linked to osteoporosis and research suggests that vitamin K supplements can reduce loss of bone calcium in post-menopausal women by up to 50 per cent as well as strengthening bones that are already weakened.

Deficiency

Symptoms that may be due to lack of vitamin K include prolonged bleeding time, easy bruising, recurrent nose bleeds, heavy periods and diarrhoea.

Dose

No EC RDA for vitamin K is currently set, but requirements are thought to be around 1 mcg per kilogram of body weight per day: 25-300 mcg. Higher doses may be suggested for treating osteoporosis.

Vitamin K is best taken with meals for optimum absorption.

Note: anyone who is taking warfarin treatment should seek medical advice before taking supplements containing vitamin K. Significant changes to dietary intake of vegetables can affect blood control in patients on warfarin: eating 250 g broccoli or cauliflower daily has a notable effect. A fairly constant intake of these foods needs to be maintained, therefore, to ensure that blood-clotting control remains stable.

Kava kava
(Piper methysticum)

Kava kava is native to Fiji where it is known locally as the 'nourishment of the gods'. Its botanical name, *Piper methysticum*, was given to it by the explorer Captain James Cook, and literally means intoxicating pepper. This refers to a 3000-year-old native custom of fermenting fresh kava kava roots to make a potent alcoholic drink used during a variety of rituals to induce relaxation and mild euphoria, to enhance dreams and to heighten sexuality. The dried root is not intoxicating however, although a few people find that it produces a pleasant, dream-like state.

Benefits

Kava kava root is widely used to combat anxiety, panic attacks and insomnia due to stress. It is mildly sedative, promotes feelings of relaxation and calm, relieves muscle tension and is helpful in the alleviation of mild to moderate pain – especially where this is due to muscle spasm as with menstrual cramps. It also has a mild diuretic action.

Kava kava seems to work in the part of the brain known as the amygdala, which regulates feelings of fear and anxiety and which is one of the areas in which benzodiazepine tranquillizers have their effect. Kava kava does not interact with benzodiazepine receptor sites however, and its exact action is not yet understood. Unlike tranquillizer drugs, tests suggest that kava kava does not impair driving skills, co-ordination, visual perception or judgement at therapeutic doses. Exceeding recommended doses may cause problems, however.

A trial involving 101 people with generalized anxiety, tension, agoraphobia, social phobia, insomnia and panic attacks found that kava kava helped most participants within two months. By three months, the average anxiety score had dropped from 30.7 to 13.4, and down again to 9.9 by six months. Other studies suggest that it's as effective as some prescription drugs in treating mild to moderate anxiety, and that it can significantly improve anxiety, depression and insomnia in women with menopausal symptoms.

Kava kava can also improve memory and is helpful for people trying to give up smoking or alcohol. It is currently being investigated as a treatment for epilepsy and to improve recovery after a stroke.

Kava kava is sometimes used with St John's Wort for a combined anti-anxiety and anti-depressant action. Anxiety and depression often go together, and anxiety can also lead to depression so it is sometimes a good idea to treat both conditions at the same time. St John's Wort needs to be taken daily for its anti-depressant effect, while kava kava may be taken on an 'as-needed' basis, which for some people may be every day. For example, a single tablet can be used to produce an immediate calming effect before a stressful event, or to help relieve insomnia associated with anxiety, while for someone with persistent anxiety, kava kava should be taken daily for 10–14 days to reach its full potential.

There is no evidence of tolerance to the herb (so that it becomes less effective with time) and no evidence of addiction.

Dose

120 mg kava pyrones a day.

Products standardized to 30 per cent kavalactones: 250 mg, three times a day.

Products standardized to 70 per cent kavalactones, 100 mg, three times a day.

The anxiolytic effects may be noticed with just a single dose, taken as required, while the other effects are usually noticeable within about ten days of starting treatment and will continue to bring about improvements over the next month.

Some kava kava teas may provide over 200 mg kavalactones per cup, so do not over-indulge.

Excess

Excessive use of kava kava at greater than recommended doses can cause dizziness, grogginess, muscle weakness and visual disturbances. High doses (equivalent to 400 mg or more of purified kava lactones per day) may result in a temporary yellow discoloration of the skin or a reversible scaly skin rash known as kani. Excess can also affect liver function and is not recommended.

Contraindications
Kava kava should not be taken:
- with alcohol (may cause nausea, stomach upset or sedation), other tranquillizers, or illegal drugs
- during pregnancy or when breast-feeding
- by Parkinson's disease sufferers as it may affect dopamine levels and produce abnormal movements.

Due to reports of adverse liver reactions in people taking Kava Kava, this herb was voluntarily withdrawn from sale by manufacturers in the UK in December 2001 pending further investigations.

Kelp
(Laminaria sp., Fucus vesiculosus)

Kelp supplements are obtained from long-leaved seaweeds and form a nutritious supplement containing 13 vitamins, 20 essential amino acids and 60 minerals and trace elements. It is a particularly rich source of calcium, magnesium, potassium, iron and iodine.

Benefits
Its main use is as a source of iodine to improve production of thyroid hormones, which in turn boosts the metabolic rate and may aid weight loss where obesity is related to

reduced thyroid function as a result of low iodine intake. The alginates present in kelp also help to promote feelings of fullness and to reduce appetite.

Other benefits of kelp include reducing hair loss, and improving the quality of hair, skin and nails where iodine intakes are low, and it can help to relieve arthritis. It also acts as a chelating agent, to remove heavy metal toxins from the intestines. Some studies suggest that a kelp-rich diet lowers blood pressure and cholesterol, boosts immune function and wards off cancer but more research is needed.

Dose
Depends on the product – follow manufacturer's guidelines. Skin patches containing iodine derived from kelp extracts are also available. Up to 3 per cent of people are allergic to iodine, and taking kelp supplements can cause sensitivity reactions.

Kudzu
(Pueraria lobata)

Kudzu is a traditional Chinese food whose starchy root is used in soups and stews as a thickening agent similar to cornstarch. It contains beneficial plant hormones (betasitosterol and isoflavones such as daidzein and formononetin) similar to those found in soya.

Benefits
The main medicinal use for kudzu involves its ability to dramatically decrease alcohol cravings, and extracts are widely recommended to treat those under the influence of

alcohol – both to sober them up, and to reduce their alcohol intake. Interesting studies have shown that daidzein and daidzin could suppress ethanol intake in the golden hamster, a species that would otherwise voluntarily increase intakes of alcohol and reduce intakes of water when given a free choice. This reaction was similar to that seen when hamsters were tested with anti-alcoholism drugs.

As a nutritional supplement with little risk of toxicity, and a traditional history of successful use in alcohol-dependent humans, kudzu is certainly well worth trying.

Dose

150 mg, three times a day.

Lapacho
(Tabebuia avellanedae)

Lapacho, also known as pau d'arco, taheebo, ipe roxo and the 'divine tree', is native to South America. It has unusual, carnivorous flowers that feed on insects, keeping it free from parasites and infections.

Benefits

Lapacho contains both naphthoquinones and anthraquinones, which rarely occur together in the same plant elsewhere. It grows at high altitudes where few other plants survive. It has adapted to this environment by developing a unique enzyme system which uses ozone to help synthesize lignin, an important constituent of woody tissues. As the reactions involved generate large quantities of free radicals, it has also developed a powerful antioxidant system based around carnosol, which contributes to the renowned anti-cancer actions of lapacho.

The inner bark of lapacho is also rich in other unique substances: lapachol and ß-lapachone, which interfere with the oxygen metabolism of tumour cells so that free radicals accumulate inside to trigger cell death. It also has an additional anti-viral action against viruses, including those associated with some forms of cancer such as leukaemia.

Lapacho also has anti-inflammatory, antibacterial, anti-fungal and anti-parasitic actions and is widely used to help treat Candida (thrush), skin infections with Gram positive bacteria, colds, warts, herpes cold sores, polio, influenza, boils, urinary tract infections, prostatitis and malaria.

Lapacho's anti-viral actions appear to be due to its ability to block enzymes involved in synthesis of viral genetic material (DNA and RNA) so that replication cannot occur. With other infections, it interferes with oxygen metabolism so pathogens cannot produce enough energy to reproduce. When taken by mouth, lapacho is secreted on to the skin surface in sweat and can even help to treat fungal skin infections, although it is also applied topically as a tincture or infusion.

Dose

1–2 g powdered bark a day for general use.

For anti-cancer activity, up to 5 g daily may be recommended by a medical herbalist – often combined with vitamin K to reduce blood thinning that has been noted when high dose extracted lapachol alone (but not whole lapacho) is taken. Select products standardized to contain at least 3 per cent naphthoquinones or at least 2 per cent lapachol.

Side effects
Very few side effects occur but lapacho may cause nausea or diarrhoea at very high doses.

Contraindications
Lapacho should not be taken by pregnant or breast-feeding women.

Lecithin
See **Choline**

Lemon Balm
(Melissa officinalis)

Lemon balm is an aromatic herb native to the Mediterranean whose leaves contain a variety of aromatic essential oils. It has been used since ancient times as a healing, soothing herb with calming properties.

Benefits
Lemon balm has sedative, anti-spasm and antibacterial actions and was also known as the 'scholar's herb' as it was traditionally taken by students suffering from the stress of impending exams. It is widely used to ease a number of stress-related symptoms including digestive problems, nausea, flatulence, depression, tenseness, restlessness,

irritability, anxiety, headache and insomnia. Lemon balm tea is also used to stimulate appetite.

When combined with valerian, the two herbs work in synergy to reduce symptoms of tension, stress and mild depression. They also have a gentle lowering effect on the raised blood pressure that often accompanies stress.

Dose
650 mg, three times a day.

Contraindications
● Lemon balm should not be taken with prescribed sleeping tablets; this may cause mild drowsiness which will affect ability to drive or operate machinery.
● Lemon balm should not be taken by pregnant or breast-feeding women.

Linseed Oil
See Flaxseed Oil

Liquorice
(Glycyrrhiza glabra)

Liquorice is native to the Mediterranean and its root has been used since ancient times to soothe coughs and upset stomachs. The rhizome contains a substance known as glycyrrhizin (also known as glycyrrhizic or glycyrrhizinic acid) which makes up 5-9 per cent of its weight, and which is 50 times sweeter than sucrose. Liquorice root also contains phytoestrogens and antioxidant flavonoids.

There are two forms of liquorice extracts available: those that contain glycyrrhizin, and deglycerrizhinated liquorice (DGL) which have different uses.

Benefits

Traditional uses for DGL extracts include speeding the healing of mouth ulcers and sore throat (lozenges), peptic ulcers (by increasing production of thin mucus to line the stomach), improving upper abdominal bloating, intestinal spasms and indigestion, relieving flatulence, and as an expectorant to thin phlegm so it is easier to cough up.

Glycyrrhizin-intact liquorice is mainly used to stimulate the adrenal glands, which is especially helpful in times of stress, convalescence and for those with chronic fatigue syndrome or fibromyalgia. A breakdown product of glycyrrhizin, known as glycyrrhetenic acid, is thought to be responsible for its action in blocking the inactivation of hydrocortisone hormone. This also results in the most well known side effect of liquorice, which is sodium retention and an increase in blood pressure (pseudoaldosteronism) with prolonged use and at high doses.

Glycyrrhizin-intact liquorice also stimulates immunity by increasing production of the anti-viral substance interferon, making this form of liquorice doubly effective against respiratory tract infections such as viral bronchitis and the common cold. It also has anti-inflammatory actions and is sometimes recommended to help treat eczema (as a cream), asthma, inflammatory bowel disease and hepatitis.

As glycyrrhizin has a weak oestrogen-like action, and, like isoflavones, helps to balance both high and low oestrogen states in the body, it may therefore be suggested to help pre-menstrual syndrome, endometriosis and menopausal symptoms.

Glycyrrhizin-intact liquorice needs to be stopped slowly rather than suddenly to prevent a rebound effect if used in high doses.

Dose

5–15 g per day of cut or powdered root.

Extracts: 200–600 mg a day (standardized to 22 per cent glycyrrhizin)

DGL: 760–1520 mg, three times a day.

Glycyrrhizin-intact liquorice should not be used by people with liver disease, low potassium levels, kidney failure or high blood pressure, by those taking diuretics or digoxin, or during pregnancy. This form of liquorice should not be taken long term (e.g. more than a month) except under supervision from a medical herbalist.

Maca
(Lepidium meyenii)

Maca is a root vegetable, related to the potato, which grows in the Peruvian Andes at heights of more than 4000 metres above sea level. It has been used as a dietary staple since before the time of the Incas as it is a good source of carbohydrate, amino acids, fatty acids, vitamins B1, B2, B12, C and E plus the minerals calcium, phosphorus, zinc, magnesium, copper and iron.

Benefits

Maca's tubers contain a number of steroid glycosides with oestrogen-like actions and is used to increase energy and stamina. It has also been used by some athletes as an alternative to anabolic steroids, without the side effects. It has long been reputed to act as an aphrodisiac for men and women, an aid to female fertility and a treatment for male impotence. It helps to relieve menopausal symptoms and other gynaecological problems related to hormonal imbalances. Some researchers believe maca to be superior to red Korean ginseng, and it is sometimes even referred to as Peruvian ginseng.

Dose

1 g, twice or three times a day.

Magnesium

Magnesium is the fourth most common metal found in the body, with 70 per cent stored in the bones and teeth. It is responsible for the function of over 300 enzymes, and is vital for every major metabolic reaction from the synthesis of protein and genetic material to the production of energy from glucose. Few enzymes can work without it and magnesium is now known to help maintain healthy tissues, especially those in the muscles, lung airways, blood vessels and nerves. Lack of magnesium leads to cell death due to depletion of energy stores.

Benefits

One of the most important functions for magnesium is to maintain the integrity of ion pumps that control the flow of sodium, potassium, calcium, chloride and other salt components across cell membranes. By moving ions against gradients, these pumps allow cells to hold an electrical charge and, in the case of nerve cells, to pass electrical messages from one neurone to another. Magnesium is essential for maintaining a cell's electrical stability and is especially important in controlling calcium entry into heart cells to trigger a regular heartbeat.

Magnesium is a co-factor in the metabolism of essential fatty acids, and for the interaction of sex hormones with cell receptors to switch on the genes they regulate. It is involved in the production of brain chemicals (such as dopamine) and helps to maintain normal moods.

Dietary sources of magnesium include soy beans, nuts, whole grains (although if these are processed they lose most of their magnesium content), seafood, seaweed products, meat, eggs, dairy products, bananas, dark green, leafy vegetables, chocolate and drinking water in hard-water areas. Mineral seasoning salt and Brewer's yeast are also important sources.

Deficiency

Lack of magnesium is common and may affect as many as one in ten people. Symptoms that may be due to magnesium deficiency include loss of appetite, nausea, fatigue, weakness, muscle trembling or cramps, numbness and tingling, loss of co-ordination, palpitations, hyperactivity and low blood sugar. It can also lead to diarrhoea (in early deficiency) and constipation (in later deficiency).

People with low magnesium levels are at risk of spasm of the coronary arteries (linked with angina or heart attack), sudden death (due to abnormal heart rhythms), high blood pressure (including that associated with pregnancy) and spasm of airways leading to asthma attacks. These effects seem to be more pronounced during times of stress. Magnesium treatment is sometimes given immediately after a heart attack to help prevent dangerous abnormal heart rhythms. It also helps to widen coronary blood vessels, and reduces the formation of platelet blood clots.

High blood pressure and heart attacks are less common in hard-water areas where water has a higher calcium and magnesium content. The use of low sodium, higher magnesium, higher potassium table salt in Finland was associated with a lower incidence of high blood pressure in the population. As many people have sub-optimal dietary intakes of magnesium, some scientists have now suggested that soft drinking water supplies should be also fortified with magnesium.

As magnesium regulates the movement of calcium in and out of cells, it is important for bone health and the prevention of osteoporosis. In one study, taking magnesium supplements (250–750 mg a day) for two years increased bone mineral density. In another study women who took magnesium supplements instead of calcium for eight months increased their bone density by 11 per cent compared with those not taking magnesium.

Low levels of magnesium are linked with chronic fatigue, fibromyalgia and pre-menstrual syndrome (PMS). Magnesium supplements are especially helpful for reducing PMS-associated symptoms of irritability, depression, anxiety, tiredness, fluid retention, weight gain, bloating, and breast tenderness. In one study, 204 women aged 18–50 with

PMS kept daily records for three consecutive menstrual cycles. Taking a magnesium supplement produced moderate, good or excellent improvements in over 70 per cent of women. When over 800 women took a magnesium-containing supplement for 90 days, at least 66 per cent showed improvements in irritability, depression and anxiety/tension.

Lack of magnesium has been linked with attention deficit hyperactivity disorder in children, and magnesium supplements can reduce hyperactivity. Other conditions in which magnesium supplements have proved helpful include restless leg syndrome, nocturnal grinding of teeth, facial tics and migraine – in one study, taking 600 mg magnesium daily helped to prevent migraine attacks in some people.

People with low magnesium intakes are almost twice as likely to develop type 11 diabetes but it is not yet known whether magnesium supplements are protective.

As magnesium levels decrease with age, magnesium deficiency may even play a role in the ageing process.

The EC RDA for magnesium is 300 mg, but people who are physically active need more than those who are not as large amounts are lost in sweat.

Dose
150 mg to 500 mg a day, taken with food to optimize absorption. Magnesium citrate is most readily absorbed, while magnesium gluconate is less likely to cause intestinal side effects such as diarrhoea at higher doses.

If taking magnesium supplements, it is important to ensure a good intake of calcium.

Magnolia vine

See **Schisandra**

Maitake
(Grifola frondosa)

Maitake is a rare, edible mushroom found in Japan growing on the trunks of deciduous trees. It forms large clusters that typically weigh around 20 pounds and is commonly known as cloud mushroom, monkey's shelf or the King of Mushrooms.

Benefits

Maitake contains powerful immune-stimulating substances known as beta-glucans.

Whereas most medicinal mushrooms contain a polysaccharide substance known as beta 1,3 glucan, that found in maitake is a unique, complex version known as beta 1,6 glucan (referred to as the D-fraction).

This increases the activity of immune chemicals (lymphokines, interleukin-1 and interleukin-2) that help to control white blood cells, leading to increased activity of immune scavenger cells (macrophages) and natural killer cells.

Maitake is taken as a general health tonic, having many of the same adaptogenic actions as Korean ginseng, reducing the effects of stress and normalizing blood pressure and blood glucose levels. Maitake is also used as an immune stimulant against viral infection and cancer. When given during chemotherapy, it has been shown to reduce the dose of toxic drugs needed, and it is believed to be more effective at inhibiting tumours than either reishi or shiitake mushrooms.

A clinical study in Japan involving 165 people with cancer found that when patients were given a combination of D-fraction and whole maitake powder, a significant improvement in symptoms occurred in 11 out of 15 patients with breast cancer, 12 out of 18 with lung cancer and 7 out of 15 with liver cancer. In those whose treatment included maitake plus chemotherapy, results were improved, and usual side effects of chemo- such as loss of appetite, nausea, low white blood cell count were reduced.

It may also be helpful in HIV and AIDS, as laboratory studies suggest that maitake enhances the activity of T-helper cells to reduce their destruction when infected with HIV. A preliminary study involving ten AIDS patients suggested that taking 5 g maitake powder daily for three months significantly increased T-helper cell count and improved symptoms such as dry cough, dermatitis and difficulty in sleeping.

Maitake is also used in the treatment of high blood pressure, diabetes, chronic fatigue syndrome, hepatitis B, glandular fever, and rheumatoid arthritis.

Dose

Extracts: 600 mg a day.

Dried mushroom: 1–4 g a day for general health, and 4–7 g to treat specific conditions.

Vitamin C improves absorption and effectiveness of maitake mushroom.

Should ideally be individually prescribed by a qualified medical herbalist.

Contraindications

As a food, maitake seems to have no toxic side effects, but none the less it is sensible to avoid taking it during pregnancy and breast-feeding.

Manganese

Manganese is an essential mineral involved in many metabolic functions, including the production of amino acids, carbohydrates, sexual hormones, blood-clotting factors, cholesterol and some brain transmitters. It also acts as an antioxidant.

Benefits

Manganese is essential for normal growth and development, as it is needed for the synthesis of cartilage, collagen and structural molecules known as mucopolysaccharides. It is especially important for healthy bones, and women with osteoporosis have been found to have manganese levels that were four times lower than those who do not.

Manganese in the diet

Foods containing manganese include black tea (one cup of tea contains 1 mg manganese), whole grains (although processing removes much of their manganese content), nuts, seeds, fruit, eggs, green leafy vegetables, offal, shellfish and milk.

Deficiency

The significance of manganese deficiency is currently unknown, but possible cases have been linked with reddening of body hair, scaly skin, poor growth of hair and nails, disc and cartilage problems, poor blood clotting, glucose intolerance, poor memory and worsening intellect. It may also contribute to reduced fertility.

Industrial workers exposed to inhalation of manganese dust have experienced toxicity with nervous system effects similar to Parkinson's disease.

Dose

No EC RDA is currently set for manganese. Up to 4 mg manganese is lost in bowel motions each day, and needs to be replaced, so intakes of 5 mg a day are suggested as safe and adequate. Some researchers suggest that up to 7 mg are needed daily for optimum bone health.

Manuka honey

See **Bee Products**

Mastic gum
(Pistacia lentiscus)

Mastic gum is a resin derived from a pistachio-like tree grown on the Greek island of Chios. It contains a number of unique constituents including masticonic, mastinininc and masticolic acids.

Benefits

Laboratory studies have shown that mastic gum has a powerful antibiotic action against *H. pylori* (a stomach infection associated with peptic ulcers and gastric cancer) – even including the antibiotic-resistant strains.

In one study, seven strains of *H. pylori* (including three that were resistant to the antibiotic metronidazole) were incubated with a dilute solution of mastic gum, which was found to kill the bacteria at concentrations as low as .06 mg per ml.

In a clinical trial involving 38 people with duodenal ulcers, 20 were given mastic gum while 18 were given a placebo. Sixteen taking mastic and nine taking placebo obtained symptomatic relief, while at endoscopy, proven healing of the duodenal ulcers was shown to have occurred in 70 per cent taking mastic gum compared with only 22 per cent on the placebo which was highly statistically significant.

Mastic gum is used to maintain healthy digestion, and to overcome symptoms such as indigestion, heartburn and dyspepsia associated with *Helicobacter* infection.

Dose

Begin with 1 g before bedtime with water for two weeks at start of symptoms. Continue with maintenance dose of 500 mg nightly.

Methyl-sulphonyl-methane or MSM-Sulphur

Sulphur is essential to health and is the fourth most abundant mineral in the human body after calcium, phosphorus and magnesium. Sulphur is involved in the production of energy in body cells, and the formation of antibodies. It is also needed for the formation of detoxification enzymes, and the production of glutathione, one of the most important antioxidants found in the body.

MSM is a sulphur compound that is made naturally in the body from the amino acids, methionine, cysteine and taurine. MSM and DMSO (unrefined MSM which is oxidized to produce MSM) are produced synthetically but are identical to those found in nature.

MSM-sulphur in the diet

Good nutritional sources of sulphur include eggs, meat, fish, onions, garlic and vegetables – especially cabbage, kale, broccoli and Brussels sprouts.

Benefits

MSM-sulphur is used to help a number of conditions, including allergies, acid indigestion, constipation, and degenerative bone diseases.

Like glucosamine sulphate, another sulphur-containing substance produced in the body, MSM seems to be important for healthy joints, cartilage, tendons and ligaments. It is also vital for healthy connective tissue containing the structural protein, collagen. With increasing age, skin tends to lose its elasticity due to the formation of cross-linkages within collagen so it becomes more fibrous. Some researchers believe that MSM helps to maintain suppleness of tissues by blocking the formation of these abnormal cross-linkages.

In a small double-blind, placebo-controlled trial involving 16 patients with osteoarthritis, those taking MSM experienced an 82 per cent reduction in joint pain after six weeks, compared with an average improvement of only 18 per cent in those on the placebo. Researchers are unsure exactly how MSM works against arthritis, but it is thought to reduce pain and swelling due to inflammation in a similar way to aspirin.

Dose

There is no EC RDA for sulphur.

Usual recommended dose: 1–2 g a day in divided doses although larger amounts may be taken under supervision.

Excess

Toxicity is low, but excess may produce gastrointestinal side effects.

Minerals

The word mineral literally means 'mined from the earth'. Minerals can be divided into two main groups of elements: metallic and non-metallic.

Carbohydrates, fats, proteins and vitamins are all based on the element carbon, and are known as organic substances. Minerals do not contain carbon and are said to be inorganic. In nutritional terms, the word mineral refers to inorganic substances of which we need to obtain more than 100 mg per day from our diet. Those needed in amounts much less than 100 mg are referred to as trace elements.

Around 20 minerals and trace elements are essential for the biochemical reactions occurring in human metabolism. The average adult contains around 3 kg of minerals and trace elements, most of which are found in the skeleton.

Minerals in the diet

In general, the mineral content of foods depends on the soil in which produce is reared or grown. This is in contrast to the vitamin content of food, which is usually more similar wherever it comes from. Acid rain and food processing can also reduce the mineral content of foods enough to cause deficiency.

Although some vitamins can be synthesized in the body in tiny amounts, minerals and trace elements can only come from the diet. As a result, mineral deficiency is more common than vitamin deficiency, especially amongst slimmers, the elderly, pregnant women, vegetarians and those eating vegetables grown in mineral-poor soils.

Benefits

Minerals have a number of different functions in the body.

- They act as antioxidants e.g. selenium, manganese.
- They are important structurally – calcium, magnesium and phosphate strengthen bones and teeth.
- They maintain normal cell function e.g. sodium, potassium, calcium.
- They act as a co-factor for important enzymes e.g. copper, iron, magnesium, manganese, molybdenum, selenium, zinc.

- They are involved in oxygen transport e.g. iron.
- They are important for hormone function e.g. chromium, iodine.

Some trace elements such as nickel, tin and vanadium are known to be essential for normal growth in only tiny amounts, although their exact roles is not yet fully understood.

See separate individual entries for all of the above.

Milk thistle
(Silybum marianum)

Milk thistle seeds contain a powerful mixture of antioxidant bioflavonoids known as silymarin, of which the most active ingredient is the flavonolignan, silibinin. The seeds contain as much as 6 per cent silymarin by weight.

Benefits

More than 300 studies have shown that silymarin can protect liver cells from the poisonous effects of excess alcohol and other toxins such as those produced by death cap mushroom and chemotherapy. It works as an antioxidant (and is at least 200 times more potent than vitamins C or E), by inhibiting factors responsible for liver cell damage – free radicals and leukotrienes – and by maintaining levels of an important liver antioxidant enzyme, glutathione. Some studies suggest that it can boost glutathione levels by over 33 per cent. Silymarin also seems to alter the outer structure of liver cell walls so poisons do not penetrate as readily – this means the liver can process toxins at a steady pace, as they enter, rather than being overwhelmed all at once.

Silymarin has been shown to stimulate liver cells regenerated after viral or toxic damage by increasing the rate at which new proteins are made and by reducing fibrosis. In addition it has recently been shown to have a protective effect on kidney cells. It is also being investigated as a possible protectant against ultraviolet-induced skin cancers and is helpful for reducing the excessive skin cell turnover seen in psoriasis.

Silymarin is mainly used to treat liver conditions such as hepatitis, cirrhosis, non-obstructive gallstones (by increasing bile flow) and to protect the liver in mushroom poisoning, after chemotherapy, and during detox programmes. In women with high oestrogen states such as endometriosis, it helps the liver metabolize oestrogen more efficiently which may reduce symptoms.

Dose

70–200 mg silymarin (standardized to at least 70 per cent silymarin), three times a day, preferably between meals.

It is best to start with a low dose and slowly increase. Liver function should start to show an improvement within five days and continue over at least the next three weeks.

Side effects

The only reported side effect is a mild laxative one in some people, due to increased production of bile.

Molybdenum

Despite its importance in plant and animal life, molybdenum is one of the world's scarcest trace elements. It acts as a co-factor for the function of three enzymes and is involved in the metabolism of iron, carbohydrate, fat and alcohol. It is also needed for the production of uric acid.

Molybdenum in the diet

Food sources include buckwheat (the richest source), whole grains, meats, dairy products and dark green leafy vegetables.

Deficiency

Symptoms that may be due to lack of molybdenum include anaemia, poor general health, increased incidence of dental caries, irritability, impotence, rapid irregular pulse, hyperventilation, visual problems and even coma due to intolerance of sulphur-containing amino acids.

A high incidence of oesophageal cancer in China has been linked with a lack of molybdenum, and this is thought to be the indirect effect of a carcinogenic fungus that can attack molybdenum-deficient maize.

Molybdenum and copper interact with one another and high copper intakes increase the rate at which molybdenum is lost from the body.

Dose

There is currently no EC RDA for molybdenum and requirements are unknown. A to Z-style vitamin and mineral formulas tend to contain around 25 mcg.

Muira puama
(Ptychopetalum olacoides)

Muira puama – popularly known as potency wood – is a small tree found in the Brazilian rain forest. Its roots, bark and wood are widely used by natives of the Amazon and Orinoco river basins to enhance sexual desire and combat impotence.

Benefits

Researchers are unsure as to how it works but it is thought to stimulate sexual desire both psychologically and physically, through a direct action on brain chemicals (dopamine, noradrenaline and serotonin) by stimulating nerve endings in the genitals and by boosting production/function of sex hormones, especially testosterone.

A clinical study of 262 patients found that muira puama was more effective than yohimbine (a pharmaceutical extract from the bark of the yohimbe tree, which is an FDA-approved treatment for impotence): 62 per cent of subjects who complained of lack of sexual desire claimed that muira puama had a dynamic effect on their sex lives, while 51 per cent who had erectile dysfunction felt it was of benefit. The researchers concluded that muira puama is one of the best herbs for treating erectile dysfunction and lack of libido.

Muira puama is also used as a general tonic for the nervous system, and is used to help treat exhaustion, neuralgia, anxiety, depression, pre-menstrual syndrome and menstrual cramps. Interestingly, it is also said to prevent some types of baldness.

Dose

1–1.5 g a day for two weeks.

Myrrh

For 4000 years, myrrh has been valued for its rich and enduring scent used in perfumes, incense and as a funeral herb in embalming. It is a gum resin produced by several species of *Commiphora*, collected mainly from wild trees in Africa, India and Arabia. The name comes from the Arabic, *murr*, meaning 'bitter'.

When the bark is cut, myrrh oozes out to form yellow-red, irregular, often tear-shaped lumps, sometimes as big as walnuts, which were said to come from the tears of Horus, the falcon-headed sun god.

Benefits

Myrrh is one of the oldest known medicines, widely used by the ancient Egyptians for mouth and throat problems, and in the Middle East for treatment of infected wounds and bronchial complaints. Ancient Greek soldiers never went to war without a pouch containing myrrh paste for first aid. It was used in traditional Indian medicine for menstrual problems and as an aphrodisiac, and was also said to improve intellect.

Myrrh's astringent, antiseptic and anti-microbial actions have been confirmed and it is now widely used in the topical treatment of mild inflammations of the mouth and throat (e.g. gingivitis, ulcers) and is often added to gargles and mouthwashes. It is one of the most effective herbal medicines worldwide for speeding healing of sore throat, mouth ulcers and gum infections. It is also used for acne, boils, bronchial, digestive and menstrual problems, including irregular or painful periods.

Myrrh has drying and anaesthetizing properties and is used in Germany to treat pressure sores caused by artificial limbs.

Dose

Gargle or rinse: add 5-10 drops of tincture to a little warm water.

Undiluted tincture 1:5 (g/ml): apply locally to affected areas of gums or mucous membranes of the mouth, twice or three times a day.

Capsules: 300 mg, twice a day.

N-acetyl cystine

N-acetyl cysteine (NAC) is an amino acid that boosts levels of a powerful antioxidant (glutathione) in the respiratory tract. Mucus dispersion can be boosted by supplements containing NAC and studies show that it can significantly reduce mucus production and associated cough in chronic respiratory conditions such as bronchitis, emphysema and sinusitis. It may also be helpful for ear infections and glue ear. Interestingly, research is currently under way to investigate observations that NAC can prevent some of the lung damage linked with lung cancer in smokers.

NAC is also thought to interfere with viral replication and may be recommended to people with viral illness, including HIV.

Dose
Up to 500 mg, three times a day.

Contraindications
NAC should not be taken by people who have peptic ulcers.

Nettle
(Urtica dioica)

Stinging nettle roots contain beta-sitosterol and a variety of other sterols and are often used together with saw palmetto.

Benefits
Nettle extracts are used to treat symptoms of male urinary retention due to an enlarged prostate gland. The ability to improve urinary symptoms of benign prostate enlargement without shrinking the gland is a relatively new finding. Nettle extracts seem to interfere with testosterone metabolism by lowering the amount bound to a blood protein (sex hormone binding globulin – SHBG) so that more testosterone is free and active in the circulation. This means that more testosterone is available for absorption into the prostate gland, so that congestion is relieved. Increased levels of freely circulating testosterone also increase sex drive.

Another possible way in which nettle extracts work is in reducing the flow of sodium and potassium ions in and out of prostate cells to reduce their metabolism and growth.

Nettle root extracts can also damp down inflammation and they are used in the treatment of rheumatoid arthritis. They may also be of benefit in treating prostatitis.

In an observational study involving 419 specialists and 2080 patients with benign prostatic hyperplasia (BPH), a combined extract containing saw palmetto berry and nettle root extracts was given. Before and after comparisons showed improvements in both obstructive and irritative symptoms, and results were described as 'very good' or 'good' in over 80 per cent of cases. Less than 1 per cent of men were suspected of having mild side effects.

Another interesting trial compared the activity of a combination of saw palmetto berry and nettle root extracts against the prescribed drug finasteride. A total of 548 men were treated for 48 weeks with either two capsules of plant extracts or one capsule of finasteride daily. The results were similar in both groups with equivalent reductions in urinary flow rate, International Prostate Symptoms Score and increased quality of life. The natural plant extracts proved superior when it came to side effects however, with fewer cases of erectile problems and headache.

Dose
250 mg extract twice a day, together with saw palmetto.

Side effects
Nettle extracts can cause mild gastrointestinal upsets. Avoid overdosage as this may cause temporary kidney problems.

Note: men with prostate symptoms should continue to have a regular medical review of their condition.

Niacin

See **Vitamin B3**

Nickel

Nickel has only been recognized as important in human metabolism within the last thirty years. It acts as an antidote to the effects of stress hormones to help offset constricted blood vessels, increased heart rate and raised blood pressure. It may therefore be important in reducing the risk of stress-related coronary heart disease.

Foods tend to contain nickel due to contamination from nickel alloys used in processing machinery and cooking utensils. Margarine is also a source where nickel is used as a catalyst during production.

In animals, nickel is also known to help the sugar-lowering effects of insulin, to have an effect on fat metabolism and to stabilize genetic material. Nickel deficiency also leads to impaired iron absorption and anaemia in animals. It is not yet known whether similar effects occur in humans.

Dose

There is currently no EC RDA for nickel.

Oats
(Avena sativa)

Extracts from the young, whole plant or unripe grain of oats are known as oatstraw or wild oats. These contain a variety of flavonoids, steroidal compounds, vitamins (especially B group) and minerals (especially calcium).

Benefits

Oatstraw is one of the most popular herbal remedies used as a restorative nerve tonic. It is used to help treat depression, nervous exhaustion and stress. It is a useful source of B group vitamins which are essential for energy production and which are needed in extra amounts during times of stress. Oatstraw soothes the nervous system and has a calming but spirited effect. It helps to reduce cravings and is helpful for those who are trying to stop smoking.

As oatstraw contains hormone building blocks, it is also recommended to women suffering from oestrogen deficiency and anyone with an underactive thyroid gland. Oat bran has been shown to help reduce high blood cholesterol levels and, taken regularly, can ease constipation.

Research in Australia found that athletes who followed an oat-based diet for three weeks showed a 4 per cent increase in stamina.

Dose

1 dropper fluid extract or tincture, twice or three times daily.

People who are sensitive to gluten (coeliac disease) should allow the tincture to settle, and decant the clear liquid for use.

Olive leaf
(Olea europaea)

The olive tree is well known around the Mediterranean where its fruits are eaten and used to make olive oil.

Benefits

As recently as 1995, olive leaf extracts became patented for their powerful antibacterial, anti-viral, anti-fungal and anti-parasitic activity. The active ingredients appear to be iridoid substances such as oleuropein and R-calcium elenolate which give the leaves of certain strains of olive tree a characteristic bitter taste. The iridoids work together in synergy to kill microbial infections by interfering with the production of certain amino acids so that they cannot grow or reproduce properly. Olive leaf extracts can also inactivate bacteria by dissolving and weakening their outer coating.

Olive leaf extracts are used to treat candida and other fungal infections, sinusitis, common colds, influenza, herpes, parasitic infections, shingles, respiratory infections, tonsillitis, pharyngitis, urinary tract infections, fibromyalgia and chronic fatigue syndrome.

A comparative trial of three products conducted by the Herpes Viruses Associate (olive leaf extract versus the cactus, *Opuntia streptacantha*, and a combined lysine, pollen and propolis capsule) found that olive leaf extracts were the clear winner. Out of 45 members taking part, 78 per cent of those using olive leaf extracts were pleased with the results in treating and preventing attacks.

Clinical studies involving 500 patients suggest that olive leaf is effective in treating 98 per cent of bacterial and viral infections – better than most prescribed antibiotics.

It has also been used in rheumatoid arthritis as olive leaf extracts also have strong antioxidant activity. Preliminary research suggests that olive leaf extracts can also lower raised blood pressure.

Dose

500 mg, twice to four times a day, between meals. For persistent problems take 1 g, three times a day. As symptoms improve, reduce back to a maintenance dose of 500 mg twice a day as necessary.

Side effects

No toxic side effects have been reported even at doses several hundred times higher than those used therapeutically. However, a few people have developed a Herxheimer reaction due to large numbers of bacteria being killed at once, which releases bacterial toxins into the system. Symptoms include fever, headache, and worsening of any current symptoms. This is usually treated with paracetamol and drinking plenty of fluids, and will resolve within 24 to 48 hours. If it occurs, cut back on the dose you are taking. Similar reactions can occur with traditional antibiotics and most people are not affected.

Contraindications

As olive leaf extracts have not been tested in pregnancy, they should not be used during pregnancy or when breast-feeding.

Olive oil
(Olea europaea)

All olives start off green. These are the unripened fruit with firm skin and a slightly bitter taste. Olives intended for producing oil are picked when unripe. They taste bitter and are totally inedible. These have a low acid content which is crucial, as the lower the acidity, the better the oil.

Extra virgin olive oil is the best quality and has not been purified. Only around 10 per cent of oil produced is of this premium grade quality. It has a distinctive green hue and often hazes at room temperature. Its flavour is superb as it comes from the first pressing of the fruit and retains the fresh, olive aroma with less than 1 per cent acidity. It also has the highest antioxidant content (vitamin E, carotenoids and polyphenols).

Virgin olive oil comes next in quality with an acidity level of not more than 1.5 per cent. Virgin olive oil is also a premium product as it is not purified and has a slightly more piquant taste. Pure olive oil is a blend of refined oils mixed with virgin oil to provide flavour and a quality suitable for cooking. Although the flavour is less pleasing, this is the most widely sold oil as it is less expensive.

Olive oil is native to the Mediterranean – an area with a low incidence of coronary heart disease.

Benefits

As well as lowering abnormally raised harmful low-density lipoprotein (LDL) cholesterol levels, its protective effects against cardiovascular disease, diabetes, arthritis and even some cancers – especially breast, prostate and colon – are now well accepted.

What is a monounsaturated fat?

The oils and fats in your diet consist of a molecule of glycerol to which three fatty acid chains are attached sideways on (triacylglycerols). This forms a molecular shape similar to a capital E. The length of the fatty acid chains and whether or not any of their carbon atoms are linked by a double bond dictate whether the fat is solid or liquid at room temperature, and how it is metabolized in your body.

Fats that contain no double bonds are referred to as saturated fats. Fats containing some double bonds are known as unsaturated fats – those with one double bond are mono-unsaturated, while those with two or more double bonds are polyunsaturated.

Most dietary fats contain a blend of saturates, mono-unsaturates and polyunsaturates in varying proportions. In general, saturated fats tend to be solid at room temperature while monounsaturated and polyunsaturated fats tend to be liquid – i.e. oils.

Foods rich in monounsaturates include olive oil, rapeseed oil and avocado. These are beneficial to health as your body metabolizes dietary monounsaturated fats in such a way that they lower blood levels of harmful LDL-cholesterol.

The health benefits of olive oil come from its antioxidants – including vitamin E – and its principle monounsaturated fat, oleic acid, which is an omega-9 fatty acid.

Oleic acid reduces absorption of cholesterol, and is processed in the body to lower the harmful LDL cholesterol without modifying desirable high-density lipoprotein (HDL) cholesterol. It also reduces abnormal blood-clotting tendencies and, as a result, in Mediterranean regions where olive oil is used liberally the incidence of coronary heart disease, high blood pressure, peripheral vascular disease, stroke and other cholesterol-related illnesses – including dementia – is low. Oleic acid also has beneficial effects on insulin levels and diabetes.

A diet rich in olive oil has been shown to reduce the risk of coronary heart disease by 25 per cent. In a study involving 605 people recovering from a heart attack, those following a Mediterranean-style diet were 56 per cent less likely to suffer another heart attack, or to die from heart problems, than those following their normal diet.

Among people with high blood pressure, using 30–40 g olive oil in cooking every day reduced their need for anti-hypertensive drugs by almost 50 per cent over a six-month period, compared with only 4 per cent for those randomized to use sunflower oil. All those on the sunflower oil diet continued to need their antihypertensive drug treatment, while 80 per cent of those using olive oil were able to discontinue their drug treatment altogether. This effect was thought related to the antioxidant polyphenols in olive oil.

Among 278 elderly people with no known memory or concentration problems, a high intake of olive oil was shown to reduce cognitive decline with age, which suggests that it plays a protective role in preserving cognition in healthy older people.

Studies looking at the link between diet and colon cancer found that populations with the highest intakes of olive oil have the lowest risks of bowel cancer. It is thought that the activity of a digestive enzyme, diamine oxidase, is reduced by olive oil so that less cancer-causing chemicals are released from the diet into the gastrointestinal tract.

Following a low-fat diet containing one tablespoon extra virgin olive oil per day can reduce the risk of breast cancer by 45 per cent over a three-year period. In post-menopausal women, those consuming olive oil more than once a day were 25 per cent less likely to develop breast cancer than those consuming it once a day (and who already had a lower risk as a result).

Pure olive oil remains stable at elevated temperatures due to its high levels of monounsaturated fatty acids and natural antioxidant, vitamin E. Refined olive oil can therefore be heated up to 210°C before chemical changes take place. Virgin and extra virgin olive oils are less stable, however, due to their higher content of heat-sensitive components. Because of this, virgin olive oil may cause unwanted smells or taste changes if heated above 180°C. Pure olive oil should therefore be used for frying, and virgin or extra virgin olive oils be kept for steaming, braising and dressing. Discard any oil that begins to smoke or smell odd during use. Ideally, cooking oils should not be re-used.

As with other oils, oxidation occurs over time. As the oil matures, extra acidity is gained which detracts from the original flavour. Most oils are best used within one year of pressing. If left longer than this, stale or even rancid flavours can develop. All types of olive oil should therefore be kept somewhere cool and dark, and used fresh – buy from outlets where turnover is high, and avoid large containers (especially those made from tin or aluminium). It is best bought in small sizes, and frequently renewed.

Dose

At least 10 g daily, and preferably 30–40 g a day. For those who do not cook their own food, or who have little opportunity to include extra virgin olive oil in their diet, extra virgin olive oil capsules are available as a supplement.

---

1 tablespoon olive oil contains 15 g total fat, 2 g saturated fat
1 tablespoon butter contains 12 g total fat, 8 g saturated fat

---

Oregano oil
(Oreganum vulgare)

Oregano is a popular herb used extensively in Mediterranean cooking. Oil of wild oregano contains essential oils (e.g. carvacrol, thymol, terpinenes, cymenes) that have powerful antimicrobial actions, and has been used to kill moulds, yeasts, bacteria and parasites even when diluted over a thousand times. It is also used to boost general immunity and to help cleanse the body during detox programmes.

Oregano oil may be used as a general immune tonic to increase resistance against infection, and to help improve symptoms due to upper respiratory tract infections, asthma, low blood pressure, tiredness, candida, irritable bowel syndrome, colitis, chronic fatigue, diarrhoea, constipation, cystitis, eczema and psoriasis.

It may also be used topically (dilute in olive oil if stinging occurs) to treat toothache, ringworm, athlete's foot, cold sores, psoriasis, eczema, warts, rosacea and wounds.

Dose
Only a small amount is needed, and doses range from 10 mg to 600 mg daily.

Peppermint
(Menthe piperitae)

Peppermint is a popular culinary and medicinal herb. It contains an essential oil that has antiseptic and painkilling properties, and it is also widely used in the treatment of fevers, colds, headaches and the discomfort of cystitis, as well as relieving tension, itching and inflammation. The essential oil is obtained by steam distillation of peppermint's aerial parts (leaves, stems and shoots). The oil is rich in menthol which may make up to 50 per cent of the oil by volume.

Benefits

It improves digestion by stimulating secretion of digestive juices and bile, and also relaxes excessive spasm of the smooth muscle lining the digestive tract. Peppermint is therefore taken to relieve indigestion, colic, intestinal cramps, flatulence, diverticulitis and irritable bowel syndrome (IBS). It may also help to dissolve gallstones.

While mild symptoms of IBS are helped by drinking peppermint tea, more severe symptoms benefit from taking peppermint oil capsules that are enteric-coated to prevent the release of peppermint oil until it has reached the large bowel.

Inhaling menthol helps to relieve nasal congestion.

Dose

Enteric-coated capsules containing 0.2 ml, one, two, or three times a day between meals.

Side effects

Treatment may produce a warm, tingling feeling in the back passage due to some of the essential oil not being absorbed. This is not harmful and will usually disappear if you cut back on the dosage you are taking.

Contraindications

- Peppermint should not be taken during pregnancy.
- Peppermint should not be taken by people who are also taking homeopathic medicines as it is believed to inactivate these.

Perilla frutescens

Perilla frutescens is an annual plant native to Asia, which has either green or purple leaves. It is also known as Chinese basil, the purple mint plant or wild coleus.

Benefits

The leaves, stems and seeds are a traditional Chinese herbal remedy whose use dates back to at least AD 500. Its main traditional use was as an accompaniment to shellfish, crab and raw seafood dishes, both as a spice and to neutralize the toxins that exist in some species and to help prevent food poisoning. In India, perilla seed oil (similar to flaxseed oil) is often added to curries.

Perilla seed oil has a high content of linolenic acid which is processed in the body to produce anti-inflammatory effects similar to those of evening primrose oil. Leaf extracts contain a number of anti-allergy and anti-inflammatory substances, including elemicine, apigenen and beta-sitosterol. Leaf extracts are believed to reduce abnormal immune reactions by inhibiting tumour necrosis factor (TNF), inhibiting immunoglobulin E (IgE) production and function as well as having antioxidant activity. Perilla has been shown to increase production of the natural antiviral substance, interferon, and is used to treat cough and lung infections. It has also been used as a sedative, to ease smooth muscle spasm, nausea, vomiting, diarrhoea and – a new indication – to reduce allergic reactions.

A cream containing perilla leaf extracts (minus the irritant, perillaldehyde) is used in Japan to treat children with atopic eczema. It has anti-inflammatory and anti-allergic actions that, in an open trial involving over 100 children, was said to have an efficacy rate of 80 per cent after three months, with improvement in itching, skin lesions and eruptions. In 20 people using both the cream and taking oral perilla extracts for two months, there was improvement in 90 per cent.

Perilla leaf extracts taken orally can reduce sneezing and runny nose due to hay fever with 85 per cent of those taking them finding them effective

Dose
3 g extracts, twice a day.

Pfaffia
(Pfaffia paniculata)

Pfaffia – also known as suma, Brazilian ginseng and Brazilian carrots – is regarded as a panacea for all ills locally, where it is called *para todo* – 'for everything'. The dried golden root of pfaffia is a rich source of vitamins, minerals, amino acids, pfaffocides and plant hormones (up to 11 per cent by weight) such as stigmasterol and sitosterol (which have oestrogen-like actions and reduce high cholesterol levels) and beta-ecdysone which increases cellular oxygenation.

Benefits

Although pfaffia is unrelated to Chinese ginseng, it has similar adaptogenic properties and can help the immune system to adapt to various stresses including overwork, illness and fatigue. It improves resistance to stress, illness and fatigue and evens out hormone imbalances. Due to its oestrogenic nature, it is used to treat a variety of gynaecological problems linked with hormonal imbalances such as pre-menstrual syndrome and menopausal symptoms.

Pfaffia has been used as a female aphrodisiac for at least 300 years, and is also used to help treat male impotence and prostatitis. It is used to boost physical, mental and sexual energy levels as well as producing a general sense of well-being. Pfaffocides are also being used to improve sleep and to treat diabetes, chronic fatigue syndrome, joint problems, high cholesterol and gout.

The Japanese have patented an extract of the root – pfaffic acid – for its potent ability to inhibit the growth of skin cancer cells (melanoma).

Dose

Extracts standardized to 5 per cent ecdysterones: 500 mg–1 g a day to combat physical and mental stress. Larger doses of 15 g a day are used in treating cancer.

Note: diabetics should monitor sugar levels closely as it seems to boost insulin production, normalizes blood sugar levels and may reduce insulin requirements.

Contraindications

● Pfaffia should not be taken by pregnant or breast-feeding women.

● Although plant-oestrogens may protect against oestrogen-sensitive conditions such as endometriosis and gynaecological tumours (e.g. of the breast, ovaries and cervix) pfaffia should not be taken by women with a history of these problems except under specialist advice.

Phenylalanine

L-phenylalanine is an essential amino acid found in many protein foods. It is involved in the synthesis of several key brain chemicals involved in regulating sex drive, such as dopamine, noradrenaline and phenylethylamine. L-phenylalanine can increase mental alertness, lift depression, boost sex drive and help to regulate the appetite.

Dose

Usual dose (capsules, powders): 500 mg–1 g a day for up to three weeks. Some nutritionists recommend taking it with B complex vitamins and high-dose vitamin C for maximum effect.

Side effects
Can cause stimulant side effects such as insomnia and anxiety.

Contraindications
- L-phenylalanine should not be taken by anyone with high blood pressure, or those taking anti-depressant drugs, except under medical supervision.

- It should not be taken by those with a history of malignant melanoma or a metabolic condition called phenylketonuria as it may make these conditions worse.

Phosphorus

Phosphorus is an essential mineral of which 90 per cent of the body's stores is found in the bones and teeth where it forms part of an important structural salt, calcium phosphate, which is also known as hydroxyapatite. The remaining 10 per cent of the body's stores serves a number of functions and is:

- involved in the production of energy-rich molecules (ATP, ADP) in muscle cells
- needed to activate the vitamin B complex which is also involved in energy production
- an important component of genetic material
- a co-factor for several metabolic enzymes and helps to keep blood slightly alkaline.

Phosphorus in the diet

Phosphorus is obtained from many food sources, including meats, eggs, dairy products, whole grains, pulses, nuts, soft drinks such as colas, and yeast extract. Vitamin D is essential for the absorption of phosphorus from the gut and for its deposition, with calcium, into bones. Deficiency can develop in people using antacids containing aluminium hydroxide long term as these impair absorption of phosphates from the gut.

Benefits

As phosphate is so important for producing energy in the body, it is needed for optimum athletic performance. Research involving endurance athletes (such as cyclists) found that taking sodium phosphate supplements for three days before a competition decreased lactic acid build-up in muscles, increased oxygen consumption by 11 per cent and prolonged the time to exhaustion by 20 per cent. Other studies suggest that sodium phosphate supplements can increase maximal power output by up to 17 per cent.

Deficiency

As phosphorus is widely found in the diet, deficiency is rare, although symptoms that may be due to phosphorus deficiency include general malaise, loss of appetite, increased susceptibility to infection, anaemia due to shortened life of red blood cells, muscle weakness, bone pain, joint stiffness and nervous system symptoms such as numbness, pins and needles, irritability and confusion.

Dose

The EC RDA for phosphorus is 800 mg.

Few people are at risk of phosphorus deficiency, and single supplements are rarely needed, although low doses are included in most A to Z-style vitamin and mineral products.

Pine bark

Extracts from the bark of the French maritime pine contain a rich blend of natural fruit acids and antioxidants (proanthocyanidins, previously known as pycnogenols) which research suggests are 50 times more powerful than vitamin E, 20 times more powerful than vitamin C and 16 times more active than grapeseed extracts, although they are generally more expensive. As pine bark extracts enhance the effects of other antioxidants such as Co-enzyme Q10, vitamin C and E, they are often combined in supplements.

Antioxidants help to mop up free radicals – harmful molecular fragments that trigger oxidation reactions and damage all components of body cells, including genetic information. Free radicals are formed as by-products of our metabolism, and are produced in increased amounts in certain conditions.

Benefits

Pine bark extracts have a beneficial effect on blood vessels which reduces hardening and furring up of the arteries, thins the blood and reduces the risk of coronary heart disease and stroke. It strengthens fragile capillaries and protects cell structures from damaging oxidation reactions. It is widely recommended to treat conditions associated with poor circulation, such as diabetes, impotence, varicose veins, thread veins, macular degeneration, peripheral vascular disease, intermittent claudication and leg cramps. As an antioxidant, it is likely to protect against cancer.

Pine bark extracts can help to protect the circulation and reduce the damage associated with smoking. Preliminary studies suggest that they are as effective at reducing abnormal blood clotting in smokers as aspirin, and might lower the risk of coronary heart disease and stroke. Pine bark extracts also have the advantage of not producing such side effects as stomach irritation, peptic ulcers or gastric bleeding, which can occur with aspirin therapy.

Pine bark extracts can help to prevent economy-class syndrome – research shows that 125 mg pycnogenol is as effective in preventing increased susceptibility to clotting as 500 mg aspirin, but without the increased stomach-bleeding time seen with aspirin. It is therefore a good alternative for those who cannot take aspirin because of a history of peptic ulcers. Pycnogenol also stabilizes capillaries so that less fluid leaks into the extracellular tissues and therefore less swelling of lower limbs and feet occurs. Pine bark extracts may be taken for several weeks before a flight to tone the circulation, or may be started in high dose the day before flying.

Dose
50–200 mg a day.

Potassium

Potassium is the main positively charged ion found inside cells, where it is present in concentrations 30 times greater than those in the extracellular fluid surrounding each cell. It is actively pumped inside cells by ion-exchange pumps found in cell walls, and in exchange, sodium ions are pumped out to make room for it.

Benefits

Potassium is essential for muscle contraction (including the heartbeat), nerve conduction, maintenance of blood sugar levels and the production of nucleic acids, proteins and energy. The kidney regulates blood potassium levels and keeps them within a fairly narrow range.

Because the sodium-potassium exchange system in cells also occurs in the kidneys, a good intake of dietary potassium helps to flush sodium from cells into the urine for excretion from the body. As excess sodium is linked with high blood pressure in some people, following a diet that is relatively high in potassium and low in sodium is linked with a lower risk of hypertension and stroke. In one study, for example, over 80 per cent of people taking anti-hypertensive medication were able to halve their dose by just increasing their dietary intake of potassium.

Most people do not need potassium supplements, unless they exercise a lot (e.g. top athletes). Low levels of potassium commonly occur in people taking certain diuretics that do not have a potassium-sparing effect in the body. Symptoms that may be due to lack of potassium include poor appetite, fatigue, weakness, low blood glucose, muscle cramps, irregular or rapid heart beat, constipation, irritability, pins and needles, drowsiness and confusion.

Excess potassium levels are rare as the body usually controls blood levels well. They can occur in people with kidney problems, or those who take excess potassium supplements however, to produce symptoms such as irregular heartbeat, and muscle fatigue.

Potassium in the diet

Foods that contain potassium include seafood, fruit (particularly tomatoes, bananas), vegetables, whole grains and low-sodium potassium-enriched salts.

Dose

There is no EC RDA for potassium. Intakes of around 3000–3500 mg daily are advised although it is estimated that one in three people get less than this.

Contraindications

Potassium supplements should not be taken by anyone who is taking a type of medication called an ACE inhibitor or who has kidney disease, except under medical advice.

Probiotic supplements

Probiotics is the use of natural 'friendly' lactic acid-producing bacteria such as *Lactobacilli* and *Bifidobacteria* naturally found in the large bowel to encourage a healthy digestive balance. It also refers to the use of food substances such as fructo-oligosaccharides (FOS) and oatmeal that promote the growth of probiotic bacteria, and which encourage colonization of the bowel with friendly microbes. FOS cannot be digested or absorbed from the human bowel, but act as a fermentable food source for probiotic bacteria in the gut. In contrast, harmful bacteria such as *E. coli* and *Clostridium* cannot use FOS as a source of energy.

The gut contains around 11 trillion bacteria, weighing a total of 1.5 kg. Ideally, at least 70 per cent of these should be healthy 'probiotic' bacteria and only 30 per cent other bowel bacteria such as *E. coli*. In practice however, the balance is usually the other way round.

Benefits

Probiotic bacteria produce lactic acid, which helps to create a healthy intestinal environment and discourage infection with potentially harmful, disease-causing organisms (viral, bacterial and fungal) known as pathogens. The presence of friendly bacteria improves intestinal health, promotes good digestion, boosts immunity and increases resistance to infection – especially during foreign travel when there are changes in food and water. *Lactobacilli* are also needed for optimum health in the vagina and to protect against recurrent candida infections, and bacterial vaginosis (a condition in which healthy vaginal *Lactobacilli* are severely depleted).

Probiotic bacteria help to reduce overgrowth of harmful yeast and bacteria in the intestines in a number of different ways. They produce lactic acid, acetic acid and hydrogen peroxide that lower intestinal pH and discourage reproduction of less acid-tolerant, harmful bacteria. They have also been shown to secrete natural antibiotics (bacteriocins such as acidophiline and bulgarican) and to stimulate production of interferon, a natural anti-viral agent which helps to protect against viral intestinal infections. They also compete with harmful bacteria for available nutrients, as well as for attachment site on intestinal cell walls. If these attachment sites are already occupied by friendly bacteria, those that are potentially harmful cannot gain a foothold in the intestines so easily and are more likely to be flushed out.

These combined actions are highly effective, and probiotic bacteria have a powerful, protective action against a number of intestinal infections responsible for traveller's gastroenteritis (food poisoning), such as *Bacillus cereus*, *Salmonella typhi*, *Shigella dysenteriae*, *Escherichia coli* and *Staphylococcus aureus*.

Over 50 trials involving more than 6000 volunteers have found probiotic supplements to be beneficial in the treatment of symptoms associated with a variety of intestinal and other disorders as well as reducing the side effects (e.g. diarrhoea) brought on by taking antibiotics. Other conditions that can be helped by probiotic supplements include diarrhoea, irritable bowel syndrome (IBS), inflammatory bowel disease, *Helicobacter pylori* infection, recurrent candida yeast infections, reduced immunity, lactose intolerance and ulcerative colitis.

In one study, 100 patients with symptomatic IBS were divided into four groups. Twenty patients were given active *L. plantarum* 299v supplements, 20 received inactivated bacteria, while the remainder received drug therapy with either mebeverin or trimebutin. The last group included 22 patients who did not improve with drug therapy alone and went on to receive the drug plus probiotic supplementation. Results showed a 75 per cent improvement in symptoms in those taking the *Lactobacilli*, compared with 23 per cent and 30 per cent in those taking the drugs trimebutin and mebeverine. When *Lactobacilli* were taken in addition to mebeverine, improvements increased to 90 per cent. In contrast, no improvement occurred in those taking an inactivated placebo solution of *Lactobacilli*.

A recent study found that infants at high risk of allergic (atopic) diseases such as eczema, asthma and rhinitis benefited when their mothers (who either had these conditions or had at least one first-degree relative or partner with atopy) took probiotic supplements of *Lactobacillus* GG during pregnancy. After delivery, the mothers had the option of continuing to take the probiotics themselves, or giving them to their infants for six months. The frequency of atopic eczema was found to be half that in the groups who had taken active probiotics than in those receiving placebo. This suggests that bowel bacteria produce a unique effect in modulating activity of the immune system, although these interactions are currently poorly understood.

Probiotic bacteria in the diet

Dietary sources or probiotic bacteria include live 'bio' yoghurts, fermented milk drinks and supplements supplying a guaranteed specified potency of bacteria in capsule, powder, liquid or tablet form – which should ideally be kept refrigerated. Dietary sources of FOS include garlic, onions, barley, wheat, bananas, honey and tomatoes.

Dose

When choosing a supplement, select one that supplies at least 1–2 billion colony forming units (CFU) of acidophilus per dose. Supplements that are enteric-coated – which improves survival of probiotic bacteria as they pass through the acidic stomach – can contain less (e.g. 10 million freeze-dried probiotic bacteria) and still achieve the same effects.

Probiotic bacteria are fragile and those found in 'bio' yoghurt that has been standing around in the supermarket or in your fridge for a week or more may contain less live bacteria than freshly made cultures.

Levels of live probiotic bacteria in bio yoghurts vary widely, from a few hundred thousand to more than 300 million live bacteria per gram. For this reason, it is best to take a probiotic supplement when aiming to reduce the risk of traveller's diarrhoea abroad.

Psyllium

See **Fibre**

Pumpkin seed
(Cucurbita pepo)

Pumpkin seeds are a popular snack food with a high oil and vitamin E content. The oil is used as a salad dressing, but due to its dark green colour and foaminess, it cannot be used for cooking.

Benefits
Some evidence suggests that pumpkin seed extracts can reduce bladder pressure and increase bladder compliance as well reducing pressure in the urethra which might be beneficial for those with urinary voiding problems. Relatively little research seems to have been carried out on humans, although there is a long tradition of using pumpkin seeds for prostate problems. Pumpkin seed extracts are often combined with other active ingredients such as saw palmetto and zinc to produce supplements aimed at improving prostate health.

Raspberry leaf

Raspberry leaf has one main specific use, and is taken in the form of tea or tablets towards the end of pregnancy to help soften the neck of the womb in preparation for delivery. It seems to reduce the duration and pain of childbirth, and is thought to work by strengthening the longitudinal muscles of the uterus to increase the force of uterine contractions. It seems to only work on the pregnant rather than non-pregnant uterus, and research has not so far isolated the active ingredients. Women who have taken raspberry leaf extracts often confirm that their contractions were relatively pain-free and that their baby was born within just a few hours of the start of labour.

Raspberry leaf has also been used to reduce pain in endometriosis, and to relieve painful diarrhoea.

Dose
1 cup raspberry leaf tea a day *or*
Tablets: 400 mg, twice or three times a day with meals.

Raspberry leaf should be taken daily during the last six weeks of pregnancy. It should not be taken during early pregnancy and is best taken under the supervision of a qualified medical herbalist or a midwife.

RDAs and RNIs

Vitamins and minerals are micro-nutrients which, although essential for health, are only needed in tiny amounts. The quantities you need are measured in milligrams (mg) or micrograms (mcg).

1 milligram = one thousandth of a gram ($\frac{1}{1000}$ or 10^{-3} grams)
1 microgram = one millionth of a gram ($\frac{1}{1,000,000}$ or 10^{-6} grams)
1 milligram therefore = 1000 micrograms.

The UK originally developed its own system of daily recommended intakes based on a unit called the Reference Nutrient Intake (RNI). It has now adopted the EC equivalent which uses the term Recommended Daily Amount (RDA). Everyone has different, individual needs depending on their age, weight, level of activity and the metabolic pathways and enzyme systems they have inherited. Some people need more vitamins and minerals, while some need fewer. The EC Recommended Daily Amount (EC RDA) is therefore an estimated intake that is believed to supply the needs of most (up to 97 per cent) of the population. The EC RDAs suggest the following intakes of each vitamin and mineral:

Vitamins

	EC RDA
Vitamin A (retinol)	800 mcg
Vitamin B1 (thiamine)	1.4 mg
Vitamin B2 (riboflavin)	1.6 mg
Vitamin B3 (niacin)	18 mg
Vitamin B5 (pantothenic acid)	6 mg
Vitamin B6 (pyridoxine)	2 mg
Vitamin B12 (cyanocobalamin)	1 mcg
Biotin	150 mcg
Folic Acid	200 mcg
Vitamin C	60 mg
Vitamin D	5 mcg
Vitamin E	10 mg

Minerals	**EC RDA**
Calcium	800 mg
Iodine	150 mcg
Iron	14 mg
Magnesium	300 mg
Phosphorus	800 mg
Zinc	15 mg

Unfortunately, food surveys suggest that only 1 in 10 people obtain all the vitamins and minerals they need from their food. As a result, more and more people are choosing to take a multi-nutrient supplement as a nutritional safety net.

See the table on page xviii for a list of the daily intakes of micro-nutrients from the diet, and upper safe levels for daily supplementation.

Red clover
(Trifolium pratense)

Red clover is one of over 70 different species of clover native to Europe and Asia. Of all the clovers, red clover is the most popular for medicinal use. The flower heads are collected when newly opened in spring, and the leaves and roots are also edible.

Benefits

Red clover contains three classes of oestrogen-like plant hormones: isoflavones, coumestans and lignans. It is one of the few plants to contain four isoflavones, and is widely used to balance oestrogen levels – either where these are too high (by competing for stronger oestrogens in the body and diluting their effect) or by providing an additional oestrogenic boost where levels are low. It is therefore widely used to treat pre-menstrual syndrome, endometriosis, fibroids and menopausal symptoms.

In one study involving post-menopausal women who took red clover for two weeks and followed an oestrogen-rich diet, significantly higher oestrogen levels were reported, which then fell again when they stopped taking the supplements. Other studies have shown reduced menopausal symptoms of hot flushes and mood swings within three to four weeks of starting to take red clover, plus a more positive outlook on life and increased energy levels. In three clinical studies involving women with menopausal symptoms, 90 per cent noticed such an improvement they chose to continue treatment after the trials were completed.

Red clover is known mainly for its oestrogenic actions, but it also has anti-spasmodic and wound-healing properties. It can be used to treat eczema, burns, psoriasis, asthma, bronchitis and some types of cancer. Interestingly, red clover is known to have a contraceptive effect in sheep, but little information is available on its effects on human fertility.

Dose
500 mg tablet (standardized to contain 40 mg isoflavones) daily.

Contraindications
Red clover supplements should not be taken during pregnancy or while breast-feeding.

Red vine leaf
(Vitis vinifera)

Red grapes are well known to contain beneficial antioxidants that have a powerful protective effect on the circulation. Less well known is that red vine leaf extracts also seem to be effective and have a similar action to Horsechestnut seed extracts (*see* **Horsechestnut**).

In a recent randomized, double-blind, placebo-controlled trial 257 people with varicose veins were randomized to take either red vine leaf extracts (360 mg or 720 mg daily for 12 weeks) or placebo. For those treated with placebo, mean lower leg volume increased by around 34 g (weight of water displaced) after 12 weeks, while those taking active treatment experienced a reduction in lower leg volume. This was equivalent to a difference between the active and placebo groups of -76 g with the lower dose, and -100 g with the higher dose. Changes in calf circumference showed a similar pattern and reductions in swelling were at least equivalent to those reported for compression stockings. There were also clinically significant reductions in symptoms such as tired, heavy legs, sensations of tension, tingling and pain.

Red vine leaf extracts are thought to work by reducing inflammation, and by reducing the permeability of small blood vessels (capillaries) so that fluid cannot leak into the extravascular tissues so easily.

Dose
360 mg or 720 mg daily

Reishi
(Ganoderma lucidum)

Reishi is one of seven different varieties of *Ganoderma* mushroom, each of which has differing colours. Reishi is the red *Ganoderma lucidum* and is regarded as superior. The Japanese name 'reishi' means literally 'spiritual mushroom, while the Chinese call it 'ling zhi' ('the mushroom of immortality') – and classify it as a superior herb equal in importance to ginseng. Reishi has been used medicinally for over 3000 years. It is too woody and fibrous for culinary use, but is widely consumed in tablet form as a herbal supplement.

Benefits

Reishi contains ganodermic acids which have a structure similar to steroid hormones. It also contains lentinan and a nucleotide, adenosine, which forms part of the body's energy regulation and storage system. The effects of Reishi are enhanced by vitamin C, which increases absorption of the active components.

Reishi is a powerful adaptogen, tonic and antioxidant. It is traditionally used to strengthen the liver, lungs, heart and immune system, to increase intellectual capacity and memory, boost physical and mental energy levels and to promote vitality and longevity. It is now also used to speed convalescence, regulate blood sugar levels and to help minimize the side effects of chemo- or radiotherapy. Reishi has antibacterial, anti-viral, anti-histamine, anti-allergy, anti-inflammatory (equivalent to hydrocortisone) and anti-cancer properties that are under further investigation. It also reduces blood clotting and can lower blood pressure and cholesterol levels. It has recently been shown to increase the flow of blood and oxygen uptake in the brain in people with Alzheimer's disease.

Reishi enhances energy levels and promotes a more restful night's sleep. In one Chinese study it was found to relieve feelings of weariness in 78 per cent of patients, cold extremities in 74 per cent and insomnia in 78 per cent. In a Japanese study of over 50 patients with essential hypertension, taking reishi extracts for 6 months lowered average blood pressure from 156/103 to 137/93. Chinese studies involving over 2000 people found that reishi extracts were helpful in treating bronchitis.

Dose
500 mg twice to three times daily.

Side effects
No serious side effects have been reported even at 300 times the therapeutic dose. A few people have experienced diarrhoea (often disappears if tablets are taken with food), irritability, thirst, dry skin rash or mouth ulcers during the first week of taking the reishi.

There is no cross-reaction with traditional 'button' mushrooms and reishi can usually be taken by those allergic to field mushrooms.

Contraindications
● Reishi should only be used under medical supervision by anyone taking immunosuppressive drugs, anticoagulants or cholesterol-lowering medication. Reishi may increase the sedative effects of certain drugs (Reserpine, chlorpromazine) and inhibit the action of amphetamines.

It should also not be taken by anyone on anti-coagulant drugs due to its blood-thinning effect.

● Although used as a food, it is sensible to avoid taking Reishi during pregnancy and breast-feeding except under supervision.

Rescue remedy

Rescue remedy is a composite of five flower essences – rock rose, impatiens, clematis, star of Bethlehem and cherry plum – preserved in brandy. It is excellent for use in emergencies (such as panic attacks, just before public speaking) and whenever you feel stressed. The flower remedies are prepared either by infusion or boiling. In the infusion method, flower heads are placed on the surface of a small glass bowl filled with pure spring water. This is left to infuse in direct sunlight for three hours then the flowers are discarded and the infused spring water preserved in grape alcohol (brandy). This resultant solution is called the 'mother tincture' and is further diluted five times to create the individual stock remedies. In the boiling method, short lengths of twig-bearing flowers or catkins are boiled in pure spring water for 30 minutes. The plant material is then discarded and the water allowed to cool before being preserved in grape alcohol. This solution (the mother tincture) will be further diluted for use.

Dose

Add 4 drops to a glass of liquid and sip slowly every few minutes until symptoms subside. Hold each sip in your mouth for a moment before swallowing. Alternatively, rescue remedy may also be dropped directly on to the tongue or rubbed on to the lips, behind the ears or elsewhere on the body.

Rhodiola
(Rhodiola rosea)

Rhodiola is an alpine plant growing more than 3000 metres above sea level. It is also known as golden or Arctic root and has been used as a medicine for over a thousand years.

Benefits
Rhodiola contains a number of active constituents, including rosavin, which together have an adaptogenic action. It helps to enhance performance during times of physical and mental fatigue, and is used to improve alertness, concentration, memory, stamina, sleep and to relieve depression (by boosting serotonin levels by as much as 30 per cent). It supports the actions of the adrenal glands and also seems to normalize hormone secretion through a direct action on the hypothalamus gland.

Dose
Take as recommended on specific packs.

Riboflavin

See **Vitamin B2**

Rye pollen
(Secale cereale)

Extracts from the pollen of certain plants, especially rye, can reduce symptoms caused by prostatitis and benign prostate enlargement. They reduce prostate swelling, pain, irritation, inflammation, spasm and residual urinary volume and strengthen urinary flow. Their precise mode of action is unknown, although studies suggest that they damp down inflammation and inhibit 5-alpha-reductase enzyme activity to encourage shrinking of the prostate gland.

Rye pollen extracts also have an anti-inflammatory pain-killing effect similar to that of aspirin and ibuprofen as they have been shown to inhibit the enzyme responsible for production of inflammatory chemicals (cyclo-oxygenase). They also seem to increase the zinc content of the prostate gland. Studies are currently under way to investigate whether pollen extracts interfere with the production or action of growth factors responsible for stimulating the increased growth of prostate cells that occurs in BPH.

First signs of improvement of prostate symptoms usually show within three months of treatment (78 per cent of men) and there is a progressive improvement over a six-month period.

A study of 60 patients with BPH showed that the pollen extracts improved prostate symptoms by 69 per cent over six months, compared with only 29 per cent for those taking a placebo. Night-time urination (nocturia) decreased significantly by 60 per cent compared with 30 per cent with the placebo, and a decrease in the amount of urine remaining in the bladder after voiding by 57 per cent. There was also a significant decrease in the diameter of the prostate when measured by ultrasound.

An open trial of 15 patients with chronic non-bacterial prostatitis and prostatodynia showed that 13 patients gained complete and lasting relief of symptoms or a marked improvement. Only two failed to respond.

Another study divided 100 patients with chronic prostatitis and prostatodynia into two groups – those with and without complicating factors such as narrowing of the urinary outlet (urethral stricture, stones in the prostate gland (prostatic calculi) and thickening of the bladder neck (sclerosis). From the data collected, the researchers concluded that any man with prostatitis whose symptoms fail to improve after taking flower pollen extracts for three months should be investigated for suspected complications.

Dose

252 mg tablets, one or two a day for up to eight weeks, after which dose should be reduced to one tablet per day for as long as required.

Side effects

No significant side effects have occurred and, despite being derived from pollen, no allergic reactions were noted even in those highly sensitive to grass pollen. Monitoring of over 3000 patients found only three subjects who had what were described as light symptoms of allergy. The reason for low allergenicity is that, during the extraction process, the long-chain chemicals usually associated with allergy are broken down by enzyme action.

Sage
(Salvia officinalis)

Sage is a well-known culinary herb whose leaves – especially those from the red purple-tinged varieties – contain a number of essential oils such as borneol and camphor. It is a native Mediterranean evergreen perennial shrub, whose name, *Salvia*, comes from the Latin salvere which means 'to be saved'. It was also known as *herba sacra* – sacred herb – by the Romans. Sage was traditionally used as a medicine by the ancient Egyptians, Greeks and Romans to stop wounds bleeding, and to clean ulcers and sores. In the first century, the Greek physician Dioscorides prescribed a mixture made by boiling sage, rosemary, honeysuckle, plantain and honey in water or wine, as a gargle to treat sore mouths and throats.

Benefits
Sage is known today for its antibacterial, anti-fungal, anti-viral, astringent, secretion-promoting and perspiration-inhibiting properties. It is widely used internally for indigestion, and externally for inflammation of the mucous membranes of gums, mouth, nose, throat and tongue. Sage is a popular herbal remedy for menopausal hot flushes and night sweats. Sage extracts (Menosan), for example, were found in a recent, randomized, double-blind placebo-controlled study involving 39 women to decrease the

frequency of hot flushes by 56 per cent over a period of 8 weeks, versus a 5 per cent increase in frequency among those taking inactive placebos.

Sage is also used to reduce the flow of breast milk during weaning, reduce excessive salivation and perspiration and to ease intestinal infections such as diarrhoea and vomiting. It can help respiratory infections such as laryngitis and tonsillitis, relieve indigestion (dyspepsia) and is said to boost memory and concentration and act as a mental stimulant. It can also be applied as a compress to promote wound healing.

Dose

Sage tea: add 1 tablespoon dried sage to a cup of boiling water and infuse for 20 minutes.
Tincture: 2–5 ml.

Contraindications

● Sage stimulates uterine contractions, and should therefore be avoided during pregnancy, although small amounts are safe for use in cooking. It should not be used during breast-feeding other than for its ability to dry up milk.

● Sage should be avoided by those with epilepsy.

St John's Wort
(Hypericum perforatum)

St John's Wort is found in many parts of the world. When held up to the light, numerous pinpoint red dots may be seen in the yellow petals; these are glands containing the fluorescent red dye, hypericin. Hypericin, pseudohypericin and hyperforin are effective anti-depressants that are thought to work by prolonging the action of a brain neurotransmitter, serotonin, slowing its re-uptake once it has been released.

Another possible action is that it damps down the production of pituitary hormones that kick-start the adrenal glands. People who are depressed usually have high levels of adrenal hormones such as cortisol and *Hypericum* is thought to help reduce this stress response. It also increases nocturnal production of melatonin hormone (the brain's own natural sedative), to improve the quality of sleep – after four weeks' treatment, it increases the amount of time spent in deep sleep.

Benefits

St John's Wort can lift low mood in at least 67 per cent of those with mild to moderate depression and is as effective as many antidepressant drugs in such cases. Studies involving over 5000 people show that *Hypericum* can lift mild depression within two weeks of starting the course – the optimum effect being reached within six weeks. Three out of four people showed a marked improvement after only five weeks, with one in three becoming symptom-free.

When compared with sertraline, an antidepressant belonging to a group known as the Selective Serotonin Re-uptake Inhibitors (SSRIs), standardized extracts of St John's Wort were found to be at least as effective in the treatment of mild to moderate depression, with at least a 50 per cent reduction in the total score on the depression rating scale used over the seven-week period of the trial. Both treatments were well tolerated.

Hypericum is also effective for seasonal affective disorder (SAD) and field trials have shown that standardized extracts were as effective in treating SAD when used alone as when combined with light box therapy.

Low sex drive is an early feature of depression, and *Hypericum* can significantly boost low libido where this is associated with depression. Research in Germany involving 111 post-menopausal women (aged 45-65 years) with low sex drive plus physical exhaustion found that *Hypericum* for three months helped 60 per cent of them to become interested in sex again, to feel sexy and to enjoy or even initiate sex with their partner. Eighty-two per cent also suffered less irritability, anxiety, low mood, hot flushes, sweating and disturbed sleep. Before the trial, 60 per cent said they were too exhausted for sex. At the end of the trial, none of them felt that way. They also reported increased self-esteem, as well as a marked increase in self-confidence and self-respect.

Pre-menstrual syndrome (PMS) is often associated with low mood, and in a pilot study of 25 women with severe PMS, there was a reduction in the incidence of crying of 92 per cent, low mood reduced by 85 per cent and nervous tension by 71 per cent compared with baseline pre-menstrual scores. Although a third still suffered from some symptoms of PMS, all women in the study reported great improvement.

Other beneficial effects of St John's Wort include anti-viral, antibacterial and anti-cancer activity which are all currently under further investigation.

Dose

Extracts standardized to 0.3 per cent hypericin: 300 mg, three times a day; one-a-day formulas are also available.

St John's Wort is best taken with food, and alcohol should be avoided.

Side effects

Side effects are significantly less likely than with standard anti-depressants. Those reported include indigestion, allergic reactions, restlessness and tiredness/fatigue each in fewer than 1 per cent of people.

Those who are sun-sensitive or on medications that cause photosensitivity (such as Tetracycline, Chlorpromazine) should avoid direct skin exposure to sunlight, especially if fair-skinned. There are no reports of skin sensitivity on exposure to sunlight (photosensitization) in therapeutic doses.

Contraindications

● St John's Wort should not be taken together with other anti-depressants except under medical supervision. Research in Germany has shown that plasma levels of amitriptyline-like antidepressants are reduced by taking *Hypericum*, and conversely blood levels of pseudohypericin (one of the active ingredients in St John's Wort) is reduced by amitriptyline. The clinical significance of this interaction is not known. Other interactions currently recognized between *Hypericum perforatum* and prescribed drugs are with warfarin, cyclosporin, oral contraceptives, anti-convulsants, digoxin, theophylline, HIV protease inhibitors, triptans and SSRIs.

● St John's Wort should not be taken during pregnancy or when breast-feeding.

Despite this seemingly long list, St John's Wort is a safe and effective treatment and when taken alone (and even combined with many drugs) it causes no harm. The risks are low, as for example, only 11 cases of breakthrough bleeding have occurred with women taking the oral contraceptive pill yet over 200 million packs of St John's Wort have been sold in Europe alone!

Sarsaparilla
(Smilax officinalis, S. sarsaparilla)

Sarsaparilla – also popularly known as *Smilax* – belongs to a group of climbing perennial vines found in tropical and subtropical parts of the world. Its dried, thick rhizomes and slender roots contain a wide range of hormone-like steroids (including sarsapogenin, smilagenin) and glycosides (e.g. sarsaponin) that have been used commercially as the basis for synthesizing sex hormones, particularly testosterone.

Benefits

It is used by many males – especially body builders – to improve virility, vitality and energy levels. No studies have shown sarsaparilla to have an anabolic effect that increases muscle mass in humans, however, and the reactions needed to convert these plant steroids into testosterone are unlikely to occur in the body. It is therefore not as virilizing as one might expect – it is even used to treat acne which is a condition usually associated with increased androgen activity.

Sarsaparilla is mainly used as a tonic and blood purifier – it is thought to bind bacterial toxins and cholesterol in the gut so fewer are absorbed into the circulation. It also acts as a diuretic and promotes sweating and expectoration of catarrh. It is said to hasten regeneration and to have anti-inflammatory properties. It is used to treat cystitis, psoriasis, eczema, acne, rheumatism, arthritis and gout, as well infections such as syphilis, herpes, gonorrhoea and the common cold.

Sarsaparilla is used to increase low sex drive in males and to help overcome impotence and infertility. It is also used in lower doses in women to boost a low sex drive and to improve menopausal symptoms.

Dose

Capsules: 250 mg, three times a day.

Some dried roots labelled Mexican sarsaparilla may actually contain so-called Indian sarsaparilla, which is a different type of plant (*Hemidesmus indicus*) with entirely different uses. *Hemidesmus* is dark brown and smells of vanilla, while dried Smilax roots have a light colour (often orange-tinged) and are odourless.

Side effects

No serious long-term side effects have been reported, although sarsaparilla can cause indigestion and, if excess is taken, may temporarily impair kidney function.

Contraindications

Because of its possible testosterone-boosting properties, some practitioners caution against its use in women with a tendency towards excessive unwanted hair.

Note: sarsaparilla saponins seems to affect the way in which the body handles some prescribed drugs. In particular, it increases uptake of digitalis and increases the excretion of hypnotic drugs.

Saw Palmetto
(Sabal serrulata, Serenoa repens)

The saw palmetto is a small palm tree native to North America and the West Indies. Its fruit contains a variety of fatty acids and hormone-like sterols that are widely used as a male tonic and sexual rejuvenator.

Benefits

Saw palmetto is a popular and effective herbal remedy for benign prostatic hyperplasia (BPH) – a condition in which the number of cells in the male prostate gland starts to increase in middle age. As the gland increases in size, it often constricts the flow of urine as it passes through the middle of the gland. This causes typical urinary symptoms of hesitancy, frequency, urgency and poor flow which are embarrassing and can have a major effect on quality of life.

One of the best ways of evaluating the mixed results of a number of studies is a meta-analysis which pools data from comparable trials to give an average of the results from as many patients as possible. A total of 18 studies involving 2939 men found that, compared with men receiving an inactive placebo, saw palmetto fruit extracts improved urinary tract symptoms by 28 per cent, night-time frequency by 25 per cent, urinary flow by 28 per cent and reduced the amount of urine remaining in the bladder after voiding by 43 per cent. No significant side effects were reported. In trials where saw palmetto extracts were compared with a variety of drugs prescribed to improve prostate symptoms, the herbal extracts were found to be at least as effective – but with fewer unwanted side effects such as erectile dysfunction.

The exact way in which saw palmetto works is unknown. Research suggests that saw palmetto extracts produce a significant anti-oestrogen effect within the prostate gland and this is probably important in reducing swelling. Also, while saw palmetto fruit extracts do not alter the circulating level of testosterone hormone, they significantly affect testosterone metabolism in cells taken from prostates affected by BPH. Although it has been suggested that saw palmetto may block the action of a prostate enzyme, 5-alpha-reductase, which converts the male hormone, testosterone, to another more powerful hormone, dihydrotestosterone (DHT), this is controversial. While it does not seem to affect circulating levels of DHT, studies have found it is a powerful inhibitor of 5 alpha-reductase in the laboratory, reducing the enzyme's activity by as much as 45 per cent. Significant reductions in the production of DHT have also been found in prostate biopsies from men who had taken Serenoa repens extracts for 3 months. This was most noticeable in prostate tissues in the centre of the gland, directly surrounding the urinary tube. It is therefore possible that saw palmetto fruit extracts mainly act on this central portion of the prostate, and only shrink this area, which would explain why studies do not show appreciable shrinking of the whole gland despite significant improvements in urinary flow and obstructive symptoms.

Researchers have also recently discovered that saw palmetto extracts can interact with a type of nerve ending known as an alpha receptor. This triggers relaxation of smooth muscle cells in the prostate gland to reduce spasm and improve urinary symptoms by widening the urinary outlet.

Saw palmetto is also used in women with polycystic ovary syndrome due to its ability to inhibit the formation of dihydrotestosterone, which plays a role in this condition.

Saw palmetto and nettle root are frequently combined.

Dose

Fruit extracts: 150 mg–3 g a day in divided doses.

Products standardized for 85 per cent–95 per cent fat-soluble sterols: 320 mg a day.

A beneficial effect usually starts within two to six weeks.

Schisandra
(Schisandra chinensis)

Schisandra – also known as magnolia vine – is a popular Chinese tonic herb also known as wu wei zi or five-flavoured fruit as it simultaneously tastes salty, sweet, bitter, sour and pungent.

Its dried berries contain lignans such as schizandrin, phytosterols and several antioxidants.

Benefits

Like ginseng, schisandra has powerful adaptogenic properties and helps the body to adapt and cope during times of stress. It has been found to increase oxygen uptake of cells and improves mental clarity, irritability, forgetfulness and prevents emotional and physical fatigue. It is regarded as a calming supplement and also boosts liver function, enhances immunity and heart function and improves allergic skin conditions such as eczema.

Schisandra is a well-known sexual tonic that reputedly increases secretion of sexual fluids in men and vaginal lubrication in women.

Dose

250–500 mg, once to three times daily.

Schisandra is traditionally taken for 100 days to boost sexual energy, vitality and produce radiant skin.

Selenium

Selenium is an essential trace element that is needed for normal cell growth, to regulate the production of thyroid hormones, and for optimum immunity against infections and cancer.

Selenium enters the food chain through plants and is found in Brazil nuts (one of the richest sources), fish, poultry, meats, whole grains, mushrooms, onions, garlic, broccoli and cabbage. The mineral content of crops depends on the soils in which they are grown, and selenium levels are low in many parts of the world including New Zealand, China, Egypt, and much of Africa.

High selenium levels are found in bread made from high-protein Canadian and American wheat grain. Because of changes in policy, most Europeans now eat bread made from varieties of wheat grown within the EC, which are low in selenium. As a result, there is widespread concern that a healthy diet can no longer provide adequate intakes of selenium in many parts of Europe. Selenium intakes have dropped significantly in Britain, for example, and between 1975 and 1994, they almost halved.

Benefits

Selenium is a powerful antioxidant. It also acts as a co-factor in the action of many antioxidant enzymes, including glutathione peroxidase which neutralizes harmful chemicals such as hydrogen peroxide before they can damage cells. Selenium therefore helps to protect against a wide variety of degenerative diseases such as hardening and furring up of the arteries, emphysema, liver cirrhosis, cataracts, arthritis, stroke, heart attack and cancer.

Deficiency

In parts of the world where soil selenium levels are low, the incidence of cancer increases by two to six times. Those with the lowest selenium intakes have the highest risk of developing leukaemia or cancers of the colon, rectum, breast, ovary, pancreas, prostate gland, bladder, skin and lungs. These risks seem to be even higher if intakes of vitamin E and vitamin A are also low. Selenium has been shown to prevent the growth of cancer cells in the laboratory, and some evidence suggests that it is involved in triggering programmed cell death (apoptosis) of abnormal cells.

Selenium also enhances the action of a liver enzyme (P450) involved in detoxifying cancer-causing chemicals (carcinogens), and plays a part in the repair of damaged genes (DNA).

A randomized study of 1312 patients showed that those receiving 200 mcg selenium a day had a 52 per cent lower risk of cancer death compared with those receiving a placebo, while another study looking at the effects of 200 mcg selenium supplementation in patients with previous skin cancer found significant reductions in total cancer deaths. The trial was therefore stopped early as it was considered unethical to withhold selenium from those in the placebo groups. In this study, selenium was found to reduce total cancer incidence by 37 per cent, lung cancer by 46 per cent, colon cancer by 58 per cent, liver cancer by 35 per cent and prostate cancer by a massive 63 per cent. This protective effect against prostate cancer was also supported by a fascinating study in which toenail clippings were collected from over 33,700 men for analysis. Those with the highest levels of selenium were found to be 65 per cent less likely to develop prostate cancer over a five-year period than those with low levels.

Selenium stimulates the production of natural killer cells which fight viral and bacterial infections, and is also needed for antibody synthesis. The production of antibodies increases by up to thirty times if supplements of selenium and vitamin E are taken together, and relatively harmless viruses become more virulent on passing through a selenium-deficient host. Exactly why this happens is unknown, but it is thought that viral mutations are encouraged due to the higher level of free radicals present in a host whose antioxidant levels are reduced through lack of selenium. This has been suggested as an explanation for the first appearance of the human immunodeficiency virus (HIV) in Zaire, and for the fact that many new strains of influenza virus seem to develop in China – both parts of the world where selenium deficiency is widespread. The risk of

HIV progressing to AIDS also seems to be less in populations where selenium intakes are high.

Other studies have shown that in carriers of hepatitis B and/or hepatitis C infection, the chance of developing liver cancer was significantly greater in those with low circulating levels of selenium, and this risk was most striking in cigarette smokers and in those with lower levels of another important antioxidant, vitamin A.

Selenium is important for healthy muscle fibres, including those found in the heart. In parts of China, selenium intakes are low enough to cause a form of heart failure (Keshan disease) and an unpleasant, deforming type of arthritis known as Kashin-Beck disease. These risks seem to be even higher if intakes of the antioxidant vitamins A, C and E are also low.

The thyroid gland has the highest concentration of selenium in the body. This is because enzymes containing selenium (thyroxine deiodinases) are needed to regulate the production of the active form of the thyroid hormone, tri-iodothyronine. It is also needed as an antioxidant, as the thyroid gland generates large quantities of potentially harmful chemical fragments (free radicals) which selenium helps to neutralize. Where iodine levels are high enough to allow normal thyroid activity, lack of selenium leads to damage and in some cases fibrosis (scarring) of thyroid tissues as the free radicals generated cannot be neutralized properly.

A study in Egypt, where iodine intakes are adequate, found that selenium levels were significantly lower in patients with an enlarged thyroid gland (multinodular goitre) compared with those whose thyroid was of a normal size. As goitre is endemic in some parts of Egypt, the researchers recommended wide-scale epidemiological studies to examine the possible preventive role of taking selenium supplements or of enriching soils with organic fertilizers containing selenium-rich yeast.

Where selenium and iodine intakes are both low however (e.g. Zaire) there is a high risk of severely underactive thyroid function (myxoedema) which may affect children to produce an illness known as cretinism (*see also* **Iodine**). Low selenium levels also increase the risk of thyroid cancer.

Abnormally low levels of selenium occur in certain types of skin cancer, and selenium has been shown to reduce the percentage of skin cells that die in the laboratory after exposure to UVB light from 79 per cent to 13 per cent. A recent study in which people took an antioxidant supplement containing selenium and vitamins A, C and E showed that this helped to protect the skin against the effects of UV irradiation. This protection was greatest if taken prior to UV exposure. Lack of selenium has also been linked with psoriasis.

Selenium is needed for normal testosterone metabolism and testicular development. A unique selenium-containing protein found in sperm cells is essential for sperm motility, and subfertile men with low selenium levels can significantly improve their chances of conception by taking selenium supplements. In one study, 69 men were divided into three groups, one of which received selenium alone, one took selenium plus antioxidants and the other took inactive placebo for three months. In both groups receiving selenium, sperm motility doubled, and 11 per cent of men receiving selenium successfully fathered a child compared with no change, and no conceptions in the placebo group.

Low selenium levels also seem to increase the risk of miscarriage. Forty women with miscarriage occurring within the first three months of pregnancy, were significantly more likely to have low selenium levels than similar women who did not experience miscarriage.

Studies have also found that selenium levels are around 10 per cent lower in people with chronic inflammatory conditions such as rheumatoid arthritis. Whether this plays a role in triggering these conditions, or whether it is a result of long-term inflammation is not fully clear, but as the incidence of rheumatoid arthritis is similar in areas of low and high selenium intakes, it is likely to be a result rather than a cause.

An international research programme is currently under way in five countries (Denmark, Finland, Sweden, the UK and the USA), known as the Precise Trial (Prevention of Cancer through the Intervention of Selenium). The study aims to assess the effects of taking selenium supplements on cancer risk in over 40,000 participants who will be randomized to receive selenium (100 mcg, 200 mcg or 300 mcg daily) versus an inactive placebo. In animals, selenium supplementation significantly improves health and prolongs life – whether or not it can do the same for humans remains to be seen. The results of the Precise study are expected to influence public health guidelines on optimal selenium intake for cancer prevention worldwide.

Problems that may be due to selenium deficiency include age spots, pale fingernail beds, increased susceptibility to infection, premature wrinkling of skin, poor growth, subfertility, arthritis, high blood pressure, coronary heart disease, cataracts, pancreatitis, muscle weakness, some cancers and Keshan disease.

Dose

100–200 mcg a day.

Intakes of up to 450 mcg daily are considered safe, but toxicity can occur above 800 mcg daily, leading to a garlic odour on the breath (from dimethyl selenide), fragile or black fingernails, a metallic taste in the mouth, dizziness, nausea and hair loss.

Supplements in which selenium is organically bound to yeast are readily bioavailable.

Shiitake
(Lentinus edodes)

Shiitake is a golden brown, umbrella-shaped Chinese mushroom found growing on fallen tree trunks. It is a popular gourmet mushroom whose medicinal use dates back over 600 years.

Benefits

Shiitake is used to treat raised cholesterol levels, gallstones, stomach ulcers, diabetes, the common cold and as a general tonic to increase the life-force energy known in traditional Chinese medicine as *chi*.

Shiitake contains a powerful immune-stimulating substance, lentinan, which is believed to boost the body's own defences against cancer, viral and fungal infections. It increases production of the body's anti-viral substance, interferon, and increases activity of a powerful, antioxidant enzyme known as superoxide dismutase (SOD).

In Japan, lentinan is extracted and given by injection to treat upper respiratory tract problems, poor circulation, liver disease, and chronic fatigue. Clinical use suggests that it improves survival of patients with advanced and recurrent cancers especially of the stomach, colon, rectum and breast. Lentinan injections have also been shown to help people with hepatitis and with HIV infection, but further research is needed.

Dose
Extracts: 400 mg, three times a day.
Dried mushroom: 5–15 g a day.

Note: shiitake should ideally be prescribed by a qualified medical herbalist if used to treat a serious medical condition.

Side effects
No serious side effects have been reported at standard doses. Larger doses may cause diarrhoea and bloating.

Contraindications
Shiitake should be avoided by women who are pregnant or breast-feeding.

Siberian ginseng
(*Eleutherococcus senticosus*)

Siberian ginseng is a deciduous shrub native to eastern Russia, China, Korea and Japan. Its root has similar actions to that of Korean and American (*Panax*) ginsengs, but it is not closely related.

Benefits

Siberian ginseng has been used for over 2000 years and, although it is often regarded as an inexpensive substitute for Korean ginseng, many researchers consider it to be the more remarkable adaptogen with a higher activity and wider range of therapeutic uses. Some users prefer it to Korean ginseng as they find it more stimulating, while others find it too strong and prefer to take the gentler American ginseng.

Siberian ginseng contains triterpenoid saponins known as eleutherosides, some of which are similar in structure to the saponins in *Panax ginseng*. Comparative studies suggest that there is little qualitative difference between Siberian and *Panax* ginsengs, but *Eleutherococcus* has the advantage of being more abundant and easier to cultivate, hence it is cheaper.

Over 1000 scientific studies show that Siberian ginseng helps the body to adapt and cope during times of stress. It is used extensively to improve stamina and strength, particularly during or after illness and when suffering from other forms of stress and fatigue. A study involving 36 volunteers who received injections of Siberian ginseng extract three times a day for four weeks recorded a dramatic increase in numbers of immune cells, especially T-cells. Russian research suggests that as a result of boosting immunity, those taking it regularly have 40 per cent less colds, 'flu and other infections compared with previous winters, and take a third less days off work due to health problems than those not taking it. Siberian ginseng is taken by 20 million Russians every day to improve performance, health and adaptation to stress or change.

Siberian ginseng is also used to counter genital herpes, jet lag, and has been shown to help normalize high blood pressure, raised blood sugar levels and abnormal blood clotting. It is therefore used to protect against (and treat) heart disease and to promote a healthy circulation.

Siberian ginseng has been shown to have antibacterial properties and is also used to help in recovery from radiation exposure, improve memory and low mood. It is particularly popular with athletes as it can significantly improve performance and reaction times by decreasing lactic acid build-up in muscles, increasing glycogen storage by as much as 80 per cent, boosting energy levels, maximizing oxygen usage and speeding production of new red blood cells. In a study of 12 male athletes, those taking Siberian ginseng increased their total exercise duration by 23.3 per cent compared with only 7.5 per cent for those taking a placebo.

Siberian ginseng has oestrogen-like activity and has been shown to relieve hot flushes, vaginal dryness, night sweats and anxiety. It is also said to improve fertility by enhancing overall vitality and by normalizing levels of sex hormones. In men, it gives higher sexual energy levels and improves their ability to achieve and maintain an erection.

Some practitioners maintain that Siberian ginseng is good for women, while Korean is better for men, but it is really a question of trial and error as to which suits who the best.

Dose

1–2 g a day. Occasionally up to 6 g a day is recommended.

Choose a brand that is standardized to contain more than 1 per cent for eleutherosides.

Start with a low dose in the morning at least 20 minutes before eating. If increasing the dose, work up slowly and take two or three times per day.

As with *Panax ginseng*, Siberian ginseng is best taken cyclically by those who are generally young, healthy and fit.

It should be taken daily for two to three months, then left for a month. Most people begin to notice a difference after around five days, but it should be continued for at least one month for the full restorative effect. Older and weaker people, or those who are unwell may take their doses continuously.

Siberian ginseng should be taken on an empty stomach unless its effects are too relaxing, in which case it can be taken with meals.

Side effects

No serious side effects have been reported. Unlike *Panax ginseng*, Siberian ginseng does not seem to produce over-stimulation or a stress-like syndrome if excess is taken. A few people do find Siberian ginseng too strong, however, and it may affect their ability to sleep. If this is the case, the last dose of the day should be taken before the mid-day meal.

Contraindications

Siberian ginseng should not be used (except under medical advice) by:

- sufferers of high blood pressure
- people with a tendency to nose bleeds or heavy periods
- anyone suffering from insomnia, rapid heartbeat (tachycardia), high fever or congestive heart failure
- women who are pregnant or breast-feeding.

See also **Ginseng**

Silicon

Silicon in its pure form is biologically inactive, but it is now recognized as an essential trace element. In its soluble (colloidal) state it forms silicic acid, which is vital for normal growth. The highest concentration of silica (silicon oxide) is found in connective tissues, cartilage and skin, where it strengthens collagen and elastin fibres and contributes to tissue elasticity. The silica acid content of skin and bones decreases with age as tissues become increasingly inelastic and brittle.

Benefits

Supplements containing silica strengthen bone by cross-linking collagen strands. Silica has been shown to increase mineralization in growing bones, especially in people whose calcium intakes are low. It is also needed for the formation of cartilage.

Silica supplements are widely taken to boost hair, skin and nail growth. In one study involving 50 women, there was an average increase of 29 per cent in skin thickness, and 50 per cent of women with thin or brittle hair or nails reported significant improvements after three months treatment.

Foods containing silicon include rice bran, whole grains, green leafy vegetables, potatoes, capsicum peppers, parsnips, nuts and seeds. The herb horsetail (*Equisetum arvense*) is also a rich source.

Deficiency

Symptoms that may be due to lack of silicon include premature skin ageing, brittle hair and nails, hardening of arteries, abnormal bone formation and osteoporosis.

Dose
There is currently no EC RDA for silicon. Intakes of 20–30 mg a day have been suggested.

Sodium

Sodium is the main positively charged electrolyte found in the extracellular fluids bathing all body cells. A pump in the cell membrane maintains high levels of sodium inside cells to offset that in the extracellular fluid.

Sodium in the diet
Food sources of salt (sodium chloride) include table salt, salted crisps, bacon, salted nuts, tinned products (especially those canned in brine), cured, smoked or pickled fish/meats, meat pastes, pâtés, ready-prepared meals, packet soups and sauces, stock cubes and yeast extracts. As sodium is widespread in foods, deficiency is unlikely.

Excess
Research suggests that at least one in two people is genetically programmed to develop high blood pressure if their intake of salt (sodium chloride) is excessive. New research suggests that people with the highest blood levels of the kidney hormone renin are most likely to respond to a low-sodium, high-potassium diet.

Not adding salt during cooking or at the table will lower systolic blood pressure by a modest amount, and if everyone who was hypertensive did this, it is estimated that the incidence of stroke in the population would be reduced by as much as 26 per cent and coronary heart disease by 15 per cent. Salt is very easily replaceable with herbs and spices, and it doesn't take long to retrain your taste buds.

Data from the Intersalt study involving 10,000 people in 32 countries suggested that the link between salt intake and rising blood pressure with increasing age may have been stronger than previously thought. Against this, however, a study involving over 11,000 American adults found that, after adjustment for age and sex, the mortality rate from any cause was highest among people who reported the lowest sodium intake, and lowest among the group with the highest sodium intake.

Other factors are undoubtedly involved and good intakes of potassium, calcium and magnesium, for example, are important for blood pressure control, while antioxidants and essential fatty acids are important for maintaining a healthy circulation.

Although not everyone is sensitive to the effects of excess dietary sodium, it is worth cutting back on salt intake if you suffer from hypertension. In one study, those taking anti-hypertensive medication were able to halve their dose (under medical supervision) just by increasing the potassium content of their food.

If you have high blood pressure, try following a low-salt diet for a month, then have your BP rechecked to see if it has made any difference. If you suffer from kidney problems as well as hypertension however, you should follow a low-salt diet as you may not be able to excrete as much salt as normally, so that it builds up in your body and contributes to your blood pressure problem.

Unfortunately, most dietary salt (around 75 per cent) is in the form of hidden salt, added to processed foods including canned products, ready-prepared meals, biscuits, cakes and breakfast cereals. This makes it difficult to influence salt intake without checking labels of bought products and avoiding those containing high amounts of salt. When checking labels, those giving salt content as sodium need to be multiplied by 2.5 to give their true salt content. For example, a serving containing 0.4 g sodium actually contains 1 g salt.

Dose

The EC RDA for sodium is 1600 mg daily but most people obtain more than twice this amount from their diet.

Ideally, you want to obtain no more than 4–6 g salt a day. Average intakes are higher than this, however, with some people eating as much as 12 g salt daily.

For those without hypertension, perhaps the best compromise is to use low-sodium, potassium-enriched salts that also contain potassium, magnesium and beneficial trace elements such as selenium.

South African star grass
(Hypoxis rooperi)

S. African star grass is a rich source of beta-sitosterol which makes up to 70 per cent of the dried extracts used to treat symptoms due to benign prostatic hyperplasia (BPH).

In a multi-centre study of 200 men with symptoms due to BPH, those given S. African star grass extracts (providing 20 mg beta-sitosterol, three times a day for six months) showed significant improvements in their symptoms. No severe side effects were reported, although one patient developed erectile problems and another reported loss of libido after two months.

The results of this trial showed that extracts of S. African star grass were at least as effective as drugs commonly prescribed for prostate problems, but without the frequent side effects that can occur with them.

Dose

Equivalent to 20 mg beta-sitosterol, three times a day.

Strontium

Strontium is closely related to calcium and behaves in a similar way in the body, so that 99 per cent of strontium stores (around 320 mg) are found in bones and teeth. The amount of strontium in biological tissues is usually around one thousandth of the concentration of calcium.

Benefits

Strontium seems to strengthen teeth – and therefore presumably bone – as research shows that people living in areas where the strontium content of drinking water is high have fewer dental caries. Excess may damage teeth however (*see* **Fluoride**).

One study found that strontium may be beneficial in the treatment of established osteoporosis. Six volunteers received supplements of strontium (600–700 mg a day) for six months. Biopsies showed bone formation to have increased by over 170 per cent. Furthermore there were reports of a reduction in bone pain. The response was better in younger people.

Foods containing strontium include dairy products, Brazil nuts, bran and root vegetable peelings.

Dose
There is currently no EC RDA for strontium. Intakes of 3 mg–1 g a day have been suggested.

Note: the stable mineral, strontium, is non-toxic but is often confused with radioactive strontium-90, produced in radioactive fallout from atomic bombs which is long-lived and hazardous when incorporated into bone. Stable strontium may, however, help to replace strontium-90 in bones, and is therefore beneficial.

Thiamin

See **Vitamin B1**

Tin

Tin is a trace element needed in tiny amounts for normal growth, including transcription of the genetic code and protein synthesis.

Food sources are unknown because it is difficult to measure tin content. Canned foods contain higher levels than fresh or frozen foods, but this is due to contamination.

Deficiency of tin is thought to lead to poor growth.

Dose

There is currently no EC RDA for tin, but A to Z-style vitamin and mineral supplements tend to contain around 10 mcg.

Tribulus terrestris

Tribulus terrestris is an Indian plant – also known as ci ji li – used in Ayurvedic medicine. Its fruit contains furostanol saponins that are widely used to treat male genito-urinary problems, low sex drive and impotence.

Benefits

Taking *Tribulus* for just five days has been shown to increase testosterone levels in some healthy men by around 30 per cent. A trial involving 50 male patients with low sex drive due to lethargy, fatigue and lack of interest in daily activities showed a 45 per cent improvement in symptoms with *Tribulus*. It has diuretic actions and in addition to its traditional use as a general male tonic, it is also taken to reduce high blood pressure and as a liver stimulant.

Dose

250 mg capsules standardized to contain 40 per cent furostanol saponins: 1–2 capsules a day.

Turmeric
(Curcuma longa)

Turmeric is native to Asia, and its orange-yellow spicy root is widely used in curry dishes. It is also a traditional Ayurvedic and Chinese herbal medicine for treating liver problems such as jaundice and bloating, and as a topical treatment (in poultices) for treating inflamed joints.

Benefits

Turmeric contains an anti-inflammatory antioxidant, curcumin, that stimulates secretion of bile and boosts liver function by increasing levels of two liver enzymes: glutathione-s-transferase and glucuronyl transferase. It also supports liver regeneration, increases bile flow, relieves bloating and indigestion, reduces blood clotting and helps to lower raised cholesterol levels.

The anti-inflammatory action of turmeric is stronger than that of hydrocortisone, and its antioxidant action more powerful than that of vitamin E. It is currently under investigation for anti-cancer properties. It is thought to interfere with viral replication and may be recommended in the treatment of viral infections including HIV. (*See* **Anosmia** in A–Z of Problems and Solutions).

Dose

Two level teaspoons of powder twice a day, or as capsules 500–1200 mg a day, standardized to 95 per cent curcuminoids.

It may be combined with pineapple extracts (bromelain) to improve absorption.

Tyrosine

L-Tyrosine is a non-essential amino acid found in many protein foods. It can also be made in the body from another amino acid, L-phenylalanine. It also plays a part in the synthesis of several key brain chemicals involved in regulating sex drive, and the prosexual claims for L-tyrosine are therefore similar to those for L-phenylalanine.

Dose

500 mg–1 g, twice or three times daily before meals, for up to three weeks. Some nutritionists recommend taking it with B complex vitamins and high-dose vitamin C for maximum effect.

Side effects

Can cause stimulant side effects such as insomnia and anxiety.

Contraindications

● L-tyrosine should not be taken by anyone who has high blood pressure, or who is taking anti-depressant drugs, except under medical supervision.

● It should not be taken by those with a history of malignant melanoma or schizophrenia as it may worsen these conditions.

Uña de gato

See **Cat's claw**

Valerian
(Valerian officinalis)

Valerian is one of the most calming herbs available. Its roots have been used as a sedative since mediaeval times to calm nervous anxiety, reduce muscle tension, stimulate appetite and induce a refreshing night's sleep.

Benefits

Valerian contains a number of unique substances (such as valeric acid, valepotriates) that are thought to act together in synergy to produce significant, positive effects on stress. It is thought to work by raising levels of an inhibitory brain chemical, gamma-aminobutyric acid (GABA), that damps down the over-stimulation occurring during anxiety.

Trials involving people with emotional symptoms due to stress showed that it helped to overcome low mood, loss of initiative, feeling unsociable, irritability, anxiety and difficulty in sleeping. It is also used to relieve cramps, period pains, intestinal colic, irritable bowel syndrome, migraine and rheumatic pains.

Of 125 people in one trial, those taking valerian extracts fell asleep more quickly and woke up less frequently during the night than those taking a placebo.

A randomized, double-blind, placebo-controlled study involving 16 patients with primary insomnia found that 300 mg concentrated dry extract (equivalent to 1800 mg fresh herb) produced beneficial effects on slow wave sleep latency and duration with, according to the researchers, 'an extremely low number of adverse events'.

Dose

250–800 mg, twice or three times a day.

Select standardized products containing at least 0.8 per cent valeric acid.

Valerian is often used together with other calming herbs such as lemon balm and hops to ease nervous anxiety, insomnia and to help avoid a panic attack. It may also be used together with St John's Wort for depression, or with kava kava for anxiety.

Side effects

Valerian is non-addictive, and does not produce a drugged feeling or hangover effect, as it promotes a natural form of sleep whose architecture is preserved. However it may cause mild drowsiness which will affect your ability to drive or operate machinery.

Contraindications

● Valerian should not be taken by anyone using prescribed sleeping tablets.

● Pregnant or breast-feeding women should not take valerian.

Vanadium

Vanadium is a trace element whose exact biological function remains unclear. It seems to be involved in growth and fat metabolism as low levels cause increased blood cholesterol and triglyceride levels.

Benefits

Vanadium is thought to be of value in protecting against coronary heart disease and possibly cancer. It may also have a role in regulating the activity of the sodium-potassium pump in cell walls, but this is not yet proven.

In rats, vanadium has an effect that mimics insulin, and can be used to reverse artificially induced diabetes.

Foods containing vanadium include parsley, black pepper, seafood (especially lobster and oysters), radishes, lettuce, whole grains, sunflower seeds, soy beans, buckwheat, carrots and garlic.

Dose

There is currently no EC RDA for vanadium but A to Z-style vitamin and mineral supplements tend to contain around 10 mcg.

Vitamins

Vitamins are naturally occurring substances that are essential for life, although they are only needed in tiny amounts. There are 13 major vitamins that must all be obtained from the diet as most cannot be synthesized in the body (e.g. vitamin C) or can only be made in minute amounts (e.g. vitamin D, niacin), too small to meet our needs.

Vitamins are involved in all the body's metabolic reactions from digestion, energy production and immunity to cell division, growth, tissue repair, hormone secretion and reproduction. They are involved in the transportation of oxygen and wastes in the circulation, vision, sensory perception and mental alertness.

Lack of vitamins is common, and if intakes are consistently below recommended levels, a variety of non-specific ailments may appear including dry, itchy skin with poor wound-healing properties, tiredness, lack of energy, lowered immunity and difficulty in conceiving.

How quickly a particular vitamin deficiency will cause problems depends on how much is stored in the body, and how quickly supplies run out. In general, vitamins that are fat-soluble are stored more easily in the body (e.g. in the liver) than those that are water-soluble and easily lost in the urine. The highly fat-soluble vitamins are A, D, E and K, and the water-soluble vitamins are the B group and C whose levels (with the exception of vitamin B12) must be continually replenished from the diet.

Lack of water-soluble folic acid may develop quite quickly (e.g. during pregnancy, to cause certain developmental abnormalities in the foetus), while in contrast, stores of the more fat-soluble vitamin B12 are large, and it can take years for deficiency to develop into pernicious anaemia.

Wheatgrass

Wheatgrass is a green food supplement, similar in action to blue-green algae. Wheatgrass juice is prepared from three-to-four-day old germinated wheat grain sprouts which are naturally rich in vitamins, minerals, trace elements and enzymes – including the important antioxidant superoxide dismutase. It is said to boost energy levels and immunity, help heal ulcers and to reduce body odours – including bad breath. It is mainly taken for its nutritional benefits, however. According to one estimate, 1 kg fresh wheatgrass juice is nutritionally equivalent to over 20 kg vegetables. Converts tend to grow their own in the kitchen and harvest the grass when it is 6–7 cm high for home-juicing. It needs to be drunk immediately before it oxidizes (e.g. 30 ml plus water to dilute at least 1:1) but it is an acquired taste. Organically grown, vacuum-dried juice extracts are therefore popular, although purists say that this destroys some enzyme activity.

A dose of around 5 g dried wheatgrass juice is nutritionally equivalent to an average portion of dark-green leafy vegetables such as spinach or kale.

Wild yam
(Dioscorea villosa)

Wild yam is a Mexican vine whose root is rich in steroidal saponins, including diosgenin, a hormone-like substance originally used in the laboratory to synthesize a synthetic form of progesterone (norethisterone) used in the first oral contraceptive pills. It is important to realize that wild yam does not contain progesterone, however, although it does seem to have progesterone-like actions and is widely used as a female remedy.

Benefits
Wild yam acts as a general tonic and will improve mood and general feelings of well-being. It is also known as the colic root as it can relieve painful spasms, including painful

periods, uterine contractions during labour and pain due to gallstones. Wild yam is also used to help treat endometriosis. It has anti-inflammatory actions and is used to treat rheumatoid arthritis and diverticulitis. Research suggests that it has an antioxidant action that prevents breakdown of fatty molecules in the body (lipid peroxidation) and increases beneficial levels of HDL-cholesterol.

Dose
Capsules: 250–500 mg once or twice a day.

Excess
Excess may cause nausea or diarrhoea.

Contraindications
- Wild yam should not be taken in pregnancy except under medical supervision.

- Wild yam should not be used for the prevention or treatment of osteoporosis.

Yerba maté
(Ilex paraguariensis)

Yerba maté is a tree that only grows in the rain forests of Paraguay. Its leaves are used to make a nutritional supplement rich in vitamins and minerals, especially vitamin C. Missionaries have been said to go for months at a time in the rain forests subsisting only on yerba maté tea, with no ill effects other than some weight loss. The plant must be allowed to dry for at least 12 months before use.

Benefits

The leaves of yerba maté contain xanthine alkaloids – related to those in coffee and guarana – which increases mental alertness and acuity without side effects of nervousness or sleep disturbance. It may even improve sleep architecture by normalizing the amount of time spent in REM (rapid eye movement) and deep, delta-wave sleep. Because yerba maté promotes a deeper, more relaxing sleep, some users find they actually need less sleep when taking it.

Yerba maté stimulates the adrenal glands to boost production of corticosteroids. It may therefore be classed as an adaptogen, helping the body to adapt and cope with stressful times. It is mainly used as a general energy boost, overcoming physical exhaustion and mental fatigue, especially when linked with stress. It is a popular digestive remedy which relieves indigestion and improves constipation, by both softening hard faeces and gently stimulating bowel movements. It can also act as a detoxifying agent that helps the elimination of wastes and toxins through both bowels and kidneys partly through a mild diuretic action.

Yerba maté is a calming tonic for anxiety, poor concentration and nervousness, lifting a low mood and relieving headaches, migraine and neuralgia. Other popular uses include strengthening heart function, lowering high blood pressure, boosting immune function and disease resistance and drying up excessive nasal secretions such as in allergic rhinitis or sinusitis. It also acts as a substitute for alcohol, and to help liver regeneration, especially when trying to reduce alcohol intake.

Those who take it also claim other benefits such as increased energy levels, reduction in allergic symptoms such as hay fever, firmer and smoother skin tone and improved circulation.

Dose
2–3 cups yerba maté tea a day.

Note: Yerba maté contains high levels of tannins, so it is best not taken with meals as it may impair the absorption of nutrients.

Zinc

Zinc is an important co-factor for over 200 metabolic enzymes. It forms an integral part of the enzyme which switches on genes to produce specific proteins in response to hormone triggers. It plays a major role in the sensitivity of the tissues to circulating sex hormones and is vital for growth, sexual maturity and wound healing. Zinc also plays a central role in immunity and helps to protect against infections such as the common cold.

Zinc in the diet
Dietary sources of zinc include red meat, seafood (especially oysters), offal, brewer's yeast, whole grains (although processing removes most of their mineral zinc), pulses, eggs and cheese.

Deficiency
Low intakes of dietary zinc (less than 5 mg per day) are associated with low testosterone levels and, in some parts of the world, dietary zinc deficiency is common and results in

delayed male puberty. Zinc is so important for sperm health that each ejaculate contains around 5 mg zinc – one third of the daily requirement (EC RDA). Men who are sexually active are therefore more at risk of zinc deficiency than women. Zinc is mixed with sperm via prostate secretions, and helps to keep mature sperm in a quiet state so that they do not release the enzymes needed to drill a hole through the egg during fertilization too soon. Once in the female reproductive tract, where zinc levels are low, sperm become more active and start releasing the enzymes (acrosome reaction) so fertilization can occur. Zinc is also needed to keep the genetic material tightly packed within the sperm head. Men who are zinc deficient may be sub-fertile because their sperm have released their egg-boring enzymes too soon.

The prostate gland has the highest concentration of zinc in any body tissue. Lack of it is associated with an increased risk of prostatitis (inflammation of the prostate gland). Recently, it was discovered that measuring the zinc content of prostate biopsy samples could help to determine whether or not prostate cancer was present, as prostate cancer cells lose their ability to concentrate zinc so levels are much lower in abnormal tissue.

Benefits

Sucking lozenges containing zinc gluconate, zinc acetate or zinc citrate is thought to stimulate immune cells in the throat to give local immunity a boost. This has been shown to reduce the duration and severity of symptoms due to the common cold in some trials, but not in others. In one study involving 100 people with early symptoms of a common cold, those sucking zinc lozenges every two hours recovered three days earlier than those using placebo lozenges. In another, in which 48 people took 12.8 mg zinc acetate or a placebo every two or three hours while awake (starting within 24 hours of developing cold symptoms), the average duration of symptoms was 4.5 days for those taking zinc, compared with 8.1 days for those on placebo. There was also a significant reduction in cough which was reduced to 3.1 days for those on zinc, and 6.3 days for those taking the placebo. Those taking zinc were more likely to develop side effects of dry mouth and constipation, but there was no higher risk of bad taste or mouth irritation.

It seems to be important to start treatment within 48 hours of the onset of symptoms, and to suck zinc lozenges supplying at least 13.3 mg elemental zinc every two hours while awake.

Women with osteoporosis have been found to have blood and bone levels of zinc that are up to 30 per cent lower than in women with healthy bones.

Many people only obtain half the EC RDA of 15 mg zinc from their diet and zinc deficiency becomes increasingly common with age. Lack of zinc is thought to be one of the commonest causes of loss of taste (ageusia) and smell sensations (anosmia). This can be tested for by obtaining a solution of zinc sulphate (e.g. 15 mg/5 ml) from a chemist. Swirl a teaspoonful in your mouth; if the solution seems tasteless, zinc deficiency is likely. If the solution tastes furry, of minerals or slightly sweet, zinc levels are borderline, and if it tastes strongly unpleasant, zinc levels are normal.

Loss of taste occurs in some people with anorexia nervosa. Zinc supplements may stimulate appetite and improve food intake. Some people with pica – an odd craving for non-nutritive substances (e.g. coal, soil, paper) – have zinc deficiency, and this should always be checked for.

Lack of zinc may play a role in gum inflammation that occurs in periodontal disease. There is also an association with an increased risk of coronary heart disease and diabetes. Some people with tinnitus have low levels of zinc, and their symptoms significantly improved with zinc supplementation. Zinc also seems to be a promising addition to treatment for acute diarrhoea in children in the Third World.

Lack of zinc is suspected of contributing to brain abnormalities (neurofibrillary tangles) such as those seen in neurological conditions such as Alzheimer's disease. It also leads to poor wound healing, skin problems such as eczema, psoriasis and acne, poor growth of hair and nails, loss of taste and smell sensation, poor appetite and eating disorders.

Dose

15–50 mg a day. Occasionally higher doses are recommended under medical advice – but need to be taken together with copper. Do not take more than 30 mg daily long term except under supervision from a qualified nutritionist or doctor.

PART 2:

A–Z OF PROBLEMS AND SOLUTIONS

Acne

Acne is an inflammatory skin disease associated with over-sensitivity of sebaceous (oil) glands to the effects of the male hormone, testosterone. Only sebaceous glands that open into hair follicles are affected, and these are found on the face, back, chest, groin and outer ear canal. In severe cases, acne may spread down the arms, lower trunk, buttocks and even the upper legs. Sebaceous glands found on hairless skin such as the eyelids and foreskin are unaffected. Although most sufferers are in their teens, one in 20 is in their 30s or 40s.

Acne is linked with:

● greasiness due to increased production of sebum (oil) which may be thicker than normal

● blackheads (comedones) formed when thickening of the duct leading from the hair follicle/sebaceous gland to the skin traps secretions inside

● infection – due to increased number of bacteria (*Propionibacterium acnes*) that also become trapped inside the follicle and sebaceous glands

● inflammation – due to bacterial enzymes which break down the oil down into a range of free fatty acids and inflammatory chemicals that attract white blood cells into the area which makes inflammation worse

● nodules, cysts and scarring if not treated properly – always seek medical advice; up to 50 per cent of women with acne beyond their teens have increased circulating levels of testosterone which can usually be treated.

Treatment

There is no evidence that acne is solely caused by a poor diet, although poor nutrition can make symptoms worse. A healthy, wholefood diet full of fresh fruit and vegetables that supply antioxidant vitamins and minerals should be eaten, including nuts, seeds, oily fish and whole-grain cereals; these contain essential fatty acids (EFAs) that have an anti-inflammatory action. Also eat more zinc-rich foods and consider testing for zinc deficiency (*see* **Zinc**). Where zinc deficiency is present, oral zinc picolinate supplements can be more effective than antibiotics. These are best taken under the supervision of a nutritional therapist, as extra copper and selenium will also be needed.

Vitamin A is required for healthy skin and deficiency can lead to scaliness, raised pimply hair follicles and increased susceptibility to acne. Vitamin A supplements therefore sometimes help and, in fact, drugs derived from vitamin A are now used to treat severe acne. Antioxidants such as vitamins E (400 IU a day) and C (1000 g a day) can also help to damp down inflammation, as can grapeseed or pine bark extracts.

Products containing dilute, antiseptic tea tree oil, aloe vera or silicol gel are often effective. A recent field trial of silicol skin gel involving members of the Acne Support Group found that an 86 per cent improvement occurred after six weeks use. No significant difference occurred between members using silicol skin gel only, and those using it in addition to prescribed oral medication. Silicol gel is applied twice a day for around 15 minutes, as a mask, to absorb excess sebum, skin cell plugs and bacteria. Once dried it is rinsed off with warm water.

Herbal remedies containing sarsaparilla are used to treat mild to moderate symptoms.

Picking or scratching spots may make scarring worse.

Note: vitamin A should be avoided by women who are either planning a pregnancy or who are already pregnant.

Adenomyosis

See **Endometriosis**

Age spots

Age, or 'liver' spots, are the result of a lifetime's accumulation of sun damage.

Every time skin is exposed to the sun, it is damaged by ultraviolet rays. This generates free radicals which set up an inflammatory reaction known as heliodermatitis. This inflammation damages skin structures and interferes with normal cell division. Enzymes released during the inflammatory process are also thought to dissolve elastin and collagen fibres leading to premature wrinkles and areas of pigmentation commonly known as age spots. These are most often seen on the backs of the hands, face and neck, and are related to damage from previous sunburn.

Dermatologists estimate that 30–40 per cent of the UK population who are fair-skinned have appreciable photo-damage caused by chronic exposure to sunlight. Studies by the American Academy of Dermatology reveal that by the age of 18, we have already received half of our lifetime's quota of sun damage – much of it while playing outdoors as a child.

Treatment

As an antioxidant, selenium provides important skin protection against sun damage, and those with low intakes are most likely to develop age spots and certain types of skin cancer. Taking selenium supplements has been shown to decrease damage of skin cell membranes (lipid peroxidation) following UV exposure. Taking supplements containing selenium and vitamins A, C and E showed systemic protection against UV irradiation. The protection was greatest if taken before exposure to UV light.

Creams containing co-enzyme Q10 (CoQ10) have been shown to reduce oxidation and wrinkle depth in human skin and to suppress production of collagenase following UVA irradiation. Researchers suggest that oral CoQ10 can also prevent many of the detrimental effects of photo-ageing.

Photo-damage may be treated with a cream containing the vitamin A derivative, tretinoin, which is available on private prescription from a doctor (patients pay the full cost of treatment). This stimulates skin collagen production and oxygenation to fade pigmented age spots. In a clinical trial involving almost 300 people, 57 per cent noticed improvement in fine wrinkling, 63 per cent reported decreased mottling and 42 per cent noticed a lessening in skin roughness after six months. Alternatively, over-the-counter fade creams may help. *See also* **B5**

Note: photo-ageing significantly increases the risk of developing skin cancer. Always seek medical advice if any skin lesion starts to get bigger, turns darker, becomes scaly, itchy, weepy, crusts over or scabs without healing, develops a raised, rolled edge or ulcerates.

Alcohol intake – excessive

In December 1995, the Department of Health suggested revised levels for safe drinking, and stated that 'Men who drink three to four units a day, and women who drink two to three units do not face a significant health risk.' This was widely interpreted to mean that the upper limit was no more than 28 units a week for men and no more than 21 for women. Strictly speaking, however, the original limits of 21 and 14 units have not been changed as the revised guidelines say that ' . . . consistently drinking four or more units a day (men), and three or more units a day (women) is not advisable because of the increasing health risk it carries.' Furthermore, it is important that women who are pregnant or planning to be should either avoid alcohol altogether, or drink no more than one or two units, once or twice a week.

The form of alcohol that seems most beneficial to health, in moderation, is red wine, mainly due to the powerful antioxidant pigments it contains. Wine should ideally be drunk with food rather than on its own, however, as this provides the best protection by protecting dietary fats from oxidation. While a low to moderate intake is beneficial in reducing stress and possible coronary heart disease, excess is harmful to health.

Alcohol is metabolized in the liver to acetaldehyde – a cellular poison – that can damage liver, brain and heart muscle cells. If alcohol intake remains excessive, fatty degeneration occurs as liver cells drop their normal housekeeping metabolic reactions and work overtime to eliminate alcohol from the body. Because liver enzymes are diverted from their normal tasks to metabolize alcohol, fewer dietary fatty acids are processed and liver cells start to swell from the accumulation of unprocessed globules of fat.

The impaired metabolic reactions inside liver cells generate large numbers of damaging free radicals. This increases the damaging effects of a continued excessive alcohol intake and liver cells accumulate more and more fatty globules so that the liver enlarges and takes on a yellow appearance. If high alcohol intake continues, cirrhosis eventually develops. If you are worried about your alcohol intake, it is important to have a blood test to check liver function.

Treatment

Extracts of milk thistle (*Silybum marianum*) – known as silymarin – have been shown in more than 300 studies to protect liver cells from the poisonous effects of excess alcohol. They can even improve liver function when cirrhosis is present.

Other herbal remedies beneficial to the liver include dandelion root (*Taraxacum officinalis*), globe artichoke (*Cynara scolymus*), gotu kola and turmeric (*Curcuma longa*).

For those who find it difficult to go without alcohol, the herb kudzu can dramatically decrease alcohol cravings.

Kudzu (*Pueraria lobata*), is a traditional Chinese food whose starchy root is used in soups and stews as a thickening agent similar to cornstarch. It contains beneficial plant hormones (betasitosterol and isoflavones such as daidzein and formononetin) similar to those found in soya. Extracts have been used to treat those under the influence of alcohol – both to sober them up, and to reduce their alcohol intake.

Kava kava and evening primrose oil are also helpful for people trying to give up alcohol by reducing anxiety and cravings. Yerba maté tea is an energizing tonic that is also used as a substitute for alcohol, and to help liver regeneration, especially when trying to reduce alcohol intake. *See also* **B1, Glutamine**

Alopecia

Alopecia areata is a non-scarring, inflammatory condition in which the hair follicles switch off and lie dormant. The exact cause is unknown, although an imbalance of enzymes responsible for the production of hair fibre and an abnormal T-lymphocyte immune response are implicated. Occasionally alopecia is linked with iron-deficiency anaemia, or with an underactive thyroid gland. Stress plays a major role as it reduces blood supply to the scalp, and also seems to increase production of oily secretions by the sebaceous glands connected to each hair follicle.

There are four main types:

● alopecia areata in which hair is lost in patches, usually on the scalp

- alopecia totalis, in which there is total loss of scalp hair
- alopecia universalis – loss of hair over the entire body, including eyebrows and eyelashes
- diffuse alopecia, a condition sometimes known as alopecia androgenetica in which widespread hair loss affects the whole scalp, causing a 'moth-eaten' appearance.

In half of all cases, the hair follicles start to recover within a year so that the hair grows back, and altogether, four out of five people regrow their hair within five years, although some people always retain a small bald area. In around one in ten people affected, the condition progressively worsens.

Treatment

Several herbal, vitamin and mineral supplements designed to help hair loss are now widely available. Nutrient deficiencies – especially of iron – can play a role in hair loss, and several supplements designed to counter this problem are now widely available in health food shops or chemists. These usually include vitamins such as B5 and biotin, minerals such as iron and silica, and may also include herbs such as ginkgo (which increase peripheral blood circulation) and seaweed extracts as a source of iodine. Evening primrose oil is also useful for hair problems as it supplies essential fatty acids needed for healthy cell membranes within hair follicles. The amino acid L-cysteine is also important for hair construction. A herbal solution known as Calosol 4H is currenly undergoing clinical trials (*see* **page 570 for more information**).

Alzheimer's disease

Alzheimer's disease is the most common form of dementia, whose symptoms vary from person to person. The first inkling that something is wrong is usually forgetfulness and loss of memory. Long-ago occurrences from childhood are often recalled while more recent events such as a television programme just the previous evening are not. It then becomes increasingly difficult to concentrate, add numbers and to find the right words when describing something. Although mild versions of these symptoms are perfectly normal with increasing age, overwork and stress, it soon becomes apparent that problems are more severe in someone suffering from this condition. Mood swings and personality changes occur and eventually, a person with Alzheimer's becomes very disorientated and confused.

Treatment

Alzheimer's is associated with the deposition of beta-amyloid plaques and proteinaceous tangles in brain tissues. Recent studies suggest that cat's claw may help to prevent this action, but this is still under investigation.

Women taking oestrogen hormone replacement therapy for at least one year after the menopause are less likely to develop Alzheimer's disease. Women who take oestrogen (HRT) for ten years or more seem to be 30 per cent less likely to develop the condition – and if it does occur, onset tends to come later than usual.

Although there is no cure for Alzheimer's disease at present, research is currently looking into the use of drugs that can change brain chemicals and so-called smart drugs that help to boost brain function. Some people are helped by taking supplements of choline or lecithin, which boost brain levels of a neurotransmitter, acetylcholine. Volunteers taking a 10 g dose of choline were found to remember a list of words more rapidly than before. Lecithin is one of the most important dietary sources of choline. Foods rich in lecithin include soya beans, sunflower oil, maize, egg yolk and liver.

Faulty memory is occasionally due to thiamine (vitamin B1) deficiency, especially in people who drink a lot of alcohol. This is treated with high doses of around 50 mg vitamin B1 a day. Foods rich in thiamine include: brewer's yeast, brown rice, wheat germ, whole-grain bread and cereals.

Garlic tablets improve blood flow in the brain and may help to improve memory.

Ginkgo supplements also boost blood supply to the brain and have been shown to improve memory and concentration. In one study, people with Alzheimer's were twice as likely to experience a delay in the progression of their illness if they took ginkgo supplements compared with those not taking them.

Colloidal silicic acid (silicol gel) has been found to bind aluminium and may reduce the risk of Alzheimer's disease. Recent research suggests that tap water containing more than 30 mg silicon per litre significantly reduces the risk of Alzheimer's disease.

Antioxidants such as vitamins C, E, grapeseed or pycnogenol (in pine bark) extracts will also help to reduce free radical damage that may be linked with brain cell damage.

See also **Reishi, Zinc**

Anaemia

Anaemia due to low concentrations of the red blood pigment haemoglobin is associated with weakness and profound exhaustion. Haemoglobin is needed to transport oxygen to body tissues, without which muscle and brain cells in particular cannot function properly.

There are three main causes of anaemia:

- reduced or defective production of red blood cells in the marrow (due to lack of iron, vitamin B12, folic acid, or to bone marrow disease, for example)

- excessive destruction of red blood cells (haemolytic anaemia due to malaria, for example, and immune or genetic conditions such as sickle cell anaemia)

- excessive blood loss (such as that in heavy frequent periods, peptic ulceration or occasionally a bowel tumour).

Treatment

It is vital to determine the underlying cause of anaemia before beginning any sort of treatment. Iron supplementation may be recommended once the cause is established, but not before, as it may mask deficiency.

Studies suggest that up to 20 per cent of menstruating women are iron deficient although fewer than half of these cases are severe enough to cause anaemia. Iron intakes can be boosted by eating iron rich foods such as shellfish, red meats, sardines, wheatgerm, wholemeal bread, egg yolk, green vegetables and dried fruit. The form of iron found in red meat (heme iron) is up to ten times more easily absorbed than non-haem iron in vegetables, and overboiling vegetables decreases their iron availability by a further 20 per cent. Vitamin C (found in citrus and berry fruits, blackcurrants, kiwi fruit and green leafy vegetables) increases the absorption of inorganic (non-haem) iron by keeping it in the more easily absorbed ferrous form. Phytate fibre, calcium, tea and coffee decrease iron absorption so iron supplements are best taken on an empty stomach unless it causes irritation.

Ferrous fumarate or ferrous gluconate are usually better tolerated and less constipating than ferrous sulphate. Iron-rich spa water is available as a liquid iron tonic, whose iron is at least twice as easily absorbed as that found in food and solid supplements. Floradix Liquid Iron Formula and Floradix tablets provide iron-rich yeast combined with fruit concentrates to improve absorption. The supplement is usually well tolerated – and may be taken in pregnancy – but a yeast and gluten-free form is also available for those with allergies.

Lack of vitamin B12 (pernicious anaemia) is treated with B12 injections although high-dose oral supplements are becoming more accepted. Wash down iron tablets with vitamin-C rich juice to increase absorption. Naturopaths recommend beetroot and beetroot juice to help increase haemoglobin concentration. Co-enzyme Q10 supplements help to increase oxygen uptake in cells.

Echinacea is also believed to promote formation of red blood cells.

Angina

Coronary heart disease (CHD) is the biggest killer in the West, killing more people than any other single disease. It is due to hardening and furring up of the coronary arteries so heart muscle is starved of oxygen-rich blood. This triggers pain (angina) which is usually:

● felt behind the chest bone
● tight and crushing – like a bear hug
● described as spreading through the chest and may radiate up into the neck, jaw or down the left arm
● brought on by exertion and relieved by rest.

If heart muscle cells die due to prolonged oxygen starvation, a heart attack occurs. Heart attack pain is similar to angina but:

● lasts longer
● is more intense
● is usually accompanied by sweating, breathlessness and paleness
● can come on at any time and is unrelieved by rest.

Sudden chest pain should always be taken seriously and medical assistance sought without delay.

Treatment

The number of deaths attributed to CHD is slowly falling as more people are taking stock of their lifestyle. Taking a few steps such as stopping smoking, losing excess weight and taking regular exercise can, together with improving diet, significantly lower the risk of CHD.

Try to ensure that you:

- *eat at least five portions of fresh fruit, vegetables and salads per day*: fruit and vegetables contain important vitamins, minerals, antioxidants and beneficial plant hormones that protect against CHD. Eating at least five servings per day reduces the risk of premature death from any cause (but especially from coronary heart disease) compared with those who eat less.

- *watch the fats in your diet*: one in three heart attacks is linked with an unhealthy diet with too much fat and not enough starchy foods or fruit and vegetables. The average adult needs to reduce their fat intake by at least a quarter. Concentrate on obtaining beneficial fats such as olive, rapeseed, walnut, fish and evening primrose oils rather than saturated fats found in donuts, chips and cream. Choose reduced fat foods where possible. Grill rather than fry. Eat red meat only once or twice a week and have more vegetarian meals instead. The effects of a high-fat diet can be offset by taking antioxidant supplements (see below) that protect circulating fats from oxidation and reduce the risk of hardening and furring up of the arteries (atherosclerosis).

- *eat more fish*: fish oils can thin the blood, lower blood pressure and – if you suffer from heart disease – can reduce your risk of a fatal heart attack by a third. Aim to eat fish – especially oily fish (salmon, herrings, sardines, mackerel) two or three times per week. If you don't like fish, consider taking an omega-3 fish oil supplement instead. Emulsified products are available that improve absorption from the gut so you don't get 'fishy' burps.

- *eat more fibre*: dietary fibre absorbs fats and slows their absorption so your body can handle them more easily. Eating 3 g or more of soluble oat fibre (roughly equal to two large bowls of porridge) every day has been shown to lower harmful blood cholesterol levels by a small but significant amount.

- *cut back on salt*: if everyone reduced the amount of salt in their diet, at least one in seven heart attacks would be prevented. Although only an estimated one in two people are sensitive to the effects of sodium chloride, it is worth avoiding obviously salty foods (such as products tinned in brine) and to stop adding salt during cooking or at the table. A good compromise is to use potassium-enriched salts or to obtain flavour from herbs, spices and black pepper instead. Adding lime juice reduces the need for salt flavour.

In addition to the above, it is sensible to keep alcohol intake within safe limits, avoid excess stress, have regular blood pressure, blood fat level, and urine checks.

As well as any supplementation recommended above, the following are worth considering.

- *Garlic tablets*: taking garlic tablets can lower high blood pressure, reduce high blood fat levels and thin the blood enough to reduce the risk of heart disease by up to 25 per cent. Garlic powder tablets have been shown in a number of clinical trials to reduce cholesterol levels by an average of 11 per cent and up to 25 per cent. A recent study followed 152 patients for over four years and found that garlic tablets could reduce and even reverse hardening and furring up of the arteries compared with those not taking them. Other interesting studies have found that garlic powder tablets can lower a raised blood pressure and increase the elasticity of the aorta so the heart has to work less hard to pump blood out into the body.

- *Antioxidant supplements*: those with high blood levels of the antioxidant vitamins C and E (usually through taking supplements) are three times less likely to have a heart attack than those with low levels. Vitamin E gained widespread medical acceptance following results of the Cambridge Heart Antioxidant Study (CHAOS) in 1996 (*see* E). Antioxidant supplements are especially important for smokers and people with diabetes.

- *Folic acid supplements*: around one in ten people has inherited high blood levels of the amino acid homocysteine. This damages artery linings and more than triples the risk of a heart attack. One in 160,000 people has extremely high levels with 30 times the risk of premature heart disease. High levels of homocysteine can be reduced by taking supplements of folic acid (400–650 mcg per day). Vitamins B6 and B12 also have a beneficial effect. Foods rich in folic acid include green leafy vegetables (spinach, broccoli, Brussel sprouts) and whole grains.

- *Drink more tea*: drinking four cups of tea per day may halve your risk of a heart attack. Both green and black tea are rich sources of antioxidants known as flavonoids. Other important sources of flavonoids include garlic, onions and apples.

Other helpful supplements include: **Arginine, Astralagus, Bromelain, Calcium, Carnitine, Co-enzyme Q10, Essential fatty acids, Grapeseed, Gynostemma, Hawthorn, Olive Oil, Magnesium, Pine bark** and **Siberian ginseng.**

Anosmia

Every day, we breathe over 23,000 times, bringing up to 10,000 different aromas into our noses. Smell receptors are located at the top of the nasal cavity and depend on tiny, hair-like nerve endings detecting aromatic substances dissolved in overlying mucus. Complete lack of smell (anosmia) is commonly related to chronic rhinitis in which inflammation and increased production of mucus block smell receptors. Two types – perennial allergic rhinitis and vasomotor rhinitis – are both associated with nasal polyps and loss of smell. It is worth undergoing investigations into either of these conditions to pinpoint dietary or environmental allergies.

Treatment

Curcumin (extracted from the spice turmeric) has powerful anti-inflammatory actions equivalent to those of some steroids. High-dose vitamin C also helps to reduce inflammation (this should be taken in the form of Ester-C by sufferers of indigestion). The amino acid, N-actylcysteine makes mucus less viscous and may improve symptoms.

Taking a daily multi-nutrient supplement containing 10–15 mg zinc may be helpful as poor sense of smell is often linked to zinc deficiency (*see* **Zinc** for information on a zinc deficiency test). Zinc is best taken in a supplement that also provides potassium, magnesium, calcium and vitamin B12 which are important for smell/taste sensation.

Anxiety

Anxiety is a common symptom of stress and is associated with feelings of apprehension, dread, panic and impending doom. While short-lived anxiety is appropriate in some situations (such as when going for an interview) those with morbid anxiety worry excessively about trivial matters and frequently experience other typical stress symptoms such as restlessness, palpitations, tremor, flushing, dizziness, hyperventilation, loose bowels, sweating, muscle tension and insomnia.

Treatment

Valerian is one of the most calming herbs available and can help to relieve anxiety, muscle tension and promote tranquillity. It is often used together with other herbs with similar effects such as lemon balm and hops to ease nervous anxiety, insomnia and to help avoid panic attacks.

Kava kava is also widely used to combat mild anxiety as it promotes feelings of relaxation and calm. Some studies suggest it to be as effective as some prescription drugs in treating mild to moderate anxiety. Kava kava may be taken in a single dose, as necessary, or taken regularly.

Where anxiety is associated with depression, St John's Wort will help to lift a low mood, but medical advice should be sought by anyone taking prescribed medications or anti-depressants.

Many people also find Bach Rescue Remedy helpful – place a few drops under the tongue whenever panic rises.

Supplements containing calcium, magnesium and B group vitamins are also important for healthy function of the nervous system, while chamomile has a gentle anxiety-reducing action.

See also **Ashwagandha, Gotu kola, Gynostemma, 5-HTP, Muira puama, Oats, Yerba maté**

Arthritis

The word 'arthritis' means inflammation of a joint. There are many different forms of which the most common, osteoarthritis (OA), causes symptoms in at least half of people over the age of 60, while most others will have some X-ray evidence of the disease. OA usually affects the larger, weight-bearing joints such as the hips, knees and spine but smaller joints such as the fingers and elbows can be involved too. The exact cause of OA is not fully understood. It used to be thought of as a degenerative disease due to wear and tear on the smooth cartilage lining the joints, but is now believed to result from an active disease process. One theory is that imbalances occur in normal repair mechanisms so that damaged cartilage is broken down and not properly replaced. This allows underlying areas of bone to rub together so that affected joints become increasingly painful and stiff.

Treatment

A number of supplements can relieve the pain and stiffness of arthritis. In general, these supplements tend to help at least two out of three people, but it is difficult to predict in advance which will suit a particular person – it is a question of trial and error to find the best one for each individual sufferer.

Eating a diet rich in the antioxidant vitamins C and E seems to slow the progression of osteoarthritis and reduce pain by damping down inflammation. Eat at least five servings of fruit or vegetables per day, and consider taking an antioxidant supplement too. Antioxidants such as vitamin C help to quench inflammation, and are therefore remarkably effective in reducing cartilage loss and in slowing the progression of osteoarthritis.

Research shows that people with moderate to high intakes of vitamin C are three times less likely to develop knee pain or to see their knee osteoarthritis worsen than those with low intakes. This effect is seen less strongly with betacarotene, and also with vitamin E but so far, only in men. Interestingly, another study found vitamin E was twice as effective as a placebo or simple analgesics in reducing pain levels in osteoarthritis.

Omega-3 fish oils have an anti-inflammatory effect to reduce pain in osteoarthritis. They are rich sources of beneficial essential fatty acids needed to produce anti-inflammatory substances in the body to reduce pain and swelling. Try to eat oily fish (e.g. salmon, herrings, mackerel, sardines) twice or three times a week, and consider taking an omega-3 fish oil supplement. Cod liver oil also contains omega-3 fish oils plus vitamins A and D which are beneficial for bones. Choose a cod liver oil described as 'high strength' or 'extra high strength' for the most effective anti-inflammatory action. A recent study investigating the relationship between dietary supplementation with cod liver oil and the intensity of pain in people with joint problems found that those taking cod liver oil seemed to experience less pain overall.

Glucosamine sulphate is rapidly gaining a reputation for helping to boost joint healing and relieve pain due to sports injuries or arthritis. Its effects may be improved by combining it with chondroitin, another substance needed for cartilage repair. Another form of sulphur – known as MSM (methyl-sulphonyl-methane) – is also becoming increasingly popular for joint problems.

Extracts of New Zealand green-lipped mussel (*Perna canaliculus*) have been taken for arthritis and rheumatic pain since 1973. They help to reduce inflammation in joints and can reduce the pain and swelling of osteoarthritis. They contain substances known as glycoproteins, which are thought to work by preventing white blood cells from moving into the joints, where they would have released powerful chemicals making pain and swelling worse.

Some evidence suggests that extracts may help to reduce the pain and swelling of osteoarthritis by 35–45 per cent and have been shown to outperform non-steroidal anti-inflammatory drugs (NSAIDs) such as ibuprofen and indomethacin. In a trial of 86 patients, 67 per cent of those with rheumatoid arthritis and 35 per cent of those with osteoarthritis benefited. As a bonus, green-lipped mussel extracts seem to have a protective action to reduce the incidence of ulcers when combined with NSAIDs.

Extracts from the root of a South African creeping plant devil's claw (*Harpagophytum procumbens*) contain anti-inflammatory chemicals that help to reduce pain and improve mobility in many people with OA.

Aloe vera contains anti-inflammatory chemicals that can help to relieve pain, swelling and stimulate regeneration of damaged tissues.

Feverfew, a herb traditionally used to relieve migraine has also been found to help reduce the pain of arthritis. Its leaves contain an anti-inflammatory agent called tanetin which seems to interfere with the production of inflammatory compounds.

Bromelain has a good anti-inflammatory action, while some people find boswellia helpful.

Other self-help measures to consider include:

- losing any excess weight
- taking regular, gentle exercise such as walking, cycling or swimming within the limits of discomfort, to maintain your strength and mobility
- applying hot or cold compresses – packs that are warmed in the microwave or cooled in the fridge are widely available from chemists
- ensuring that your mattress is not overly hard or too soft as either can make joint pain worse.

See also **B3, CMO, Copper, Evening primrose oil, Flaxseed oil, Hempseed oil, Histidine, Maitake, Nettle, Olive leaf, Olive oil, Sarsaparilla, Selenium, Wild yam**

Asthma

Asthma is a long-term, inflammatory disease of the lungs. Researchers are uncertain as to what exactly causes it, but the inflammation is thought to be linked to an abnormal immune response. The lining of the airways becomes red and swollen and produces increased amounts of mucus. This triggers airway spasm producing symptoms of cough, wheezing and shortness of breath. Once irritation has set in, the airways become increasingly sensitive to a wide range of triggers such as viral infections, exercise, emotion and exposure to the cold. Even between attacks, when symptom-free, the airways are still red and inflamed. This inflammation produces irritation and spasm of the airways that triggers wheeze and difficulty breathing. It also increases production of secretions that block the airways and interfere with breathing – even if the tubes are fully dilated. To relieve this, an inhaler such as salbutamol is needed more than once a day, and normally a preventer inhaler (such as cromoglycate, nedocromil or inhaled steroids) is used every day as well. The preventer inhaler is needed to damp down hidden inflammation in the lungs as the reliever can only open up the airways to make it easier to breathe – it can't tackle the underlying inflammation that causes the irritation in the first place.

Treatment

General measures in the treatment of asthma include avoiding cigarette smoke, and keeping the home as dust-free as possible by dusting with a damp cloth and using a vacuum cleaner with a special filter. Special covers over mattresses, pillows and duvets are recommended to overcome bed mites, and any foods that seem to trigger attacks should be avoided.

Some researchers believe that the increased incidence of chronic inflammatory diseases such as asthma is linked with an imbalance of dietary fats. Dietary polyunsaturated fats (PUFAs) are of two main types, omega-3 PUFAs derived from fish oils and omega-6 PUFAs derived from vegetable oils. Ideally, we need a balanced intake of omega-3s and omega-6s, but the average British diet currently contains seven times more omega-6s than omega-3s. Eating more fish may be beneficial – aim for 100 g oily fish twice or three times a week, or try omega-3 fish oil, flaxseed or hemp seed oil supplements.

Asthma has also been linked with low dietary levels of selenium, magnesium or B6 in some studies, while those with high intakes of antioxidants (vitamin E or vitamin C) seemed to have the lowest risk – possibly because these antioxidants help to protect omega-6 PUFAs from the oxidation that is thought to trigger inflammation. At least seven studies have shown that people with asthma have reduced symptoms and improved breathing when taking 1–2 g vitamin C daily, and vitamin B6 supplements may help to improve asthma by reducing the severity and frequency of attacks. Boswellia is used to treat chronic inflammatory conditions such as asthma, and has recently been shown to have anti-inflammatory properties, while red clover, known mainly for its oestrogenic actions, also has anti-spasmodic properties and is used to treat asthma.

Other supplements that can be helpful include bromelain, magnesium, oregano, antioxidants such as the flavonoids in quercetin and green tea, and the anti-inflammatory action of liquorice.

Atherosclerosis

Healthy arteries are elastic to even out the peaks and troughs of blood pressure produced as the heart pumps blood around the circulation. Atherosclerosis, or hardening and furring up of the arteries, starts early in life, usually in the teens, and is triggered by normal wear-and-tear damage to the artery walls, which reduces their elasticity. Once the damage occurs, small cell fragments in the bloodstream – known as platelets or thrombocytes – stick to the damaged area and form a tiny clot. These platelets release chemical signals to stimulate healing of the damaged area, but if excessive damage continues (e.g. as a result of high blood pressure, raised cholesterol levels or lack of antioxidants in the diet) the area becomes infiltrated with a fatty porridge-like substance that builds up to form a plaque (atheroma).

Antioxidants protect dietary fats in the circulation from oxidation, and it is only oxidised fats that are taken up by scavenger cells and transported into the blood vessel lining where they become 'stuck'. Although the main culprits were thought to be saturated (animal) fats, increasing evidence suggests that an imbalance of polyunsaturated fatty acids (PUFAs) plus lack of antioxidants are to blame.

Unlike saturated fats, polyunsaturated fatty acids have a molecular structure containing spare double bonds. This makes them highly reactive and more susceptible to chemical changes such as oxidation. This chemical change produces toxic substances known as lipid peroxides that are linked with atherosclerosis.

There are two main types of polyunsaturated fat:

- omega-3 PUFAs mainly derived from fish oils
- omega-6 PUFAs mainly derived from vegetable oils

The body handles omega-3 and omega-6 oils in different ways so that omega-3 fish oils have a thinning effect on your blood and are good for the heart and circulation, while excess omega-6 PUFAs are thought to be linked with inflammatory processes in the body. Saturated (animal) fats traditionally thought of as the baddies when it came to coronary heart disease are now thought to be less important – especially if your intake of antioxidants is high .

Two types of cholesterol are found in the circulation: low-density lipoprotein or LDL-cholesterol is the harmful form that is linked with hardening and furring up of the arteries (atherosclerosis), and high-density lipoprotein or HDL-cholesterol is the beneficial type which protects against coronary heart disease by transporting LDL-cholesterol away from the circulation. Although total cholesterol levels may be raised, it is the ratio of total cholesterol to beneficial HDL-cholesterol which is important. It is only a total cholesterol/HDL ratio of above 4.5 that is thought to be associated with increased risk of coronary heart disease. Even then, it is not so much the raised cholesterol that is harmful, but a lack of dietary antioxidants which protect circulating fats from oxidation. Only oxidized fats are thought to enter vessel walls to cause atherosclerosis.

Another type of fat, triglyceride, also increases the risk of circulatory problems if it is raised. The levels of these blood fats are related to diet and exercise levels, but heredity also has a significant role.

A raised level of the amino acid homocysteine damages artery walls to trigger atherosclerosis and is now recognized as an important risk factor for coronary heart disease and stroke. Normally, homocysteine levels are tightly controlled by three different enzymes that convert homocysteine to cysteine – a safe end product that promotes cell growth. Two of these three enzymes depend on adequate intakes of folic acid, vitamins B6 and B12 for optimal activity. When these nutrients are lacking, homocysteine levels rise. Genetic mutations also affect enzyme activity and an estimated one in ten people inherit levels of homocysteine that triple the risk of cardiovascular disease. One in 160,000 inherit extremely high homocysteine levels with 30 times the risk of premature heart disease, and post-menopausal women seem less able to process homocysteine so their levels also build up.

Treatment

High levels of homocysteine can be reduced by taking folic acid supplements (400–650 mcg a day) plus vitamins B6 and B12. Although diet should always come first, synthetic forms of folic acid found in supplements and fortified foods (e.g. breakfast cereals) are more bioavailable than those found in natural food sources (such as green leafy vegetables) which are in the less easily absorbed polyglutamate (folate) form.

Antioxidants (vitamins A, C and E for example) protect circulating cholesterol molecules from oxidation which increases the risk of atherosclerosis. Vitamin C is a powerful antioxidant in body fluids. Many studies, including one lasting ten years and involving 11,000 people, found that men with the highest intakes of vitamin C had a 40 per cent lower risk of developing coronary heart disease and a 35 per cent lower risk of dying from it. For women with the highest intakes of vitamin C, there was a 25 per cent lower risk of coronary heart disease.

A recent study suggested that people taking high-dose vitamin C supplements may experience increased arterial thickening in some parts of the body – especially the neck.

This was initially interpreted with alarm, but independent experts feel this is probably a reversal of the thinning that occurs with age, and is actually beneficial – it is one of the benefits associated with taking hormone replacement therapy (HRT), for example.

Vitamin E is a powerful antioxidant in body fats, and helps to protect fats in the circulation from oxidation. Researchers believe this slows the progression of atherosclerosis and reduces the risk of fatty plaques in the coronary arteries rupturing and triggering the formation of a blood clot (coronary thrombosis). Vitamin E gained widespread medical acceptance following results of the Cambridge Heart Antioxidant Study (CHAOS) in 1996 (*see under* E). As a result, many physicians now recommend high-dose vitamin E supplements for those at risk of a heart attack.

Garlic powder tablets have been shown in a number of clinical trials to reduce harmfully raised cholesterol levels by an average of 11 per cent (and up to 25 per cent), and triglyceride levels by an average of 13 per cent (and up to 32 per cent). The trials used doses of 600–900 mg garlic powder tablets a day for between three and 16 weeks. Garlic powder tablets seem to be more effective than garlic oil capsules – in one randomized trial of 80 patients, garlic powder tablets reduced cholesterol levels by 11 per cent and garlic oil by only 3 per cent over four months. Other interesting studies have found that garlic powder tablets can lower a raised blood pressure and increase the elasticity of the aorta so the heart has to work less hard to pump blood out into the body. An important recent study followed 152 patients for over 4 years and found that garlic tablets could reduce and even reverse atherosclerosis.

Omega-3 fish oil supplements also have beneficial effects on blood fats by raising beneficial HDL-cholesterol and lowering harmful LDL-cholesterol.

Ginkgo biloba extracts can improve peripheral circulation due to atherosclerosis by up to 50 per cent. Ginkgo is particularly useful for atherosclerosis that causes poor blood flow to the legs so that calf pain develops on exercise (intermittent claudication).

Ginkgo leaves contain unique chemicals – ginkgosides – that improve blood flow throughout the body to help offset the effects of atherosclerosis. It is particularly useful for those with pain in one or both calves brought on by exercise (intermittent claudication due to lack of blood and oxygen reaching the calve muscles).

The flowering tops and berries of the hawthorn (*Crataegus oxycantha* and *C. monogyna*) contain chemicals that normalize the cardiovascular system, and can:

- relax peripheral blood vessels
- dilate the coronary arteries, improving blood circulation to heart muscle
- discourage fluid retention
- slow and possibly even reverse the build-up of atheromatous plaques.

Hawthorn also increases the strength and efficiency of the heart's pumping action. Hawthorn preparations are so effective in helping angina and hypertension that it is being researched in the search for new drugs.

All the usual health guidelines also apply. These include:

- stopping smoking, which is a powerful trigger for atherosclerosis

- following a healthy, low-salt, low-fat, high-fibre diet
- maintaining a healthy weight
- taking regular brisk exercise (prolonged brisk walking, for example, has been shown to significantly reduce blood fat levels following a high-fat meal compared with not exercising; this effect was noticed even when exercise was taken as much as 15 hours before the meal, and when exercise was taken 90 minutes after the meal).

See also **Arginine, Carnitine, Grapeseed, Silicon**
Related entry: **Cholesterol – raised**

Attention deficit hyperactivity disorder

Attention deficit hyperactivity disorder (ADHD) – also known as hyperactivity and hyperkinetic syndrome – is a persistent and severe abnormality affecting psychological development in which a child is continually inattentive, restless and impulsive so they are unable to sit down quietly even when overly tired or exhausted. Any stimulation leads to feverish excitement and attempts to calm the child frequently result in screaming fits and hysteria.

ADHD comes on in early childhood with symptoms often appearing before the age of two, usually before five, and necessarily by the age of seven for diagnosis. Four times as many boys are affected as girls, and it is estimated to affect just over 1 per cent of boys of primary school age. Some children improve at puberty, and around 40 per cent seem to 'outgrow' ADHD. Behavioural problems often persist into adolescence and adulthood however, with insomnia, abnormal thirst and difficulty in concentrating.

The exact cause of ADHD is poorly understood, but many researchers believe that diet plays a significant part – both during foetal development and in childhood. Some children with ADHD seem to be lacking in essential fatty acids (EFAs) which belong to a group of oils called long-chain polyunsaturated fatty acids (LCPs). While the body can make small amounts of EFAs from other dietary fats, these are rarely sufficient to meet our needs and dietary intakes remain important.

Children with ADHD seem to be lacking in EFAs. Boys are more commonly affected than girls, and this fits in with the observation that males in general have higher requirements for dietary EFAs than females. Another link is that lack of essential fatty acids causes excessive thirst which is a symptom commonly found in children with ADHD.

Low maternal intakes of EFAs during pregnancy have also been linked with an increased risk of the baby developing problems such as ADHD, dyslexia, autism and schizophrenia. Although lack of EFAs may not be the root cause of these conditions, it could trigger them in children predisposed through other genetic or environmental factors.

Treatment

Taking EFA supplements during pregnancy, therefore, may help to reduce the risk of a baby developing ADHD although this is not yet proven.

There are two main groups of EFAs: omega-3 fatty acids and omega-6 fatty acids. Children with ADHD seem to be deficient in both. Lack of omega-3 EFAs is linked with behavioural and learning problems, while lack of omega-6s seems to lower immunity. Omega-3s are found in highest quantities in oily fish (mackerel, herring, salmon, trout, sardines, pilchards and in certain algae on which these fish feed). Evening primrose oil and omega-3 fish oil supplements are also excellent sources and the Hyperactive Children's Support Group have found that 80 out of 96 children given evening primrose oil supplements no longer showed hyperactive behaviour. Fewer infections and improvements in allergic conditions such as asthma and eczema were also noted.

Beneficial omega-6 EFAs are found in plant oils, e.g. nuts, seeds, whole grains and dark green, leafy vegetables.

In one study, when a group of hyperactive children were given a diet free from added sugar, artificial colourings and flavourings, monosodium glutamate, preservatives, chocolate and caffeine, parents recorded a 58 per cent improvement in their children's behaviour compared with little improvement in those not on the diet.

The Hyperactive Children's Support Group suggest following a nutritional, wholefood diet containing plenty of fresh fruit and vegetables – preferably organic – which excludes as many artificial colourings, flavourings, preservatives and sweeteners as possible. Once the child is used to a wholefood diet, they recommend gradually cutting out foods containing white flour and sugar and replacing these with more nutritious foods. Food should only be sweetened when absolutely necessary, with raw Barbados sugar, muscovado sugar, honey or molasses used sparingly.

Some researchers in the USA have found that the behaviour of children and adults with attention deficit hyperactivity disorder improved when taking glutamine supplements.

See also **5-HTP, Magnesium**

Back pain

Back pain is common, and those most likely to suffer include those whose work involves heavy lifting or carrying, or people who spend long periods of time sitting in one position or bending awkwardly. Almost any day-to-day activity can bring it on, however, including housework, gardening and over-vigorous exercise. If you are overweight and unfit, with poor muscle tone, you are also at increased risk as apart from having to support a heavier load, your back will not receive the support it needs from your abdominal muscles.

Back pain most commonly affects the lower, lumbar region of the spine. Most cases are due to excessive strain on muscles, ligaments and small joints. As well as discomfort from the damaged tissues, the surrounding muscles may go into spasm so that pain and tenderness spread over a larger area. More severe symptoms will occur if the soft, jelly-like centre of an intervertebral disc ruptures through the outer fibrous coating under pressure – a condition popularly known as a slipped disc. The prolapsed centre of the disc may press on the root of a spinal nerve to cause muscle weakness, pins and needles, spasm and pain in the back. If the sciatic nerve is irritated, pain will shoot down the leg.

Non-specific back pain is usually treated with simple painkillers such as aspirin, paracetamol and codeine. If necessary, muscle-relaxant drugs can be taken to reduce painful spasms and applying hot or cold compresses will also help. Bed rest is no longer recommended routinely (except in cases of a slipped disc) as keeping active has been shown to restore sufferers to normal daily life more quickly. Early mobilization is essential to prevent the back from 'seizing up'. Manipulation from a chiropractor or osteopath is often the most effective treatment and should be performed as early as possible – preferably within six weeks of the original symptoms.

Treatment

To help strengthen bones, it is important to take a bone-building supplement containing calcium, magnesium, manganese, vitamin C and vitamin D. Boron and vitamin K are also helpful, while evening primrose oil increases calcium absorption and deposition in bone.

The following supplements also tend to help two out of three people.

- Omega-3 fish oils contain essential fatty acids that act as building blocks for hormone-like substances (prosta-glandins) that help to damp down inflammation. Taking omega-3 fish oils, or extra-high-strength cod liver oil supplements can help to improve back stiffness and pain.

- Glucosamine sulphate or MSM-sulphur can relieve pain and stiffness and improve symptoms related to a prolapsed intervertebral disc by strengthening the central nucleus pulposus of the disc.

- Back pain due to inflammation is often helped by supplements containing raw extracts of New Zealand green-lipped mussel. Research suggests that these contain substances (glycoproteins) that prevent immune cells from entering inflamed joints and releasing powerful inflammatory chemicals that would make pain worse.

- Devil's claw and bromelain are also helpful in relieving pain.

Bacterial vaginosis

Anaerobic or bacterial vaginosis (BV) is due to an imbalance in the bacteria normally found in the vagina. Healthy *Lactobacilli* are reduced, or lost, and other bacteria that do not need oxygen to survive (anaerobes) start to flourish. In some studies, BV was found to affect as many as one in four women and has been linked with increased risk of miscarriage during the first three months of pregnancy, and with pre-term labour. The exact cause of BV is unknown, and while it is not classed as a sexually transmissible disease, it is more common in sexually active women.

BV often seems to arise spontaneously around the time of menstruation and then resolves mid-cycle. Because of their strange metabolism, anaerobic bacteria produce chemicals that can cause irritation, an unpleasant fish odour – especially after sex – soreness, and a heavy discharge, although 50 per cent of women do not notice any appreciable symptoms. BV can also irritate male sexual partners if condoms are not used.

Medical treatment is with antibiotics (metronidazole tablets/gel or clindamycin cream) but unfortunately, it often seems to recur.

Treatment

Replenishing levels of healthy *Lactobacillus acidophilus* bacteria by smearing on live, bio yoghurt (natural flavour!) inserted on a probiotic pessary and by taking a probiotic oral medication may help to prevent recurrences.

If general immunity is low, a vitamin and mineral supplement providing around 100 per cent of as many micro-nutrients (including iron) as possible should be helpful. It is also worth considering taking an immune-supporting supplement such as echinacea to boost white cell function.

See also **Probiotic supplements**

Bell's palsy

Bell's palsy is a weakness of muscles on one side of the face due to temporary paralysis of the facial nerve. The exact cause is unknown, but it is believed to be due to a viral infection which causes inflammation and swelling of the facial nerve as it passes through a narrow channel in the temporal bone. Pain behind the ear is common at the onset and there may be loss of taste on the front two thirds of the tongue. Left untreated, Bell's palsy usually starts to improve within two weeks but may take up to 12 months to resolve fully. Around one in seven sufferers retain some residual, permanent weakness.

To encourage full recovery, early treatment with prednisolone or adreno-corticotrophic hormone (ACTH) may be recommended at the onset of symptoms. Anti-viral drugs are sometimes tried but their efficacy is unknown. The eyelids may need to be temporarily closed (either with a pad or by stitching) to prevent drying and ulceration of the cornea. Electrical stimulation of muscle fibres is often helpful, and can also predict which patients are unlikely to recover. In these cases, cosmetic surgery may be suggested to improve the appearance of severe, permanent paralysis. It may also be possible to rejoin some of the remaining nerves to the facial nerve to help it to start working again.

Treatment

Taking a vitamin B complex, including high-dose vitamin B12 may help to improve nerve function as it is needed for the formation of healthy myelin nerve sheaths and the conduction of messages along nerves.

Benign prostatic hyperplasia (BPH)

The prostate is a male gland found at the base of the bladder, wrapped around the urinary outlet. Once a man reaches the age of 40, the prostate gland naturally starts to enlarge – a condition known as benign prostatic hyperplasia (BPH). When this happens urinary outflow can be compressed to cause symptoms such as:

- difficulty in starting to pass water
- a weak urinary stream
- starting and stopping in mid-flow
- passing water more often, especially at night
- a feeling of not having emptied the bladder fully
- dribbling incontinence.

One in three men over the age of 50 experiences symptoms, and up to 80 per cent of all adult males will eventually need treatment.

Treatment

If diagnosis of BPH has been confirmed by a doctor (it is not advisable to self-diagnose), extracts from saw palmetto berries are a good form of treatment. Trials comparing the effectiveness of saw palmetto berry extracts with prescription drugs found the natural treatment produced similar results but with less risk of adverse side effects. The exact way in which saw palmetto works is unknown, but it seems to change the hormone environment of the prostate gland so that its muscle cells relax, and the tissue directly encircling the urinary outlet shrinks. The overall size of the gland does not change significantly, however.

The following can also be beneficial: **Lapacho, Nettle Root, Pfaffia, Pumpkin seeds, Rye pollen, South African star grass.**

Related entry: **Prostate problems**

Bereavement

Bereavement is one of the worst emotional experiences anyone has to bear. Everyone copes differently with bereavement and, in time, it usually becomes easier to accept what has happened.

Treatment

Kava kava helps to overcome anxiety and may be taken to help the bereaved get through the early days. For difficulty in sleeping, valerian and lemon balm are a good combination. Sometimes, people who have suffered a bereavement slowly sink into depression until they are overwhelmed with feelings of sadness, loneliness and despair. When this happens, anti-depressant drugs are the most effective route to recovery, by correcting imbalances of certain chemicals in the brain. St John's Wort (*Hypericum perforatum*) is a natural herbal extract that is as effective in treating mild to moderate depression as many prescribed medications. However it can interact with prescribed medications so it should be taken under medical guidance.

Black tongue

Discolouration of the tongue can result from substances in the diet (e.g. liquorice) or from certain mouthwashes containing chlorhexidine gluconate. A condition known as 'black hairy tongue' can result from the proliferation of pigment-producing (chromogenic) micro-organisms causing brown staining of elongated taste bud formations (filiform papillae) on the tongue. Why this overgrowth occurs is unknown but it has been linked with heavy smoking and the use of antiseptic mouthwashes. Soreness of the tongue (glossitis) can be due to iron-deficiency anaemia, lack of B group vitamins (especially B2, B3 or B12), and Candida yeast infections.

Treatment
Using a tongue scraper will help to reduce any build-up of bacterial colonies. Try taking a B group vitamin.

See also **Myrrh, Sage**

Blepharitis

Blepharitis is an inflammation of the eyelids whose symptoms can include redness, soreness, itching and scaling. It can be a difficult condition to treat as it often recurs, especially during times of stress.

Allergic reactions may play a role, so it is worth stopping using all creams, cosmetics, perfume/colognes and shampoos, then gradually re-introducing them one at a time to see if any retrigger the problem. Contact lenses should not be worn until the problem has resolved as some lens solutions and saline preservatives may be involved. Hypoallergenic toiletries should be used wherever possible – the gentlest shampoos, soaps and moisturizers are those formulated for newborn babies.

Treatment

Sometimes all that is needed is gentle removal of the scales around the lashes using gauze or cotton buds and warm saline solution or a very dilute solution containing baby shampoo. Herbal practitioners suggest bathing the eye with a compress soaked in dilute infusions of chamomile. Use separate compresses and eyebaths for each eye.

Aloe vera gel may be applied to damp down inflammation. It is also worth considering taking 1 g vitamin C, three times a day (non-acidic Ester-C for those who are prone to indigestion) along with an omega-3 fish oil supplement as these are helpful in reducing inflammatory skin conditions. Echinacea tablets/tincture by mouth help to boost general immunity. If eyes also feel dry, artificial tears (available over the counter) will help.

Bloating

Although bloating is commonly linked with overindulgence or eating a rich diet, it can also occur after eating relatively little in those with functional disorders of the gut such as irritable bowel syndrome (IBS). If symptoms have been present for a while, it is important to seek medical advice to find out the cause, but assuming a clean bill of health is given, symptoms may be related to insufficient bile production in the liver which is needed to emulsify dietary fats before they can be absorbed.

Treatment

Extracts of globe artichoke leaves (*Cynara scolymus*) stimulate bile production and can quickly relieve bloating without side effects. It is also helpful when bloating and indigestion are due to overly spicy food or drinking alcohol. Other natural treatments that can help to reduce bloating include dandelion leaf and root, guarana, drinking peppermint, ginger or fennel tea, taking probiotic supplements containing digestive bacteria (e.g. *Lactobacilli*), probiotic food substances (e.g. fructo-oligosaccharides), aloe vera juice or colloidal silicol gel.

Bronchitis

There are two types of bronchitis: acute and chronic.

Acute bronchitis is a relatively mild inflammation of the larger lung airways – the bronchi – and can be due to a viral or bacterial infection. Symptoms are more common in winter and often follow on from a cold. They are due to inflammation of mucous membranes lining the bronchi, which swell and secrete increased amounts of yellow-green mucus. Airway narrowing can cause shortness of breath, cough and wheeze and you may notice a hoarse voice. Feelings of soreness or rawness are often felt behind the breast bone (sternum) and a low-grade fever may occur. In most cases, symptoms come on suddenly and clear up quickly within a few days and often, it sounds much worse than it feels.

Symptoms may be relieved by steam inhalations (plain, or with added essential oils of menthol or eucalyptus) and by drinking plenty of fluids – this helps to loosen the phlegm so you can cough it up more easily.

Those most at risk include smokers, people who are exposed to atmospheric pollution, babies, the elderly and people with a pre-existing lung disease such as chronic bronchitis or asthma.

In contrast to acute bronchitis, chronic bronchitis is a long-term lung problem which is diagnosed when phlegm is coughed up:

● on most days
● during at least three consecutive months
● for at least two years.

The commonest causes of chronic bronchitis are smoking cigarettes and exposure to industrial pollution. Long-term inflammation of the bronchi results in widespread stiffening, narrowing and obstruction of the airways which, together with increased secretions, makes a secondary bacterial infection (i.e. acute bronchitis) more likely. Other symptoms of chronic bronchitis include cough, breathlessness, wheezing and sometimes chest pain or coughing up blood. The last two symptoms should always be investigated to rule out other causes.

Smoking also causes widespread emphysema (overstretching and rupturing of air sacs). When emphysema and chronic bronchitis develop together, the condition is often referred to as Chronic Obstructive Airways Disease or COAD.

Treatment

Steam inhalations are helpful and it is important to drink plenty of fluids. Zinc and vitamin C lozenges will help to boost immunity so that sore throat is less likely. Supplements containing echinacea, astragalus, lapacho, reishi, shiitake or maitake are effective in boosting immunity including the activity of white blood cells needed to fight infections. Garlic and olive leaf extracts have natural anti-viral and antibacterial actions. Eucalyptus is also helpful.

Mucus dispersion can be improved by supplements containing N-acetyl cysteine (NAC) – an amino acid that boosts levels of a powerful antioxidant (glutathione) in the respiratory tract. NAC has a pronounced mucus-dissolving action and studies show it can significantly reduce mucus production and associated cough in chronic respiratory conditions such as bronchitis, emphysema and sinusitis. *See also* **Bromelain**.

In general, to help maintain a healthy respiratory system, regular exercise throughout the year is important to improve general fitness. Smoky or polluted atmospheres which can damage airways making infection more likely should be avoided, and smokers should make every effort to stop.

Antibiotics are needed when acute-on-chronic bronchitis develops, as it frequently does. Regular sufferers from bronchitis should speak to a doctor about being immunized against influenza and pneumococcal pneumonia.

Note: a doctor should be consulted by anyone who is susceptible to chest infections (due, for example, to a lung problem such as chronic bronchitis, asthma or emphysema) or if:

- their temperature goes above 38°C
- severe breathlessness develops
- thick, green-coloured phlegm is produced
- symptoms last longer than three days
- there is a pre-existing lung problem
- there is chest pain.

Related entry: **Catarrh – excess**

Bruising

Easy bruising is common in older people, partly due to increased fragility of skin and blood vessels (known as Easy Bruising Syndrome). If this is excessive, it is important to consult a doctor as a blood test may be needed to investigate the possibility of a bleeding tendency.

Treatment
Occasionally, lack of vitamin K can be a cause of easy bruising in older people, and a doctor should be asked about taking supplements containing this. General skin quality can be improved by taking evening primrose oil capsules (at least 1 g a day). Horsechestnut, red vine leaf or gotu kola

extracts which help to strengthen connective tissues supporting blood vessels may help.

Burns

The skin is designed to protect the body from a variety of environmental insults, including excessive heat. If the skin is heated above 49°C, its cells are damaged to cause a burn. If only the top layer of skin is injured, reddening and pain occur to form a first-degree burn. This will heal quickly and the dead cells often peel after a few days (the classic example is sunburn). If the damage is more severe, cells in the deeper layers of the skin are destroyed and a blister forms. This is known as a second-degree burn. Enough live cells remain for regeneration, so the burn usually heals without scarring. If the full thickness of the skin is affected, a third-degree burn results. Extensive treatment, including skin grafts, may be needed and there is a risk of scarring. If second- or third-degree burns cover more than 10 per cent of the body, the effects often trigger clinical shock, where the pulse speeds up and blood pressure falls.

Immerse the burned area in cold, running water as soon as possible. If this isn't possible, soak a clean towel or pillow case in cold water and hold against the burn until pain disappears. Take off any jewellery before the area swells then dress with a clean, non-stick, non-fluffy material such as sterile gauze.

Do not:
- try to remove any clothing that is stuck to the wound
- use adhesive plasters

- apply butter, oil or grease
- try to burst any blisters
- use fluffy dressings (e.g. cotton wool). In an emergency, cling film will help to prevent fluid loss and infection until you can obtain urgent medical attention.

Burns easily become infected. Seek medical advice for anything more than a mild burn, or if burns result from contact with chemicals and electricity.

Treatment
Natural approaches that can help include applying aloe vera gel or neat lavender essential oil to the burns to relieve pain and inflammation. Calendula (marigold) or goldenseal cream may be used for their antibacterial actions. High dose vitamin C supplements are useful for reducing inflammation, and promoting formation of collagen fibres during healing. Vitamin E, zinc, selenium and co-enzyme Q10 can also help the healing process.

Cancer

Cancer will affect an estimated one in three to four people at some time in their life. If you are diagnosed with cancer, you should ideally seek individual advice from both a nutritionist and a herbalist to tailor a plan to your individual needs.

It is usually advisable to follow a low-fat, salt-free, mainly vegetarian diet which is as organic as possible, and to avoid junk food, alcohol and caffeine. Most practitioners advise high-dose vitamin C, (the form known as Ester-C is least likely to produce side effects such as indigestion, as it is acid free) plus other powerful antioxidants such as vitamin E, selenium, green tea, grapeseed and/or pine bark extracts. Other vitamins and minerals such as folic acid and other B group vitamins are also important. Iron is thought to suppress immunity so it may be advisable to avoid supplements containing iron except in cases of anaemia. An immune-boosting supplement such as echinacea, maitake, lapacho (*pau d'arco*) or cat's claw (*Uncaria tomentosa*) may be recommended to improve the destruction of abnormal body cells. Some researchers recommend that cat's claw is stopped two days before until two days after receiving chemotherapy.

Milk thistle is often used to protect the liver when receiving chemotherapy. Glutamine seems to enhance the effectiveness of chemotherapy and radiation treatments while reducing toxicity. Daily doses of around 0.5 g help to decrease infections, weight loss and to improve healing of radiated intestines.

See also **Astralagus, Cat's claw, Echinacea, Lapacho, Maitake, Reishi, Shiitake**

Cancer prevention

Researchers increasingly believe that there are close links between cancer and diet and lifestyle.

Fruit and vegetables are a rich source of protective antioxidants such as carotenoids, vitamins C, E, and mineral selenium. These neutralize harmful chemicals (free radicals) that form as a by-product of normal metabolism. Free radicals can damage genetic material to trigger cancer unless mopped up quickly by high circulating levels of antioxidants. Those people with high intakes of vitamin C (found in citrus and berry fruits), carotenoid pigments (e.g. betacarotene, lycopene found in yellow, orange, green and red fruit and vegetables) and selenium (found in Brazil nuts and fruit and vegetables grown in selenium-rich soils) seem to have a lower risk of developing some cancers.

Unfortunately, dietary antioxidant intakes – especially of selenium – are generally low in the UK where they have halved over the last 20 years. In parts of the world where soil selenium levels are low, the incidence of cancer increases enormously. In a randomized, placebo-controlled double-blind study looking at the effects of 200 mcg selenium supplementation in 974 men, the incidence of a number of cancers – including colon and rectum – were reduced by over 50 per cent. As a result, the blinded phase of the trial was stopped early.

Eating red meat (beef, pork, lamb, sausages, hamburgers, ham, bacon) – especially if fried or barbecued – increases the risk of certain cancers. This is thought to be as a result of chemicals (amines) produced during these methods of cooking. Anti-cancer guidelines suggest eating no more than 140 g red and/or processed meat per day.

High-dose vitamin E has also been shown to decrease the risk of colon cancer, and works synergistically with selenium to improve general immunity. It is therefore worth taking a supplement supplying these. It has also been found that those with highest intakes of folic acid have half their risk of developing colorectal polyps (a risk factor for colonic cancer) and that eating a diet high in fibre and low in sugar and fat (especially a vegetarian diet) also reduces the risk of colonic cancer. Omega-3 fish oils have an anti-inflammatory effect and can inhibit the growth of colonic polyps and may have an anti-cancer action although this is still under investigation. *See also* vitamin **D, Olive oil**.

A variety of strategies will help to reduce the risk of hormonal cancers such as breast or prostate cancer. At least seven to ten servings of fruit and vegetables per day should be eaten – preferably those that are organic. Cruciferous vegetables such as broccoli are especially important as, along with soya, they are rich sources of protective plant hormones known as phyto-oestrogens. Although it is hard to include soy in a Western diet, soya/linseed bread and muesli-style bars are available (or pulses such as chickpeas, kidney, black eye or mung beans are just as good). It is important to ensure a good intake of fibre, and it is also a good idea to take a tablespoon of flax (linseed). It is recommended to eat oily fish at least three times a week and olive oil should be used in cooking and salad dressings. Omega-6 polyunsaturated fats such as those found in margarines should be cut right back and excess sugar should be avoided. Alcohol consumption should be limited to no more than three units per week – especially for pre-menopausal women or those who are taking HRT. *See also* **Grapeseed, Green tea, Olive oil, Pfaffia, Pine bark, Oregano.**

The World Cancer Research Fund recommends the following general guidelines to help lower the risk of cancer.

- Avoid exposure to cigarette smoke (responsible for an estimated 30 per cent of all cancer deaths).
- Follow a healthy, low-fat, high-fibre diet.
- Eat more fruit, vegetables and whole-grain cereals.
- Cut back on intakes of both saturated and unsaturated fat.
- Consume salt-cured, salt-pickled and smoked foods only in moderation.
- Drink alcohol in moderation, if at all.
- Maintain a healthy weight for your height.

Always seek medical advice about any recurring symptoms, and accept invitations for health screening such as mammography and cervical screening.

Candida albicans

Vaginal thrush is common, affecting three out of four women at some time during their lives. It is caused by an overgrowth of a yeast, candida albicans, that is normally present in the vagina in many women without causing obvious harm. Candida spores are in the air and thrive in warm, moist places such as the groin and vagina. Infection can sometimes also be passed on during sexual intercourse. Thrush is more likely to occur around the time of a period due to changes in the acidity of vaginal discharge. It is also more common in women who are pregnant, have uncontrolled diabetes mellitus, or who use oral contraceptives. Candida often occurs after taking antibiotics which kill off the healthy bacteria (e.g. *Lactobacillus acidophilus*) naturally found in the vagina which help to keep disease-causing organisms such as candida at bay. An inborn error of biotin metabolism may also be involved.

Some women suffer repeated bouts, which may be due to slightly reduced levels of iron needed by white blood cells to make the chemicals used to destroy opportunistic infections such as these. This can be diagnosed by a blood test that measures serum levels of ferritin – an iron-binding protein.

Symptoms of thrush vary and can include itching, soreness or burning, a yeasty smell, vaginal discharge, which is sometimes white and cottage-cheese-like, and discomfort during urination and/or intercourse.

Diagnosing candida from symptoms and examination alone is not always accurate as other conditions such as bacterial vaginosis cause similar problems and need different treatment. For any genital symptoms, it is best to visit a genito-urinary medicine clinic for full screening and proper diagnosis.

Treatment

To help keep thrush at bay, avoid getting hot and sweaty – use panty-liners and change them as necessary throughout the day, and avoid wearing tight underwear, especially nylon tights or tight-fitting trousers. Stockings and cotton underwear are recommended. It's worth boiling cotton underwear or hot-ironing underwear gussets because modern low-temperature washing machine cycles do not kill candida spores and re-infection may occur via underclothes. Avoid bath additives, vaginal deodorants or douches which can upset the naturally acidic vaginal environment.

Eat an iron-rich diet and take a multivitamin and mineral supplement containing iron – a vitamin C source such as orange juice will also increase iron absorption from the gut. It can also be helpful if partners use an anti-fungal cream as men can harbour yeast spores and pass infection back without developing symptoms themselves. Some women find it helpful to smear the affected area with natural yoghurt containing a live Bio culture of *Lactobacillus acidophilus* or use acidophilus pessaries. This colonizes the vagina and may help to prevent overgrowth of candida. Bio yoghurt is particularly helpful if thrush is a result of antibiotic treatment. Taking a probiotic supplement to replenish intestinal levels of friendly digestive bacteria will help to suppress candida overgrowth in the gut which is believed to act as a reservoir for recurrent vaginal candida infections. Biotin supplements may also help.

One of the most successful herbal remedies for candida is lapacho – also known as *pau d'arco*. Lapacho is an unusual Brazilian tree with carnivorous flowers that feed on insects, keeping the tree free from infection. Extracts from lapacho bark can increase resistance to infection and are especially active against candida.

Other popular and effective options include grapefruit seed extract and olive leaf extracts. Siberian ginseng (*Eleutherococcus senticosus*) is useful for boosting immunity when under excess stress.

Although there is no scientific evidence to support dietary changes, some women have found it helpful to follow a yeast-free diet. Others avoid alcohol, mushrooms, sugary foods, tea, coffee and chocolate. A wholefood diet of salads, fruit, vegetables, pulses and whole-grain cereals is recommended instead.

Carpal tunnel syndrome

Carpal tunnel syndrome (CTS) occurs when the median nerve becomes pinched as it passes through a bony tunnel in the wrist.

Treatment

Some people with carpal tunnel syndrome (CTS) have a low vitamin B6 level (needed for optimum nerve functioning) and, although supplements are not effective in everyone, the pioneer of B6 treatment for CTS claims that at least 85 per cent of people respond to doses of between 50 and 200 mg daily, with improvement starting in a few weeks, and complete resolution of symptoms occurring within eight to twelve weeks. It is generally recommended that high-dose vitamin B6 is only taken under medical supervision as excess may, in itself, lead to nerve conduction problems.

Vitamin B3 also seems to be important, as are essential fatty acids found, for example in evening primrose oil, which are important for optimal nerve sheath function. Diuretic herbs such as dandelion may relieve symptoms where these are linked with fluid retention, while bromelain may help to reduce inflammation and pain especially when combined with vitamin B6 supplements.

Cataracts

A cataract is an opacity in the normally crystal clear eye lens, caused by changes in lens proteins similar to those that turn cooked egg white cloudy. This results in blurring, sensitivity to sun glare, changes in colour perception, and seeing haloes around light. Most people over the age of 65 have some degree of cataract, which progresses with age and – like macular degeneration – is linked with damaging oxidative reactions. Most cataracts are due to degenerative changes with increasing age, worsened by exposure to ultraviolet light, but sometimes they are triggered by a direct injury to the eye, especially if a foreign object becomes embedded in the lens.

Smokers and anyone who is diabetic or overweight seem more prone to cataracts than others. People with the highest dietary intakes of antioxidants (vitamins C, E, selenium and carotenoids) are less likely to develop cataracts. A major ten-year study of more than 50,000 nurses aged 45–67 found that those whose diet was rich in spinach and carrots or who had been taking vitamin C supplements for ten or more years had up to a 45 per cent lower risk of cataracts than women whose antioxidant intake was poor (i.e. they ate little fruit and vegetables and/or took no supplements).

Treatment

Bilberry extracts are rich in antioxidants and carotenoids and can help to protect against cataracts and macular degeneration of the eye, as well as reducing the progression of cataracts once they have started to appear. Antioxidant vitamins prevent damaging oxidative chemical reactions in the body by mopping up free radicals (oxidizing molecular fragments produced by the metabolism and by smoking). One consultant ophthalmologist claims to have seen cataracts improve in people taking high-dose vitamin C tablets.

See also **B2, B3, Selenium**

Catarrh – excess

Catarrh is excess phlegm, or mucus, produced by the respiratory tract, and is a very common problem.

Treatment

Excess catarrh can sometimes be helped by cutting out dairy products, red meat, wheat and excess refined carbohydrates. Try following a restricted diet for a few weeks, then re-introducing products one at a time to see if any seem to trigger your symptoms. If a particular group of foods is omitted long-term, it is important to seek nutritional advice so that important micro-nutrients such as calcium or iron are not lost.

Excess mucus can be dissolved by supplements containing N-acetyl cysteine (NAC), an amino acid that makes phlegm less viscid (do not take if you have peptic ulcers). Steam inhalations with essential oils of lavender, eucalyptus or tea-tree oil can also help. Avoid exposure to cigarette smoke and other pollutants.

See also **Bromelain, Sarsaparilla, Yerba maté**

Chapped lips

Chapped lips are due to repeated wetting and drying of the skin around the mouth (e.g. due to nervous licking) which removes natural, protective skin oils. Exposure to cold winds is another common cause.

Cracking and soreness at the corners of the mouth where the lips meet may indicate a fungal infection which will respond to an oral anti-fungal gel – ask a pharmacist for advice. Cracked corners can also be a sign of low levels of iron or B group vitamins. If you feel tired, have heavy periods or suspect you are anaemic, seek medical advice.

Treatment
A protective lip salve is essential but choose one that is non-flavoured as toffee or fruit flavours just encourage more licking. Piercing a capsule containing evening primrose oil

and gently rubbing the oil into the sore area and surrounding skin will also soothe and protect. When going out in the cold, apply a protective layer of marigold ointment (or petroleum jelly) on the skin around the lips, and cover your lower face with a scarf.

See also **B2, B6**

Chemotherapy

It is important to seek individual advice from a nutritionist and/or herbal practitioner for support during and after receiving chemotherapy. Checking levels of iron, folic acid and B12 may be recommended as anaemia can cause weakness and lack of stamina after cancer treatment.

Supplements such as milk thistle and high-dose antioxidants may be suggested to help support liver function. Siberian ginseng (*Eleutherococcus senticosus*) has been extensively investigated in Russia, and found to improve energy levels and increase sense of well-being during and following both chemo- and radiotherapy. It also had beneficial effects on immunity during convalescence. Co-enzyme Q10 can boost general energy levels by encouraging oxygen uptake in cells, but it usually takes three weeks – and occasionally up to three months – for energy levels to be noticeably improved. B group vitamins and evening primrose oil may be helpful, while St John's Wort can relieve fatigue associated with low mood.

See also **Astralagus, Glutamine, Lapacho, Maitake, Reishi, Shiitake**

Chickenpox

Chickenpox is a highly infectious illness, to which the majority of adults are immune as a result of exposure during childhood. Unfortunately, when chickenpox does occur in adults, it can be severe and may lead to complications including viral pneumonia. If an adult develops typical vesicles, it is important to consult a doctor as soon as possible, as an anti-viral drug, acyclovir, helps to reduce the duration and severity of adult chickenpox. Treatment must be started early for best results however – preferably within 72 hours of the onset of symptoms.

Treatment
Herbal extracts that boost immunity against viral infections include echinacea, cat's claw (*una de gāto*), reishi, shiitake or maitake. Antioxidants such as high-dose vitamins C, E or olive leaf extract can help to reduce inflammation. Aloe vera gel may be applied to the rash to help soothe and heal.

Related entry: **Shingles**

Chilblains

Chilblains are triggered when small arteries go into spasm on exposure to cold. This reduces the flow of oxygen and nutrients to tissues to produce the classic, itchy, inflamed lesions. Interestingly, women are six times more likely to suffer than men.

Treatment

Hands and feet should be massaged daily with a good moisturizing skin cream containing evening primrose oil and/or aloe vera. Eat plenty of oily fish (e.g. salmon, sardines, herrings, mackerel) which help to damp down inflammation as well as having a useful thinning effect on blood. Fish oil supplements may also be taken. Garlic powder tablets reduce the risk of chilblains by improving circulation through a thinning effect on blood, and by dilating small arteries in the skin. Ginkgo biloba also increases circulation to the extremities and may be taken together with garlic for additional benefit. Ginger also has a beneficial warming effect and some supplements combine all three extracts.

In addition, avoid tight, restrictive clothing, exercise regularly and, when going out in cold weather, wear several layers of thin, loose clothing to trap body heat plus gloves, thick socks, scarf and hat.

Related entry: **Splits in Fingers**

Childbirth

Many midwives recommend raspberry leaf tea or tablets to reduce both the duration and pain of childbirth. Raspberry leaf is thought to strengthen the contraction of longitudinal uterine muscles and should only be taken during the last eight weeks of pregnancy. The homoeopathic remedy, Caulophyllum 30c, is recommended to strengthen uterine contractions, soften the cervix and reduce the need for interventions such as episiotomy, Caesarian or forceps delivery. Take twice a week (but not on consecutive days) from the 37th week of pregnancy, until labour starts. Two other homoeopathic remedies, Arnica 30c and Hypericum 30c, can be taken as soon as labour is established to reduce blood loss, bruising and hasten healing.

See also **Black cohosh, Bromelain**

Cholesterol – raised

Anyone who is told that they have a raised cholesterol level, needs to find out the ratio between beneficial high-density lipoprotein (HDL) cholesterol, which protects against heart disease by transporting fats away from the arteries, and harmful low-density lipoprotein (LDL) cholesterol which is linked with an increased risk of atherosclerosis (hardening and furring up of the arteries – *see* **Atherosclerosis**). A total cholesterol/HDL ratio above 4.5 is associated with increased risk of coronary heart disease.

It is estimated that reducing the average total blood cholesterol level by 10 per cent could prevent over a quarter of all deaths due to coronary heart disease. Research shows that for every 1 per cent rise in beneficial HDL cholesterol, there is a corresponding fall in the risk of CHD of as much as 2 per cent. This seems to be due to reversed cholesterol transport in which HDL moves LDL cholesterol away from the tissues to the liver.

Treatment

Since it is not so much a raised cholesterol that is harmful but a lack of the dietary antioxidants that protect circulating fats from oxidation (only oxidized fats are thought to enter vessel walls to cause atherosclerosis), consuming more of vitamins A, C, E and mineral selenium is important. This seems to protect against atherosclerosis, high blood pressure and stroke.

Taking garlic powder tablets may prove beneficial; in a number of clinical trials they have been shown to reduce cholesterol levels by an average of 11 per cent (and up to 25 per cent), and triglyceride levels by an average of 13 per cent (and up to 32 per cent). A recent study followed 152 patients for over 4 years and found that garlic tablets could reduce and even reverse hardening and furring up of the arteries compared with those not taking them.

Omega-3 fish oils can help to increase the ratio of HDL-cholesterol and lower harmful LDL-cholesterol. Also, research suggests that eating 3 g or more of soluble oat fibre (roughly equal to two large bowls of porridge) per day can lower total blood cholesterol levels by up to 0.16 mm/l by absorbing fats in the gut. This slows their absorption so that the body can handle them more easily. This is a small, but significant change.

In addition to the above, the following supplements have all been used to help people with raised cholesterol levels:
Arginine, Artichoke, B3, Betacarotene, Carnitine, Chitosan, Choline, Chromium, Coenzyme Q10, Conjugated linoleic acid, Devil's claw, Flaxseed oil, Folic acid, Ginseng, Green tea, Gynostemma, Isoflavones, Lecithin, Lycopene, Olive oil, Pfaffia, Probiotics, Psyllium, Reishi, Royal jelly, Shiitake, Turmeric, Wild yam

Chondromalacia patellae

Chondromalacia patellae is a common but painful condition of adolescence in which cartilage behind the patella becomes roughened rather than smooth. The exact cause is unknown, but it usually resolves after a few years. Orthodox treatment is with rest, painkillers, avoiding high heels and warmth.

Treatment

Supplements containing glucosamine sulphate will ensure optimum production of synovial fluid and cartilage, and in one study it was found helpful for athletes with chondromalacia patellae. MSM-Sulphur is also helpful in reducing joint pain. Other supplements such as devil's claw and omega-3 fish oils that are beneficial in treating arthritis are also worth trying.

Chronic fatigue syndrome

Chronic fatigue syndrome, post-viral fatigue syndrome and myalgic encephalomyelitis (ME) are linked with persistent feelings of extreme weakness, tiredness and loss of energy that last at least six months but are not relieved by sleep or rest. The exact cause is unknown and many different factors are thought to be involved, including abnormal immune responses.

Treatment

Antioxidants including high-dose vitamin C and carotenoids may be recommended as well as immune-stimulating herbs such as echinacea, astragalus and lapacho which also have anti-viral actions.

A recent study provided preliminary evidence that B vitamin status, especially pyridoxine (vitamin B6) is low in people with chronic fatigue syndrome and it is therefore worth trying an oral B complex supplement to see if this helps.

Up to 80 per cent of people with chronic fatigue have benefited from taking high doses of evening primrose and omega-3 fish oils which are rich in essential fatty acids.

Levels of CoQ10 naturally start to decline from the age of 20 and taking supplements can improve fatigue – it usually takes three weeks and occasionally up to three months for energy levels to become noticeably increased, however.

St John's Wort (*Hypericum*) is helpful if mild to moderate depression is present.

Liquorice root extracts are often recommended for chronic fatigue syndrome but are not appropriate for everyone and, in some cases, can make the symptoms worse. Liquorice contains substances that reduce the breakdown of some steroid hormones made in the adrenal glands, and so increases levels of the body's natural steroids which can give you a temporary boost. This effect can wear off however, as the adrenal glands produce fewer steroids hormones to compensate. Some practitioners suggest trying liquorice root extracts for a few weeks then switching to another form of adaptogen such as Korean or Siberian ginseng.

Olive leaf extracts have a powerful anti-viral action and they are often helpful for people with chronic fatigue syndrome.

Note: liquorice root extracts should only be taken under supervision of a doctor or medical herbalist, as they can cause side effects of high blood pressure and water retention in some people when used in high doses long term. *See under* **Liquorice**.

See also **Alpha-lipoic acid, Carnitine, Catuaba, Echinacea, Ginseng, Goldenseal, Magnesium, Maitake, Pfaffia, Reishi, Rhodiola, Shiitake**
Related entry: **Tiredness All the Time**

Colds

As many as 200 different viruses can infect the upper respiratory tract to cause symptoms of the common cold. Cold viruses attack the lining of the nose, throat and sinuses which swell and produce increased amounts of mucus and fluids. At first, nasal secretions are clear, but they often turn yellow or green due to pus cells (white blood cells) rushing in to fight the infection. Other symptoms include sore throat, runny nose, watering eyes, coughing and sneezing. Often senses of smell and taste are also affected and a slight fever, headache and muscle pains may be experienced. Symptoms usually last from three to seven days unless complications such as chronic rhinitis, sinusitis or chest infection set in.

Cold viruses are highly infectious and spread through nasal droplets passed on from person to person through coughing and sneezing. If one member of a family becomes infected, it is likely that three quarters of those in the same house will suffer too. Young adults get an average of two to three colds per year while children may suffer as many as eight to 12 colds annually. Once infected with a cold, the body makes specific antibodies against that virus which are secreted into the nasal fluids for at least two years. These will protect against closely related viruses, but will not protect against the many other viruses that can also produce cold symptoms. To make matters worse, cold viruses frequently change their surface markers, so that as soon as the immune system gets to grips with one, it could mutate enough to cause problems again next time it is encountered.

Colds are common in winter but if your immune system is in the peak of health you can usually shrug them off with either no symptoms or only very mild ones. And if symptoms do strike, you can take several relatively simple steps to ensure you recover as quickly as possible.

To help prevent a cold, stress levels should be kept to a minimum. Avoid becoming overtired and avoid exposure to cigarette smoke which damages nasal linings to make infection more likely. Eat a healthy, wholefood diet including five portions of fresh fruit or vegetables every day to make sure you get enough immune-boosting vitamins, minerals and phytochemicals.

Vitamin C is one of the most popular supplements in winter when the risk of catching a cold is high. Vitamin C supplements have been shown to reduce the risk of catching a cold by as much as 30 per cent because the common cold virus cannot multiply and survive in cells containing high levels of vitamin C, so taking supplements regularly helps to lessen the chance of a cold virus taking hold. Studies involving military troops under training and participants in a 90-km running race, found that taking 600 mg–1 g vitamin C per day halved the risk of developing cold symptoms.

Treatment

Saturate your circulation with vitamin C as soon as you feel symptoms coming on to help boost your resistance and reduce the severity and duration of a cold. Take 1 g of vitamin C (e.g. non-acidic ester-C) every hour until symptoms start to improve up to a total dose of 6 g. Researchers are not certain how it works, but believe its powerful antioxidant action mops up the free radicals producing inflammation.

Sucking lozenges containing zinc gluconate may shorten duration of a sore throat.

Nasal congestion can be relieved by plain steam inhalation, but adding essential oils such as menthol, eucalyptus, cinnamon, or pine will bring immediate relief.

Elderberry extracts contain anti-viral compounds that have been shown in double-blind, placebo-controlled trials to reduce the severity and duration of common cold and influenza infections. In one trial involving 40 patients (children and adults) with viral respiratory infections, 93 per cent receiving elderberry extracts showed significant clinical improvement within two days versus six days with a placebo.

Olive leaf extracts have a powerful anti-viral action against the common cold and influenza. Other supplements used to treat respiratory infections include propolis (a natural antiseptic produced by honey bees) and Siberian ginseng (*Eleutherococcus senticosus*) which is a powerful immune stimulant and, according to Russian research, reduces the incidence of colds, flu and other respiratory infections by 40 per cent in those taking it regularly.

Echinacea may be taken as soon as symptoms start, to boost general immunity. Most studies show that this reduces susceptibility to colds by around a third. In one study of just over 100 people with a common cold, some were given echinacea and others a placebo. After eight weeks, those taking echinacea had longer intervals between recurrent infections, less severe symptoms and a quicker recovery if infection did occur than those taking the placebo. On average, it seems to lengthen the time between infections by around 60 per cent.

While diet should always come first (eat plenty of fresh fruit, vegetables and salads) a general vitamin and mineral supplement that includes selenium (needed to make antibodies) and iron (needed to make infection-fighting chemicals in white blood cells but may be low in non-meat eaters) will guard against micronutrient deficiencies.

Taking garlic powder tablets, may help to protect against viral infections.

See also **Angelica, Bee products – Propolis, Ginger, Goldenseal, Lapacho, Liquorice, Oregano, Peppermint, Perilla, Reishi, Shiitake, Yerba maté**
Related entry: **Catarrh – excess**

Conception

One of the most important times in a baby's development is the first four weeks after conception – often before an expectant mother is even aware she is pregnant. If a baby is undernourished at this critical time, it is more likely that he or she will develop certain illnesses such as coronary heart disease, high blood pressure, stroke or diabetes in later life, possibly because of the way the circulatory system is laid down.

Studies have shown a significant relationship between size of a baby at birth and maternal diet at or around the time of conception. These first few weeks of gestation are a time of rapid division of cells and a baby's brain and spinal cord are often fully developed before the pregnancy has even been recognized.

A woman needs twice as much folic acid during pregnancy as at any other time. Folic acid is essential for copying genetic material correctly during cell division and deficiency during the first few weeks of pregnancy can cause faulty development of the brain or spinal cord – a condition known as a neural tube defect (e.g. spina bifida). Lack of folic acid is also associated with chromosome abnormalities. Taking 400 mcg folic acid a day from the time of first trying to conceive (and preferably earlier) can reduce the risk of conceiving a child with a neural tube defect by as much as 70 per cent. Women with a family history of this condition are advised to take around 10 times as much (4–5 mg a day) – a doctor should be consulted for advice. Foods naturally rich in folic acid should be eaten (e.g. dark green leafy vegetables) and fortified foods (such as cereals).

Vitamin B12 works together with folic acid and deficiency seems to be an independent risk factor for neural tube defects. These are five times more common in babies whose mothers have low blood levels of vitamin B12. Some researchers now suggest that B12 supplements should be included in programmes designed to reduce the risk of neural tube defects.

To guard against other vitamin and mineral deficiencies, a varied, healthy diet should be followed, and a multivitamin and mineral supplement is also worth considering. It is important to take one especially designed for pregnancy as megadoses of some micronutrients (such as vitamin A) can be just as harmful as not enough. A supplement containing essential fatty acids derived from fish (e.g. DHA) which are important for development of your baby's eyes and brain is also helpful.

Supplements containing evening primrose oil help to keep skin in good condition during pregnancy and may reduce the risk of stretch marks.

See also **Agnus castus, Choline, Maca**

Advice for future dads

Men who are planning to father a child should stop smoking – smokers have damaged sperm and are only half as fertile as non-smokers. If they don't stop, at the very least they should take antioxidant supplements – including high-dose vitamin C and E; these are essential to help protect sperm from the damaging effects of cigarette smoke. Alcohol intake should be lowered, and preferably cut out altogether as 40 per cent of male infertility is linked with just a moderate intake of alcohol. A diet rich in natural antioxidant vitamins C, E, carotenoids, selenium and zinc is important, and a multinutrient supplement containing these should also be considered.

See also **Arginine, Astralagus, Carnitine, Co-enzyme Q10, Lecithin, Selenium, Siberian ginseng**
Related entry: **Sperm count – low**

Constipation

Most doctors define constipation as passing bowel motions less than twice a week, or straining more than 25 per cent of the time.

A number of factors can contribute to constipation, including poor fibre intake, poor fluid intake, lack of exercise and poor muscle tone, poor toilet habit (putting off going due to being busy), pregnancy, an underactive thyroid gland and depression. Old age, the side effects of some drugs (e.g. codeine phosphate) or supplements (such as iron), bowel obstruction (a bowel tumour or scar tissue) and abnormal masses (e.g. large fibroid or ovarian cyst) can also be a cause. Chronic constipation and straining at stools can lead to a number of other problems including haemorrhoids, diverticular disease, anal fissures and even rectal prolapse which will in turn make the constipation worse.

To help overcome mild constipation, a wholefood diet is recommended, containing more brown bread, brown rice, cereals, salads, fresh fruit and vegetables for roughage. Apples, bananas, pears, grapes, dried apricots or figs are good snacks, rather than crisps, cakes or biscuits. Five to six prunes soaked in water or cold tea overnight may be eaten for breakfast with natural bio yoghurt, and seeds (such as sunflower, pumpkin, fenugreek, fennel and linseed) should be added to salads and yoghurt for extra roughage.

Natural bulking agents (eg. bran, wheat husks, ispaghula taken with plenty of water) can increase the volume of bowel motions and soften them by absorbing fluid. The seed and husks of psyllium are a safe and effective remedy for constipation, increasing the frequency of bowel movements and making stools softer and easier to pass.

When taking fibre supplements, it is vital to drink plenty of fluid: at least six glasses of mineral water per day to swell up the dietary fibre and get things moving.

Other supplements that will help include probiotic bacteria, dandelion root, dong quai and aloe vera juice. Goldenseal may be recommended to help to normalize muscular action in the bowel.

See also **Oats, Yerba maté**

Coronary heart disease
See **Angina**

Corticosteroids – taking oral treatment

Oral corticosteroids are powerful drugs that damp down inflammation and abnormal immune reactions. Those taking oral corticosteroids may benefit from taking herbs that support liver function. These include dandelion extracts (which are also diuretic and help to reduce fluid retention) and milk thistle extracts (silymarin). Curcumin, which is extracted from turmeric, is also used to support liver function and has been shown to have a strong anti-inflammatory action similar to that of the corticosteroid hydrocortisone in its own right. Herbal preparations that enhance immunity such as echinacea or cat's claw may also be beneficial.

Note: it is important for each individual to consult a medically qualified herbal practitioner for specific treatments tailored to suit them.

Coughs

A cough is the most common symptom of respiratory disease, and is designed as a protective reflex that helps to bring up excess phlegm or irritant substances from the lungs, or which prevents foreign particles from being inhaled. If mucus is brought up, the cough is described as productive. If there is no phlegm, the cough is said to be dry. An irritating, repetitive cough with annoying sensations at the back of the throat is called a tickly cough, while whooping cough is due to a bacterial infection (pertussis) in which long paroxysms of coughing are followed by a desperate whoop as air is drawn back into the lungs. A smoker's cough contains mucky grey discoloured phlegm.

Coughs are usually due to irritation of the airways from dust and smoke, from mucus constantly dripping down from the back of the nose or to infection and inflammation of your upper airways. When somebody with a cold coughs or sneezes over people near by, they will be showered with droplets teeming with millions of infectious viral particles and will then be at risk of catching the infection themselves.

Treatment

In general, a dry, irritating, tickly cough that interferes with sleep may be damped down with a cough suppressant, but a productive cough should not usually be damped down with anti-cough medicines as the excess mucus needs to be brought up. An expectorant can help to bring up infected phlegm from the lungs.

Infective coughs benefit from drinking plenty of fluids (especially hot drinks) to loosen secretions, and from steam inhalations.

Liquorice or slippery elm lozenges may be used to soothe an irritating cough and sore throat, while zinc lozenges can also reduce tickling coughs.

Olive leaf extracts have a natural antibiotic effect and can help cough linked with bronchitis or other infection. Tinctures or teas containing thyme can help to reduce cough and have traditionally been used to help children with whooping cough infection. *See also* **Angelica – European.**

Note: always seek medical advice about a cough that is troublesome, recurrent or associated with coughing up blood, as it may be an important sign of chronic lung infection (e.g bronchitis), inflammation (e.g. asthma) or irritation (e.g. lung cancer).

Cradle cap

Cradle cap (*Crusta lutea*) is a form of seborrhoeic dermatitis that commonly affects newborn infants. In severe cases, a thick circle of yellow, waxy crusts build up on the scalp to resemble a cap. The face, neck, behind the ears and the nappy area can be affected, too. The cause is unknown, but sensitivity to a common skin yeast, *Pityrosporum ovale*, overactivity of sebaceous glands, lack of essential fatty acids and failure of immature skin cells to shed properly, have all been suggested as possibilities.

Treatment

Scales are traditionally loosened by gently massaging in a little warm olive oil, leaving overnight, then washing off next morning using a simple shampoo designed for use on newborns. This should be repeated until all the scales have been loosened and washed off. Brushing the hair with a clean soft-bristled brush will also help, but care should be taken not to scratch the skin. Improvements have also been seen in many babies who are given evening primrose oil drops – whether these are added into their feeds, or rubbed directly on to the affected skin. Nursing mothers can also take evening primrose oil supplements to enrich the essential fatty acid content of their milk.

Cramp

Cramp is the popular name for the painful, excessive contraction of a muscle. It is most commonly felt in the leg, but any muscle can be affected. Cramps are linked with a build-up of lactic acid and other waste products of muscle metabolism – usually during or after physical exercise. It can also be triggered by repetitive movements (as in writer's cramp) and or by sitting or lying in an awkward position. Poor circulation decreases the oxygen supply to muscles and interferes with the flushing away of lactic acids and other chemicals. This can happen at night in elderly people with hardening and furring up of their leg arteries. Night cramps are also common during pregnancy, possibly because of changes in blood circulation. After eating a heavy meal, blood is diverted away from peripheral muscles to aid digestion; this is why swimming immediately after eating is not advised. Excessive sweating, a fever, and hot weather can also cause cramps due to dehydration.

Treatment

Increasing dietary intakes of calcium (low-fat milk, cheese, yoghurt and other dairy products, dark green leafy vegetables) and magnesium (nuts, seafood, dairy products, wholegrains, dark green, leafy vegetables) can help to prevent cramps, and plenty of fluids should be drunk during the day, especially mineral water. Supplements containing calcium, magnesium and vitamin E are also beneficial. Poor circulation may be improved by taking garlic tablets, omega-3 fish oil supplements or ginkgo biloba extracts. Many sufferers also find co-enzyme Q10 – which increases oxygen uptake in muscle cells – effective, especially where circulation is poor.

Cramps can usually be relieved by vigorous massage, applying a hot or cold compress, or by gently stretching the affected muscle. Applying a warm compress will increase circulation and help to bring relief.

Note: seek medical advice if cramps last longer than an hour.

See also **Ginseng, Grapeseed, Pine bark**

Crawling sensations

A prickling sensation that resembles ants crawling over the skin is known as formication. It is a form of pins and needles (paraesthesiae) which may be due to irritation or compression of part of the nervous system. It can also occur in diabetes, liver or thyroid disease, as a side effect of some drugs (e.g. alcohol, cocaine), and from taking excessively high amounts of some supplements (e.g. agnus castus or vitamin B6). Confusingly however, it can also occur due to severe lack of certain micronutrients such as B12 or phosphorus. If sensations persist, it is best to seek medical advice.

Crohn's disease

Crohn's disease is a chronic inflammatory disease of the bowel whose origin is unknown. Some researchers believe it to be an abnormal allergic reaction – possibly to dietary components or an as-yet unidentified bacterial, viral or parasitic infection. Particular foods often exacerbate symptoms, and should be avoided to help reduce symptoms or maintain clinical remission. Unfortunately, it is not always easy to identify the culprits. In one study, the foods most commonly implicated were corn, wheat, milk, yeast, egg, potato, rye, tea, coffee, apples, mushrooms, oats and chocolate. A 19-year study in Japan found that the strongest independent dietary risk factor for Crohn's was an increased intake of animal protein.

Treatment

Malabsorption in Crohn's disease can lead to a variety of vitamin and mineral deficiencies, especially zinc, selenium, B12 and folic acid, and a high-vitamin, low-fibre, low-sugar diet is often recommended. Several studies have found that fish oils are beneficial. In one, enteric-coated fish oil capsules supplying 1.8 g of eicosapentaenoic acid (EPA) and 0.9 g of docosahexaenoic acid (DHA) a day were taken for one year. Only 28 per cent of the 39 patients taking fish oils relapsed to active disease versus 69 per cent of 39 patients receiving a placebo. Aloe vera gel, probiotic supplements containing healthy digestive bacteria (e.g. *Lactobacilli*) and herbal supplements with a natural anti-microbial action such as grapefruit seed extract, goldenseal or garlic are often helpful.

People with Crohn's disease tend to be smokers, and giving up smoking can help to improve symptoms.

See also **Glutamine, Liquorice**

Cystitis

Cystitis is an inflammation or infection of the bladder. It is more common in women than men as the passage from the bladder to the outside world (urethra) is much shorter in females than males (2 cm as compared with around 20 cm), making it easier for infection to pass up the urinary tract. As many as one in two women experiences symptoms at some time during her life.

Symptoms depend on the severity of the infection. In mild cases, only one or two symptoms may occur. In severe cases, a sufferer may develop every symptom. These include:

- burning, stinging or discomfort on passing urine (dysuria)
- a need to rush to the toilet (urgency)
- passing frequent, small amounts of urine
- low abdominal pain or backache
- unpleasant smelling urine which may appear cloudy or blood-stained.

Infection is usually due to bacteria from the vagina or bowel. Seventy per cent of cases are due to *Escherichia coli* which normally lives in the large intestines. Sexual intercourse is one of the commonest triggers of cystitis as it can push bacteria up into the urethra. This is sometimes referred to as honeymoon cystitis. Research suggests that sexual activity can multiply a woman's risk of a UTI by fourteen times. Some attacks of cystitis are thought to be caused by wearing tight trousers or nylon tights as these can increase warmth and humidity which encourage bacterial growth.

Sufferers of recurrent cystitis should be investigated for conditions such as diabetes, anaemia and anatomical abnormalities of the urinary system.

Treatment

Supplements containing natural extracts of the herbs dandelion, bearberry and peppermint can help to prevent the symptoms of cystitis. In one study, 57 women who had suffered at least three episodes of cystitis during the previous year were given either a preparation containing dandelion, bearberry and peppermint or inactive placebo tablets. After 12 months, none of the women taking the herbal product had developed cystitis during treatment, while around one in four of those receiving the placebo suffered at least one bout of cystitis.

Drinking 300 ml cranberry juice daily can almost halve the risk of developing cystitis. Studies also suggest that cranberries contain an anti-adhesin that prevents bacteria from sticking to the urinary tract wall. Concentrated cranberry extracts also seem to be beneficial.

Olive leaf extracts have a powerful antibacterial action and are often helpful for treating cystitis.

Note: Medical advice should be sought in any of the following circumstances:

- symptoms that last longer than a day or keep recurring
- pregnancy
- urine is cloudy or stained with blood
- a fever or uncontrollable shakes develop.

See also **Bromelain, Goldenseal, Lapacho, Olive leaf, Oregano, Peppermint, Sarsaparilla**

Dandruff

Dandruff is the shedding of tiny flakes of skin from the scalp which does not usually cause any discomfort. Seborrhoeic dermatitis produces an itchy, scaly rash on the scalp, and affected skin may look red and inflamed. Dry or greasy scales form around the hairline and in severe cases, a yellow-red crust appears. Seborrhoeic dermatitis is thought to be triggered by a hypersensitivity to the skin yeast,

Pityrosporum ovale. On the face, the red, scaly rash commonly affects the eyebrows and forehead, with greasy scaling of skin folds running between the nose and lips. A wide range of shampoos/lotions are available containing anti-fungal agents (such as pyrithione zinc, selenium sulphide, ketoconazole) which reduce flaking and help to control the number of yeast cells present. Corticosteroids (hydrocortisone, betametasone) may be prescribed to damp down inflammation, while products containing salicylic acid may be used to help loosen scales.

Treatment

A solution of seven drops of rosemary or tea tree essential oil diluted with 1 tablespoon (15 ml) carrier oil should be rubbed into the scalp before washing the hair with a tea tree shampoo.

Inflammation can be reduced by increasing intakes of essential fatty acids – eat more oily fish, nuts, seeds and take evening primrose, flaxseed or omega-3 fish oil supplements. Dry, scaly skin is sometimes linked with a lack of certain vitamins and minerals, especially vitamins A, B2, B3, C, biotin and the minerals iodine, manganese, selenium and zinc. A good multinutrient supplement containing around 100 per cent of the recommended daily amount (RDA) for as many vitamins and minerals as possible might be beneficial. Kelp supplements contain 13 vitamins, 20 essential amino acids and 60 minerals and trace elements, and are a particularly rich source of calcium, magnesium, potassium, iron and iodine so are often recommended to improve any associated hair problems.

Deep vein thrombosis (DVT)

See **Economy-class syndrome**

Depression

Depression is common and affects as many as one in eight men and one in five women at some time during their life. It is caused by an imbalance of chemical messengers in the brain that are responsible for passing signals from one brain cell to another. If levels of one or more fall too low, the brain does not function properly and a variety of psychological and physical symptoms can occur including:

● low mood with crying and sadness
● tiredness or exhaustion
● nervousness, anxiety and agitation
● headache, difficulty in concentrating
● loss of self-esteem and lack of confidence
● low sex drive
● loss of interest in everyday life.

Women are more susceptible to depression than men and are up to three times more likely to suffer due to hormone changes linked with menstruation, childbirth and the menopause. Sadly, at least half of all people with depression do not seek help, yet it is important to address low mood quickly before more serious symptoms set in. It is one of the commonest reasons why people consult their doctor yet it is estimated that only half of all cases are diagnosed, as sufferers either do not realize they have a depressive illness or they are unwilling to seek help. Once a diagnosis or assessment has been made, a doctor should advise on whether antidepressant drugs or referral for a psychiatric assessment are needed.

Treatment

Treatment with standardized preparations of the herb St John's Wort (*Hypericum perforatum*) are effective in treating mild to moderate depression. Standardized extracts contain active ingredients known as hypericins plus antioxidant bioflavonoids and naturally occurring vitamin C. They work at the root cause of mild depression to boost neurotransmitter function and return mood to its natural, even keel.

Research involving over 5000 patients shows that St John's Wort can lift mild depression within two weeks of starting the course – and the optimum effect is reached within six. Three out of four patients showed marked improvement after only five weeks – one in three became symptom-free.

St John's Wort extracts providing 900 mcg hypericin a day are at least as effective as prescribed antidepressants in treating moderate depression, but with much less risk of side effects.

St John's Wort does interact with some prescribed drugs, however, so anyone who is on other medication should check with a doctor or pharmacist before taking it.

Other supplements that may be helpful include 5-HTP (although this should not be taken together with St John's Wort) and kava kava (which can be taken together with St John's Wort to reduce any associated anxiety).

See also **B3, B6, Biotin, Ginkgo biloba, Gotu kola, 5-HTP, Lemon balm, Muira puama, Oats, Phenylalanine, Rhodiola, Siberian ginseng**

Diabetes

Diabetes mellitus occurs when the body is unable to make enough insulin hormone in the pancreas gland. Insulin controls blood sugar levels by helping to transport glucose into liver and muscle cells where it is used as a fuel or stored as a starchy substance called glycogen. Without insulin, glucose builds up in the bloodstream, and the way in which cells process carbohydrate, protein and fat becomes abnormal as a result. People under the age of 40 tend to get Type 1 (or insulin-dependent) diabetes in which they stop making insulin altogether. Older people tend to get Type II (or non-insulin-dependent diabetes) in which they still make some insulin, but not enough to control sugar levels properly.

Diabetes tends to run in families which suggests a heredity factor, although another trigger such as a particular viral infection, high-sugar diet, overweight, overactive thyroid, or certain drugs (e.g. corticosteroids) seems to be necessary for the condition to develop.

Symptoms of untreated Type 1 diabetes include thirst, producing excess urine and weight loss. In Type II diabetes, symptoms are often less specific and can include lack of energy, tiredness, listlessness and easy fatigue. Obesity is also common. High sugar levels also encourage recurrent infections such as cystitis, thrush and boils.

People with diabetes no longer need to follow a special 'diabetic' diet, but are advised to follow the same healthy eating guidelines as everyone else, with a diet that is high in fibre, low in fat, and avoids excess sugar. However, medical advice should always be sought as in some cases tablets or insulin treatment are needed to keep a tight control of blood glucose levels to help prevent long-term complications such as diabetic retinopathy, kidney problems, heart disease and leg ulcers.

Treatment

Bananas, barley, cabbage, lettuce, oats, papaya, turnip and sweet potato are said to help increase natural insulin production.

Garlic and fish oils help to reduce the risk of coronary heart disease, but as fish oils may affect insulin production, blood sugar levels should be carefully monitored.

A vitamin and mineral supplement that includes magnesium, chromium, zinc and vitamin B3 (niacin) – which are involved in glucose metabolism and needed to stabilize blood sugar levels – should be taken.

High-dose antioxidants (vitamins C, E, carotenoids and selenium) help to mop up the excess harmful free radicals produced during diabetes and also seem to improve glucose metabolism, especially high-dose vitamin E (e.g. 800 IU a day). Bilberry extracts may help to protect the eyes from some of the long-term retinal damage that can occur in diabetes and may lower glucose levels.

Pfaffia seems to boost insulin production, and normalize blood sugar levels.

Blood glucose levels must be carefully monitored if using herbal remedies, and they should only be used under the supervision of a medical herbalist/Ayurvedic doctor if prescribed drugs are already being taken to lower blood glucose levels as it is important to avoid hypoglycaemic attacks.

See also **Artichoke, Astralagus, B3, Bilberry, Cayenne, Chromium, Conjugated linoleic acid, Grapeseed, Magnesium, Maitake, Olive oil, Pine bark, Shiitake, Siberian ginseng**

Diarrhoea

Diarrhoea is a loose consistency of stool plus increased frequency of bowel motions.

It occurs when the bowel works overtime, to secrete increased amounts of mucus and to hasten the intestinal contents through. The problem is usually intermittent and associated with other classic symptoms such as distension, bloating, excess wind and sensations of incomplete bowel movement. Diarrhoea may be caused by bacterial, viral, yeast or protozoon infections, irritable bowel syndrome, overuse of laxatives, anxiety or stress, taking antibiotics or inflammatory bowel disease such as Crohn's or ulcerative colitis. It can also occur in bowel obstruction with overflow. Diarrhoea that lasts longer than a week should always be investigated to find out its cause. Severe diarrhoea is debilitating and can even be fatal – especially in infants for whom medical advice should be sought straight away. Large amounts of salts such as sodium and potassium as well as water can be washed out through the bowels, causing dehydration, low blood pressure and even shock.

Treatment

Drink plenty of fluids to counter dehydration, especially if urine production has slowed down and only small amounts of dark urine are passed. Avoid fruit juices and prunes and cut down on milk and dairy product consumption as sometimes temporary lactose intolerance (to milk sugar) can occur.

Enteric-coated garlic powder tablets are often used to treat infective diarrhoea, wind and indigestion. Goldenseal has a natural anti-diarrhoeal effect, helping to normalize muscular action in the bowel; it may be used to treat both constipation and diarrhoea.

Psyllium is a soluble fibre source which helps to bulk up motions and can absorb excess fluid in diarrhoea to help normalize bowel motions.

Probiotic supplements supplying friendly digestive bacteria are essential for those with diarrhoea, especially that brought on by infection or by taking antibiotics. Lack of probiotic bacteria in the intestines encourages abnormal bacterial overgrowth of less beneficial bacteria in the colon (gut dysbiosis) which has been linked with diarrhoea. Probiotic supplements and grapefruit seed extracts have a powerful, protective action against a number of intestinal infections responsible for traveller's gastroenteritis such as *Bacillus cereus*, *Salmonella typhi*, *Shigella dysenteriae*, *Escherichia coli* and *Staphylococcus aureus*.

Manuka honey, mastic gum, olive leaf extracts and lapacho have useful anti-infective actions that may help treat infective diarrhoea. Aloe vera juice and colloidal silicol gel have a useful cleansing and soothing action on the intestines. Raspberry (and blackberry) leaves are traditionally used to make an infusion (tea) that is drunk to relieve pain and spasm plus frequency of bowel movements in diarrhoea.

Slippery elm and ginger are used to sooth the intestinal lining and reduce inflammation, while goldenseal, echinacea and cat's claw help to boost general immunity against infection.

See also **Bilberry, Brewer's yeast, Cayenne, Ginger, Perilla, Raspberry leaf, Sage**

Dieting

Middle-aged spread commonly strikes after the age of 35 due to changes in both physiology and lifestyle. The most significant change is loss of lean muscle tissue, which is mostly replaced with fat. Between the ages of 25 and 70, the average woman loses 5 kg (11 lb) of muscle and her average body fat increases from 27 to 40 per cent. Over the same period, men lose around 10 kg (22 lb) muscle and their body fat increases from 20 to 30 per cent. As muscle cells burn more energy than fat, the resting metabolic rate slows by around 5 per cent for every ten years after the age 25. By the time a woman is 75, she needs around 300 kcals less per day than when she was 18, and 130 kcals per day less than when she was 50. Unfortunately, following a healthy, low-fat diet and increasing levels of physical activity are the only effective ways to beat middle-aged spread.

Exercise is the most effective way known to increase your metabolic rate (as much as ten fold), mobilize fatty acids from fat cells and increase the burning of fatty acids as fuel in muscle cells. Exercise replaces flab with denser muscle. In one study, middle-aged people following a two-month walking programme building up from two 15-minute sessions a week to two hours weekly lost a total of four inches off their waist, hips and thighs even though they ate the same as before.

Research has also shown that prolonged brisk walking will cause blood fat levels to rise much less than usual after eating as dietary fats are rapidly burned for fuel rather than added to fat stores. Aim to exercise briskly (e.g. brisk walking, swimming, cycling, jogging, gym work) for at least half an hour every day, starting off slowly and increasing effort as fitness levels rise.

A number of supplements are widely used to help weight loss, and some have research evidence to back their claims.

Trivalent chromium is needed in minute amounts to form an organic complex known as Glucose Tolerance Factor (GTF). This encourages the production of energy from glucose, and lowers blood fat levels, including harmful LDL-cholesterol. It may also suppress hunger pangs through a direct effect on the satiety centre in the brain. In one study, 233 people randomly received a placebo or chromium for 72 days, without receiving weight loss, dietary or exercise guidance – subjects could follow whichever type of weight loss programme they wished. Statistical analysis showed that those receiving placebo had an average body weight of 83.3kg before the trial, and only lost 0.4 kg over the 72 days. Those receiving chromium picolinate (at least 200 mg) had an initial weight of 84.6 kg and lost an average of 1.26 kg. There were also significant improvements in body composition (more fat lost, compared with lean tissue).

Conjugated linoleic acid (CLA) is a fatty acid that helps to regulate enzymes involved in the mobilization and transport of dietary fats so that less fat is laid down in fatty tissues, and more is transported to muscle cells. Because it affects the body's ratio of lean to fatty tissue, people taking it often experience a reduction in waist size (average loss of 1.6 inches in one study) even when they do not make any other changes to their diet or lifestyle. It is particularly useful for losing fat from troublesome areas such as the hips or tummy.

Hydroxycitric acid (HCA) is a fruit acid originally derived from the rind of an exotic fruit (*Garcinia cambogia*) that curbs appetite and blocks an enzyme responsible for converting excess dietary carbohydrate and protein into fat. Excess carbohydrate is diverted into the production of glycogen – a starchy, muscle energy store instead. In a placebo-controlled study, 50 overweight adults took either HCA in varying doses, or a placebo, and were instructed not to change their normal dietary lifestyle. After four weeks, the body weight of those in the placebo group had increased by an average of 1.3 kg, while those taking HCA had reduced by between 2.2 and 5.5 kg directly related to the daily dose of HCA taken. Subjective evaluation of appetite levels showed considerable reduction in those taking HCA, but not in the placebo group.

Chitosan is a fibre supplement derived from shellfish (crabs, shrimps) to bind 12 times its own weight of dietary fat when taken with meals, so that less is absorbed and more is excreted. Each capsule prevents up to 3 g fat from being absorbed. This helps to maintain a low fat intake and can also reduce circulating blood fat levels. In a number of randomized clinical trials with volunteers following a low-calorie diet, those taking chitosan experienced considerably more weight loss than those taking a placebo. Significant changes in blood pressure and blood fat levels can also occur.

Zotrim, a blend of three Amazonian plants, guarana, damiana and yerba maté, slows the rate of stomach emptying to help reduce food intake, and helps you feel full, faster and for longer. In a recent clinical study, 47 overweight people were divided into two groups. Those who took Zotrim lost an average of 11 lb over 45 days, compared with under one pound in those taking a placebo. *See also* **Guarana**.

Iodine is essential for the production of thyroxine, a hormone that regulates metabolism. The normal range for thyroxine hormone is wide, with the upper limit of normal three times greater than the lower. If iodine intakes are low (sources include iodized salt, seaweed and seafood) thyroxine levels may be in the lower normal range. Supplements providing iodine (e.g. kelp) act as a mild thyroid stimulant and may encourage a more efficient metabolism if your iodine intake has been sub-optimal.

In one study, nine healthy volunteers aged 32–64 were either given 2 g glutamine or a placebo. Those taking glutamine had accelerated fat burning (while preserving muscle tissue) compared to those taking the placebo and it may prove beneficial as part of a weight-loss regime.

An extract from green tea leaves (*Camellia sinensis*), known as AR 25 catechol (Exolise), was shown in clinical studies with healthy volunteers to boost the rate at which the body burns calories by as much as 40 per cent over a 24-hour period. This is due to its ability to inhibit a metabolic enzyme (catechol-methyl transferase) so that levels of noradrenaline increase to stimulate the amount of energy burned in body cells (thermogenesis). It also blocks the activity of intestinal enzymes (gastric and pancreatic lipases) needed to digest dietary fat, so that 30 per cent less fat is absorbed overall. Clinical trials involving 80 overweight men and women who took green tea extracts found they lost 3.5 kg over 3 months, with a decrease in waist circumference of 1 cm.

See also **5-HTP**

Diverticulosis

Diverticulosis, or diverticular disease, affects most older people in the Western world. The term simply means that small out-pouchings have formed in the large intestines (colon) where the lining has herniated through the muscular outer layer of the bowel. This is thought to occur due to increased pressure such as straining – most commonly from constipation.

Treatment

Fibre aids the digestion and absorption of foods, promotes a healthy bacterial balance and provides important bulk to stimulate peristalsis – the muscular, wave-like motion which transports digested food through the intestines. For every gram of fibre you eat, bowel motions increase by an estimated 5 g in weight. A fibre-rich diet helps to stimulate bowel function, avoid constipation and to reduce the chance of any pouches becoming infected and inflamed to cause diverticulitis.

Fibre from different plants varies widely in its composition. Recent research suggests that bowel bacteria adapt to the types of fibre eaten: after a few weeks of eating a fibre-rich diet, they release more of the enzymes needed to break down the different fibre types. This means that some of the benefits are lost unless the types of fibre that are eaten are regularly varied. As wide a range of fibre-rich foods as possible should be eaten from whole-grain sources, fruit and vegetables, increasing intakes slowly to avoid wind and bloating from an initial fibre overload. Similarly, fibre supplements (e.g. bran, ispaghula, psyllium, sterculia) should also be varied every month or so. A very good fluid intake is also essential as this helps fibre to swell and work effectively.

Probiotic supplements containing bowel-friendly bacteria help to maintain optimum bowel function, while aloe vera juice and colloidal silicol gel have a useful cleansing and soothing action on the intestines.

See also **Peppermint, Wild yam**

Dupuytren's contracture

Dupuytren's contracture is a painless thickening of fibrous tissues which cause gradual puckering of the skin and flexion of digits. In the hand, the ring and little fingers are usually affected, and may be drawn down onto the palm. The exact cause is unknown but abnormal activity of cell growth factors may be involved.

Treatment
Unfortunately, cortisone injections and physiotherapy do not help and surgery is the treatment of choice for advanced lesions, although recurrences are common.

Some researchers have claimed that high-dose vitamin E can improve contracture by damping down oxidative damage in affected tissues. Other antioxidants such as vitamin C, grapeseed extract, green tea extract and CoQ10 have also been used, but there is little research into their effectiveness with this condition.

Dyslexia

Dyslexia is a condition in which there is a considerable discrepancy between intellectual ability and written language skills. There is:

● an unexpected failure in learning to read and write
● an unusual anatomical symmetry in language areas of the brain, which are normally larger in the dominant cerebral hemisphere (the left side in right-handed individuals)
● microscopic differences in the way cells are organized during development in the language areas of the brain
● difficulty in processing rapid changes in visual stimulation (e.g. flicker, motion)
● impaired night vision (dark adaptation)
● poor peripheral vision
● difficulty in processing rapid changes in the sounds involved in speech.

It is now thought that dyslexia is a brain development disorder linked with deficiency of certain essential fatty acids (EFAs) in the womb. This leads to mild abnormalities in the membranes of synapses in the foetal brain that are less fluid than normal, and which transmit information more slowly. This may help to explain why dyslexia is more common in males, who have a higher requirement for EFAs than females.

Treatment

The essential fatty acid, docosahexaenoic acid (DHA), is particularly important for visual perception and research is under way to see if giving fish oil supplements (a rich source of AA and DHA) to pregnant women with a family history of dyslexia can help to prevent the condition in the early stages of their baby's development. Recent studies have confirmed that fatty acid metabolism is abnormal in people with dyslexia, with an increased turnover of two lipids – phosphethanolamine and phosphocholine. This may be a genetic difference that is worsened by lack of dietary EFAs and improved by a diet rich in EFAs. Supplements supplying DHA are often helpful in improving dyslexia in children and adults.

Dysmenorrhoea

See **Period problems**

Dyspepsia

See **Indigestion**

Economy-class syndrome

Economy-class syndrome describes the increased risk of deep vein thrombosis (DVT) associated with long-haul flights in cramped conditions on board aircraft. In spite of its name, it is not just confined to the cheaper class cabins, and can also occur in business (club) and first classes.

Treatment

Several options are available for those who wish to limit their general risk of DVT. These include:

- omega-3 fish/cod liver oils which increase bleeding time
- pycnogenol (pine bark extracts) which contains powerful antioxidants that are as effective in reducing susceptibility to clotting as aspirin (but without the same side effects)
- guarana, which lowers levels of fibrinogen (a blood coagulation factor)
- ginkgo biloba or garlic powder tablets which improve general circulation to the peripheries.

Drink plenty of fluids during the flight, avoid alcohol, walk around frequently, and ask a pharmacist to measure you for support socks to wear on the plane. An in-flight blow-up exerciser cushion that simulates the action of walking is also very effective in boosting blood flow through veins in the lower leg to minimize the risk of DVT.

A doctor should advise you on the use of aspirin or – if your risk of DVT is high and you are unable to take aspirin – prophylactic low-molecular-weight heparin (daily injection) to protect you during your flight.

Note: because of the risk of over-thinning the blood, it is inadvisable to combine different supplements without seeking advice from a qualified nutritionist/herbalist. Also, they should not be combined with heparin unless under specialist advice.

Eczema

Eczema is an inflammatory skin disease that affects as many as one in ten people. It most commonly appears on the hands, inside the elbows or behind the knees but may be found anywhere on the body. In severe cases, it may spread to affect skin covering most of the body. There are several different types of eczema, including:

- atopic – mainly affects the face, neck and inner creases of the elbows and knees; it is linked with an increased risk of asthma and allergic rhinitis and tends to run in families
- seborrhoeic – greasy crusts on the face or in the scalp (e.g. cradle cap, dandruff)
- discoid – round lesions on the legs and trunk
- asteatotic – dry, crazy-paving skin patterns in older people, often on the legs
- stasis – eczema of the lower legs due to varicose veins and poor local circulation
- pompholyx – small, itchy vesicles on the fingers, palms or soles
- lichen simplex (or neurodermatitis) due to rubbing or irritation of the skin
- allergic (contact dermatitis, e.g. due to contact with nickel)

- photoallergic – due to the action of sunlight on skin sensitized by absorbed drugs or chemicals.

Eczema symptoms vary from mild to severe and can include dry, scaly, thickened skin, redness, itching with excoriation, blisters, weeping sores which may become infected, crusting and flaky scalp.

Worsening eczema is sometimes associated with colonization of skin by a bacterium, *Staphylococcus aureus*, even in areas that do not look obviously infected. One study found that 95 per cent of people with moderate eczema were colonized with 90 per cent showing a heavy growth. This bacterium secretes superantigens that activate inflammatory cells and worsen skin inflammation. They are also thought to induce steroid insensitivity making treatment less effective, although a cream that combines steroid with a topical antibiotic (e.g. fusidic acid plus hydrocortisone or the stronger betametasone cream) may help.

Treatment

If oral antibiotics are needed, a probiotic supplement will reduce intestinal side effects.

The reason why *S. aureus* colonizes skin in atopic eczema is not known, but one suggestion is that levels of essential fatty acids (EFA) are reduced in cell membranes which might make it easier for bacteria to adhere. Therefore it is worth taking an EFA supplement such as evening primrose, flaxseed or omega-3 fish oils to see if this helps. Evening primrose oil contains essential fatty acids (e.g. gammalinolenic acid also known as GLA) which can moisturize the skin from the inside. GLA is important for the formation of healthy skin cell membranes and helps to reduce itching and dryness in people with essential fatty acid deficiency – at least 80 per cent of the population.

Evening primrose oil needs to be taken in large doses of around 3 g daily for at least three months before fairly evaluating the response to treatment. Pure evening primrose oil can also be rubbed directly on to affected skin.

Omega-3 fish oils also have an anti-inflammatory action that is helpful for improving conditions such as eczema. These oils can certainly reduce itching and inflammation but may take a few months to have maximum effect.

It's worth avoiding cows' milk products for a few weeks to see if symptoms improve. Ensure a good calcium intake from nuts, seeds, whole-grains, leafy vegetables and supplements however – especially if dietary restriction is followed long term.

Aloe vera gel is often very effective for treating eczema when applied twice a day. It may also be taken by mouth.

A multi-nutrient supplement is worth considering as lack of some vitamins and minerals (especially antioxidants and zinc) have been linked with scaly skin rashes. An A to Z-style vitamin and mineral formula, plus additional antioxidants (e.g. vitamins C, E, carotenoids, selenium, pine bark or grape seed extracts) is recommended.

Recent research suggests that probiotic supplements taken during pregnancy and in infancy may reduce the chance of eczema developing in children – possibly they have a beneficial effect on immunity.

Treatment of eczema should also include liberal application of emollient creams and soothing (non-perfumed) bath additives to soothe and moisturize the skin from the outside.

See also **Echinacea, Liquorice, Oregano, Perilla, Red clover, Sarsaparilla, Zinc**

Endometriosis

Endometriosis is one of the commonest gynaecological conditions to affect women, with as many as one in ten affected although not all with troublesome symptoms. It is the only known condition in which apparently normal, non-cancerous cells spread from one part of the body (the womb lining or endometrium) to another, take root and continue to grow – most commonly in the pelvic and abdominal cavities. Because these cells remain sensitive to the monthly hormone cycle, they may swell and bleed into surrounding tissues during each menstrual period to produce pain, inflammation and scarring. As the condition progresses, fluid-filled hollow cysts or solid nodules can develop especially on the ovaries. The four classic symptoms are painful periods that may be heavy, deep pain during sex, deep pelvic pain and subfertility.

Adenomyosis is similar to endometriosis, in that ectopic endometrial deposits are found outside their normal position, within the muscular wall of the womb itself, nestled between the muscle fibres to form diffuse patches, or a larger lump similar to a fibroid.

Treatment
Self help for both conditions includes eating a healthy, wholefood diet and avoiding salt, caffeine, sugar, fried and processed foods. Some nutritionists suggest avoiding meat and dairy products because of the potentially high level of animal oestrogens they contain, although it is important to seek dietary advice to ensure correct intakes of important nutrients such as iron or vitamin B12.

Essential fatty acid intake should be increased (e.g. linseed, sunflower, walnut oils and oily fish) and 3 g evening primrose oil daily is recommended for those essential fatty acids that help to overcome hormone imbalances and damp down inflammation. Studies suggest that women who obtain the most fish oils in their diet have the least painful menstruation.

Lack of iodine has been linked with hormonal imbalances that may lead to endometriosis, so it is a good idea to take a multivitamin and mineral supplement that includes iodine (150 mcg). Also ensure a good intake of antioxidants – at least five servings of fruit or vegetables a day – and consider supplements such as vitamins C and E, pine bark or grapeseed extracts to reduce inflammation.

Calcium and magnesium will help to reduce any associated uterine muscle spasm and pain. Agnus castus has a progesterone-like action in the body and may also help. Some practitioners also recommend using progesterone cream to balance the oestrogen dominance that is linked with endometriosis.

Herbal remedies that may be prescribed to reduce symptoms include: **Black cohosh, Dandelion, Dong quai, Liquorice, Maca, Milk Thistle, Raspberry leaves, Red clover, Siberian ginseng** and **Wild yam.**

Emphysema

Emphysema is a disease affecting the tiny air sacs (alveoli) of the lungs which become overstretched, damaged and rupture. As a result, the small sacs merge to form fewer, larger sacs with a significantly reduced surface area. This makes gas exchange less efficient and the lungs may become over-inflated.

Treatment

Almost all cases of emphysema result from smoking cigarettes, so stopping smoking is vital.

Antioxidant supplements (e.g. vitamins A, C, E, selenium, pine bark or grapeseed extracts) help to neutralize the free radicals (*see* **Antioxidants**) that have been implicated in emphysema. A trial involving over 2500 patients with respiratory illnesses found that taking the amino acid N-actylcysteine (which makes mucus less viscid) improved symptoms.

Garlic powder tablets help to loosen mucus and protects against respiratory infections. If a chest infection starts, echinacea may be taken as well, and omega-3 fish oils may help to reduce wheezing.

Energy – lack of

A number of conditions can reduce energy levels and if symptoms persist, it is important to consult a doctor to identify treatable conditions such as an underactive thyroid gland, anaemia, diabetes or depression.

Treatment

Assuming that nothing sinister is identified, treatments that might help to correct a lack of energy include an A to Z-style vitamin and mineral supplement to safeguard against any micro-nutrient deficiencies – including B group vitamins (needed to produce energy in cells) and iodine which is needed to make thyroid hormones. Co-enzyme Q10 is often helpful in overcoming fatigue, as are evening primrose oil supplements. Guarana contains a complex of natural stimulants, including a form of caffeine known as guaranine. These components are slowly absorbed to provide a stimulant action for up to six hours creating more energy without producing over-stimulation or irritability. Most people find it more gentle and calming than caffeine.

A good energizing pick-me-up can be made by mixing 5 ml each of guarana powder, brewer's yeast and wheatgerm with 15 ml pure honey and topping up to a glass with mineral water and blending thoroughly. This should be drunk every morning before breakfast.

Siberian ginseng or Korean ginseng are also useful energy boosters. Antioxidants such as Vitamin C, E, carotenoids, grapeseed or pine bark extracts will help to damp down any inflammatory processes contributing to lack of energy.

Evening primrose oil is helpful for people with chronic fatigue (see **Chronic Fatigue Syndrome**).

See also **Gotu kola, Iodine, Iron, Kelp, Oats, Reishi, Rhodiola, Schisandra, Wheatgrass, Yerba maté**

Epstein-Barr virus (EBV)

See **Glandular fever**

Exam stress

It is important to balance time spent revising for exams with time for safety-valve activities such as relaxation and non-competitive exercise to burn off the adverse effects of stress hormones. While this may seem like time wasted as exams loom, the ability to absorb information is much improved after taking a break.

Diet is very important – eating a cereal breakfast, for example, can improve concentration and increase the speed at which new information is recalled. Ginkgo biloba extracts can improve short-term working memory, while lemon balm (*Melissa officinalis*) is known as the 'Scholar's Herb' as it was traditionally taken by students suffering from the stress of impending exams. Bach Rescue Remedy (containing flower essences) is excellent for when panic rises and can be used before exams to help steady the nerves.

See also **Valerian**

Eyes – dry

Dry eyes are relatively common, especially if you forget to blink when concentrating on your work or VDU screen. Some people suffer with dry eyes all the time, however – a condition known as keratoconjunctivitis sicca – due to lack of tear production. Dry eyes become more common with increasing age. They can also result from the production of abnormal antibodies that switch off tear production. This can happen in some autoimmune disorders such as rheumatoid arthritis, systemic lupus erythematosus and Sjögren's syndrome.

Treatment
The standard treatment for dry eyes involves lubricating drops known as artificial tears. These can be successful but

may need to be used frequently to prevent burning, itching, grittiness and painful ulceration.

In some parts of the world, dry eyes are frequently due to lack of vitamin A. This is known as xerophthalmia. Although it is rare in the Western world, it may be worth taking a cod liver oil supplement (which contains vitamin A) to see if this helps. Supplements containing bilberry extracts help to stabilize tears and are often very successful – they also contain carotenoids that can be converted into vitamin A where needed.

See also **Grapeseed**

Feet – painful

A large number of conditions can cause painful feet. These include:

● flat feet
● arthritis
● tarsal tunnel syndrome (the foot version of carpal tunnel syndrome)
● plantar fasciitis (pain mainly under the heel and in the midline)
● erythromelalgia (burning feet syndrome)
● metatarsalgia (pain mainly in the ball of the foot)
● conditions affecting nerve transmission (neuropathy).

Treatment
Occasionally, burning feet are due to lack of B group vitamins and supplements may help.

Arthritis in the feet may be helped by glucosamine sulphate (with or without chondroitin), devil's claw, MSM-sulphur, green-lipped mussel extracts or antioxidants such as vitamin C.

Related entry: **Arthritis**

Fibromyalgia

Fibromyalgia is a debilitating condition from which women are five times more likely to suffer than men. It causes widespread aches and pains plus sleep disturbance, and the pains tend to move from place to place, vary in severity and are often made worse by cold and stress. Sufferers develop localized areas of tenderness known as trigger points, especially around the lower spine, between the shoulder blades, at the base of the neck, over the sacro-iliac joints, elbows and knees. In some people, these tender spots develop fibrous nodules.

In fibromyalgia sufferers, all blood tests and x-rays show up as normal, and the condition seems to be due to reduced energy production in muscle cells and an inability of muscle fibres to relax. Sufferers do have a characteristic lack of delta wave (deep non-REM sleep) when brain waves are monitored during sleep, however. They therefore feel tired and exhausted much of the time as they wake unrefreshed. Interestingly, if normal volunteers are monitored during sleep and woken periodically so that they lack delta wave sleep, similar aches and pains will appear. Sleep disturbances have been linked with low levels of serotonin (a neurotransmitter) in the brain.

Treatment

Unfortunately, painkillers and anti-inflammatory drugs are usually unhelpful although anti-depressant drugs that raise brain serotonin levels (SSRIs) sometimes improve the sleep disturbance. St John's Wort is therefore a useful alternative to try.

People with fibromyalgia often seem to be lacking in magnesium, and supplements containing magnesium malate, B group vitamins, manganese and co-enzyme Q10 (which improves oxygen utilization in cells) may help. Kava kava is excellent for relieving anxiety and promoting restful sleep as well as improving tolerance to pain.

Blood circulation to the peripheries may be improved with ginkgo, garlic or Padma 28 (a blend of over 20 different herbs). Supplements may take up to two months to produce a beneficial effect.

Olive leaf extracts have a powerful anti-viral action and they are often helpful for people with fibromyalgia.

See also **Cayenne, 5-HTP, Liquorice, Magnesium**

Fluid retention

Fluid retention may be due to a number of different problems and, if persistent or recurrent, it is important to seek medical advice to find out the cause.

Treatment

General measures to reduce fluid retention include losing excess weight, taking regular exercise, and cutting back on salt intake. Intakes should be increased of fruit, vegetables, salads and juices containing potassium salts that also help to flush excess sodium from the body.

Dandelion is a natural herbal diuretic that is widely used to flush excess fluid from the body. As well as having a powerful diuretic action, dandelion root extracts are also a rich source of mineral potassium. They should not be taken by anyone who is on other prescribed medications however.

If fluid retention is linked with premenstrual syndrome (PMS), supplements that include magnesium and vitamin B6 are especially helpful. Magnesium helps to maintain sodium and potassium balance in and out of body cells, while vitamin B6 increases cell membrane transfer and utilization of magnesium. Food sources of magnesium include fish, nuts, seeds, soy beans, whole grains and dark green, leafy vegetables.

Food poisoning

Food poisoning (gastro-enteritis) is usually associated with abdominal pain, vomiting and diarrhoea.

Treatment
Usual advice with prolonged gastro-enteritis is to replace lost fluids and minerals with an electrolyte solution (available from pharmacies).

Probiotic supplements containing healthy, digestive bacteria (e.g. *Lactobacilli*) help to keep the digestive system in balance, and keep harmful bacteria at bay through a number of mechanisms, including the production of natural antibiotics (bacteriocins), lowering the pH to discourage reproduction of less acid-tolerant bacteria and competing for available nutrients and attachment sites on intestinal cell walls.

Some herbalists recommend taking 2–3 garlic powder tablets last thing at night for their natural antibiotic action. Manuka honey and mastic gum contain natural antibiotics which may also help. Ginger is used to sooth the intestinal lining and reduce inflammation, while goldenseal, echinacea and cat's claw help to boost general immunity against infection.

Medical advice should be sought if problems continue, as one in three people with bacterial gastro-enteritis whose symptoms are still present after three months are likely to have developed irritable bowel syndrome as a result of the infection.

See also **Perilla frutescens, Sage**
Related entry: **Diarrhoea**

Frozen shoulder

Frozen shoulder is the common name for increasing pain, stiffness and immobility of the shoulder joint. It is due to inflammation and thickening in the lining of the capsule surrounding the joint (capsulitis). In most cases, no obvious cause is found, but it may come on after a fall, a task involving repetitive movements of the joint (e.g. painting the ceiling) or after unaccustomed exercise. Attacks have also been linked with other medical conditions such as chronic bronchitis, stroke or heart pain (angina), perhaps triggered by general immobility.

Treatment

During the initial, acutely painful stage of frozen shoulder, rest is usually advised along with non-steroidal, anti-inflammatory drugs to relieve pain and inflammation. Applying hot or cold packs can also help. After the pain starts to reduce, manipulation by a physiotherapist, osteopath or chiropractor will improve mobility, but it can take many months before the range of movement approaches normality again. A new osteopathic treatment for frozen shoulder, the Niel-Asher technique, involving up to eight sessions lasting 30 to 40 minutes, has shown impressive results, and acupuncture and bioelectromagnetic therapy can also help.

Supplements that can reduce joint inflammation include vitamin C, New Zealand green-lipped mussel extracts, devil's claw and omega-3 fish oils. Glucosamine sulphate is useful for improving the quality and quantity of synovial fluid – the joint's oil.

Gallstones

Most gallstones are made of cholesterol, although some contain high amounts of bile pigments or calcium salts. They are four times more common in women than men, and overall, it is estimated that one in five women develops gallstones at some time in her life. Symptoms can include severe pain (biliary colic) in the upper right abdomen which often seems to spread to the right shoulder, inflammation or infection of the gallbladder (cholecystitis) or pancreas (pancreatitis) and jaundice. Eight out of ten people with gallstones do not develop symptoms, however.

Treatment

General self-help measures to reduce gallstone formation including following a low-fat, high-fibre diet and losing any excess weight. A diet rich in soluble fibre such as pectin (e.g. found in apples, carrots) and gums found in oat bran and dried beans is recommended, as these help to bind cholesterol and bile salts in the gut so less is re-absorbed.

Lecithin (e.g. in soy beans or lecithin supplements) is an essential component of bile and keeps cholesterol emulsified to reduce stone formation, as can high-dose vitamin C supplements (e.g. 1 g three times a day; products containing ester-C are preferable to reduce acidity in sufferers of indigestion). Olive oil is a rich source of oleic acid, a mono-unsaturated fat that has a beneficial effect on blood cholesterol balance. A regular intake may help to prevent gallstones.

Flaxseed, walnut, omega-3 fish oils and garlic powder tablets also have a beneficial effect on blood cholesterol balance and a diet rich in these may reduce gallstone formation. Artichoke leaf supplements stimulate bile flow and are also beneficial, but should not be used if gallstones are obstructing bile flow or if jaundice is present. Low intakes of vitamin E and calcium have been linked with an increased risk of developing gallstones.

Milk thistle extracts have beneficial effects on the composition of bile (e.g. reduced cholesterol content) which is also thought to reduce formation of gallstones.

See also **Dandelion, Peppermint, Shiitake, Wild yam**

Gingivitis

See **Gums – receding**

Glandular fever

Glandular fever – also known as infectious mononucleosis – is caused by the Epstein-Barr virus (EBV), and mainly affects teenagers between the ages of 15 and 18. This is the time when the immune system is most vigorous and many of the symptoms are due to the body over-reacting to the infection. EBV is passed on in saliva and can be spread by coughing, spluttering, sneezing, kissing and by sharing toothbrushes. Someone who has recently had glandular fever can remain infectious for several months. Only around half the people who catch the virus develop symptoms, however. During convalescence it is common to feel tired, depressed and lacking in energy for six months or more.

Treatment

It is important to take things easy for several months after glandular fever to allow the immune system time to recover. It is also advisable to avoid alcohol.

Co-enzyme Q10, B group vitamins and evening primrose oil may be helpful for fatigue. High-dose vitamin C also helps to reduce inflammation. Herbal remedies for glandular fever (e.g. echinacea, maitake) are best prescribed individually by a qualified practitioner.

Gout

Gout is an inflammatory arthritis due to high levels of uric acid which precipitate out into joints and tissues. As most uric acid is produced in the body during the breakdown of purines released when the genetic material (DNA) of worn out cells is recycled, dietary changes can only lower uric acid levels by up to 20 per cent.

Symptoms of gout include hot, red, extremely painful swelling of a joint, most commonly involving the big toe.

Treatment

Standard dietary advice is to reduce your intake of purine-rich foods such as offal, shellfish, oily fish, game, meats, yeast extracts, asparagus, and spinach. Alcohol both increases uric acid production and reduces its excretion (especially beer which is also rich in purines) and should therefore be avoided.

A high-fibre, mainly vegetarian diet should be followed with plenty of fruit and vegetables. Dark blue-red pigmented fruits (e.g. cherries, grapes, blueberries, bilberries) contain antioxidants such as anthocyanidins that can lower uric acid levels and are said to prevent gout when around 250 g are eaten daily. Alternatively supplements containing extracts of bilberry, cherry fruit, grape seed or pine bark are recommended. An intake of at least 2 litres of fluid must also be ensured each day.

High-dose vitamin C mobilizes uric acid from the tissues and increases its excretion – the pre-digested form known as ester-C is best as it is non-acidic. High-dose folic acid supplements inhibit uric acid synthesis, but should only be taken once vitamin B12 deficiency is ruled out. Supplements containing more than the RDA (recommended daily amount) of vitamin B3 (niacin) or vitamin A should be avoided as high doses can increase uric acid levels.

Extracts of devil's claw (*Harpagophytum procumbens*) contain natural anti-inflammatory analgesics (e.g. harpagoside) that both reduce pain and also encourage excretion of uric acid, so reducing the risk of recurrent gout. Bromelain is also useful for reducing pain and inflammation in acute attacks of gout.

See also **Cat's claw, Pfaffia, Sarsaparilla**

Grave's disease

See **Thyroid gland – overactive**

Gums – receding

Receding gums are a common occurrence in old age – so much so that older people are often described as being 'long in the tooth'. Receding gums are associated with a build-up of plaque in the pockets between the gums and teeth. This leads to inflammation known as gingivitis in which gums become red, swollen and bleed during brushing. If left untreated, gingivitis can progress to infect the tissues and bone surrounding tooth roots to cause periodontitis. Both gingivitis and periodontitis can lead to bad breath, receding gums and loosening or falling out of teeth.

Treatment

To help avoid receding gums, good dental hygiene is vital. Teeth must be brushed regularly, at least twice daily – and preferably after each meal. An electric toothbrush that helps to remove plaque is worth considering, and dental floss or tape should be used regularly (this needs to be done correctly as directed by a dentist). Dentists can also offer referrals to a dental hygienist for regular cleaning of gum pockets and removal of scale, as well as advising about a new treatment, Gengigel, which contains hyaluronic acid. This is an important component of gum tissue, providing strength, elasticity, and binding 50 times its own weight of water to help plump up thinning tissues. Applied externally, it stimulates production of collagen by cells known as fibroblasts to promote new gum formation.

Liquid folic acid and powdered vitamin C supplements have also been used to stimulate healthy regeneration of gum tissue.

Diseased gums have been shown to have significantly reduced levels of Co-enzyme Q10 (CoQ10) compared with healthy gum tissue from the same patients. A double-blind trial in which the action of 60 mg CoQ10 daily was compared with that of a placebo showed that CoQ10 was able to reverse periodontal gum disease and save teeth scheduled for surgery.

A good intake of calcium is essential as dietary deficiency can also contribute to receding gums.

Research is currently looking into the plaque-reducing properties of cranberry juice which contains anti-adhesins – substances that stop bacteria sticking to body cells.

Note: dental advice should be sought for redness or swelling of the gums around the teeth, or for gums that bleed during brushing.

Haemorrhoids

Piles (haemorrhoids) are dilated varicose veins in the back passage. They often develop as a result of straining, overweight or pregnancy and can cause an unpleasant dragging sensation, itching, a mucous discharge and cause bright red bleeding from the back passage. If bleeding occurs, it is important to seek medical advice to confirm the diagnosis as more serious bowel conditions need to be ruled out.

Treatment

To reduce symptoms, a mild, non-spicy, high-fibre diet with plenty of fluids is recommended.

Glycerine suppositories will ease the passage of bowel motions and reduce straining while psyllium husks and seeds are an excellent remedy for constipation.

A bath or shower should be taken every day using unperfumed soap, and finishing by spraying the area with cold water. The area must be kept scrupulously clean to help stop itching – this means washing the area with unscented soap after each bowel motion and patting dry with a soft tissue; if necessary the area may be kept dry using a hairdryer set on gentle heat.

Sitting in a solution of 1 drop of peppermint and 2 drops of chamomile essential oils added to warm water (in a bidet or large, shallow plastic bowl) for five or ten minutes can be helpful. If the area feels sore and burning, two tablespoons of bicarbonate of soda can also be added. Cypress, lemon and Roman chamomile essential oils are another helpful combination.

Vitamin C plus extracts of horsechestnut or gotu kola may be recommended to strengthen supporting tissues around the veins (but not during pregnancy).

Take steps to reduce constipation (*see* **Constipation**).

See also **Grapeseed, Red vine leaf**

Hair loss

Hair loss seems to have become an increasingly common problem. While it is sometimes linked with scalp skin conditions, lack of iron or an underactive thyroid gland, frequently no obvious cause is found. Hair is a good indicator of general health and nutrition, and is often the first part of the body to show signs of ill health, or a dietary lack of vitamins, minerals or essential fatty acids. This is because, although hair is often thought of as a dead structure, its root – the hair follicle – is very much alive. The rate at which new hair cells are produced is second only to the speed at which new blood cells are made in the bone marrow. Hair follicles, therefore, need a constant supply of nutrients for optimum health. Unlike the marrow however, hair is a non-essential structure and the body preferentially diverts precious nutrient stores away from it in times of lack or stress.

Treatment

Research shows that levels of specific minerals laid down in the hair vary significantly with time – even from hour to hour. The majority of women who consult a trichologist about hair problems are found to be deficient in at least one nutrient as this fluctuation in supply can lead to weak, thinning hair unless steps are taken to improve hair health. The following tips will help.

- A healthy, balanced diet containing as many unrefined, wholefoods as possible, and as organic as possible, should be followed. Whole grains, fruit, vegetables and seeds are a rich source of vitamins, minerals and essential fatty acids that provide nourishment for hair roots and contribute to a healthy head of hair. Avoid eating erratically and skipping meals (especially breakfast) or the supply of nutrients to non-essential tissues such as hair follicles will be reduced. Try to eat something – for example a healthy snack such as fresh or dried fruit – at least every four hours.

- Hair has a high content of the tough, fibrous protein keratin, which is made from amino acid building blocks obtained from the diet. A source of protein, such as poultry, fish, eggs, nuts or beans, should be eaten at every meal. Vegetarians are more prone to thinning hair as some important amino acids (e.g. lysine) and micro-nutrients (e.g. vitamin B12, iron) may be lacking from their diet.

- Reduce salt intake – excess salt reduces hair follicle function and research shows that reducing salt intake can reduce hair loss and thinning by as much as 60 per cent.

- After the age of 25, the diameter of individual hairs naturally starts to decrease, especially in women. Although this often goes unnoticed, it can change the texture and body of the hair, so that by the age of 40, most people have finer hair with less body. At the same time, more follicles stay in their resting phase so less hair grows and the rate of growth decreases, resulting in progressive thinning. This effect can be minimized by massaging the scalp regularly with the fingers every day. Underlying tightness can also be loosened by holding handfuls of hair near the roots and gently moving the scalp back and forth and from side to side. Massage and scalp movement open up the circulation and stimulate the flow of blood, oxygen and nutrients to the hair follicles.

- Regular exercise and a healthy weight for height are recommended. Severe dietary restriction at any time of life, but especially middle age, can have permanent effects on hair health. Excess weight loss should be achieved slowly and sensibly as over-exercising and crash diets affect the body's hormone balance and dramatically reduces the nutrient supplies to hair follicles.

- Combs are generally kinder to hair than brushes. Choose a comb with widely spaced teeth and without mould lines down the centre of each tooth which can damage hair shafts. If using a brush, choose one with wide-spaced, plastic bristles that have smooth, blunt tips. Avoid metal prongs as these can damage the hair and scalp.

- Excess stress should be avoided as stress hormones constrict blood supply to the scalp and hair follicles, reducing their supply of nutrients. This can lead to generalized hair thinning or even patchy hair loss. In times of stress use massage and scalp movement to loosen the scalp and improve circulation to hair follicles.

● Avoid chemicals coming into contact with your scalp and follicles. Perms and colour treatments should be applied only to the hair shafts. Plastic caps can help to protect follicles when bleach is applied. Semi-permanent colour is kinder to hair than permanent.

● Consider taking a good A to Z-style vitamin and mineral supplement containing around 100 per cent of the recommended daily amount (RDA) of as many vitamins and minerals as possible (including iodine). Alternatively, choose one especially formulated for hair, skin and nails which often contains boosted amounts of B group vitamins such as biotin and B5 (pantothenic acid). Many herbal blends are also available (e.g. those including ginkgo which improves circulation).

● Essential fatty acids found in evening primrose, flaxseed, hemp seed or omega-3 fish are important for hair health. Evening primrose oil supplements (1000 mg a day) can improve the hair and nail quality within three months as new cells grow down (although as new hair only grows down at a rate of half an inch per month, it may take as long as a year for the overall improvement to show).

● Kelp supplements are widely used as a nutritional source to improve hair and nail condition.

See also **Silicon**
Related entry: **Alopecia**

Halitosis

Bad breath, or halitosis, affects eight out of ten people at some time in their life. For two thirds, it is a long-term problem. Most cases result from a build-up of bacterial plaque in the mouth or on the tongue. These bacteria produce around 300 different gases and volatile chemicals, of which over 100 smell unpleasant. Other less common causes include lack of saliva, nose problems (e.g. previous fracture, post-nasal drip, nose surgery), sinusitis and chronic lung infection. Breath odours due to eating onions and garlic, for example, are a dietary side effect and do not constitute true halitosis.

People with gum disease are four times more likely to have bad breath than others. Redness or swelling of the gums around the teeth, or gums that bleed when brushing could be signs of gingivitis (infected gums) which, if ignored, will spread to involve the jawbone around the teeth (periodontitis) after which gums will start to recede. If this in turn is ignored, teeth will eventually be lost altogether.

Treatment

Unfortunately, twice daily cleaning of teeth is not enough to solve bad breath and gum disease and standard mouthwashes only solve the problem temporarily.

Dental tape should be used regularly to clean between teeth, as well as a tongue scraper to remove bacterial accumulations on the tongue which can contribute to bad odours. An electric toothbrush designed to remove plaque should be used and gum pockets should be cleaned and descaled regularly by a dental hygienist. Saliva flow may be stimulated first thing each morning by drinking a glass of citrus juice and eating fruit. It is also important to drink at least 2 litres of fluid per day.

Some food supplements can also help. Co-enzyme Q10 has, for example, been shown to help reverse gum inflammation and promote healing of gum disease. Green tea leaves contain polyphenols that have a natural deodorizing effect and green tea is widely drunk to help reduce bad breath and suppress odours due to chemicals such as methyl mercaptan and ammonia as well as trimethylamine. Extracts of Agaricus bisporus and blue-green algae can also help.

Related entry: **Gums – receding**.

Hangover

A hangover is an unpleasant group of symptoms that include headache, nausea, dizziness, linked with excessive alcohol intake, which stresses the liver, generates toxins, and also leads to dehydration.

Prevention

Supplements containing antioxidants and milk thistle (silymarin) can help to prevent a hangover. More than 300 studies have shown that silymarin can protect liver cells from the poisonous effects of excess alcohol by maintaining levels of an important liver antioxidant enzyme, glutathione, needed to metabolize alcohol.

Before indulging in alcohol, a B group vitamin supplement (50–100 mg) plus 1–2 g vitamin C should be taken as these nutrients are used up while metabolizing alcohol and a lack of them can contribute to hangover symptoms.

Always drink on a full stomach – this slows alcohol absorption so it is metabolized before it reaches your brain; if you are going out to a party and don't expect to eat until later, have a substantial snack before going out.

Drink according to your size. Slender souls weighing nine stone cannot handle as much alcohol as someone weighing 18 stone. Women also handle alcohol less well than men, as they tend to have a higher body fat percentage, which soaks up the alcohol (so it is less available for breaking down) then slowly lets it back out again.

Drinking more slowly means that alcohol is metabolized before it can build up in the circulation. Alternating alcohol with non-alcoholic drinks and/or drinking cocktails containing plenty of non-alcoholic mixers is a useful technique. Avoid too many sparkling alcoholic drinks (such as champagne or rum and coke) as the bubbles speed up alcohol absorption causing intoxication more quickly. Drinks containing congeners – substances that add flavour and colour to alcohol – are also best avoided. Among the spirits, vodka and gin are kindest, while cognac, brandy and whisky trigger the worst hangovers. Red wine contains tyramine, a chemical that can produce a severe headache in some people.

Drink at least half a litre of water or fresh orange juice before going to bed to help overcome the dehydrating effects of alcohol. It's also worth taking another 1 g vitamin C.

Treatment

A pint of water should be drunk on waking and a good fluid intake maintained throughout the day. Electrolyte solutions (made up from sachets or effervescent tablets) available from pharmacies should be taken to replenish potassium and other important salt levels. A good substitute for these is clear consommé soup (if necessary, made from stock or cubes).

A large glass of fresh orange juice contains fructose, a fruit sugar that will help to accelerate the removal of any remaining alcohol in the system. Yeast extract or honey on toast for breakfast will help; honey is a concentrated source of fructose that will also raise your blood sugar level. Baked beans on toast is another good combination.

Extracts of globe artichoke (*Cynara scolymus*) have liver-regenerating effects similar to those of the milk thistle. *Cynara* also stimulates bile production and can quickly relieve symptoms due to insufficient bile production such as nausea, bloating and indigestion – often within an hour.

Antioxidants are also needed to mop up harmful free radicals produced when metabolizing alcohol, so 1 g vitamin C should be taken three times a day. A vitamin B complex will replace B vitamins used up while metabolizing alcohol.

Hay fever

Hay fever is an allergic response triggered by sensitivity to plant pollens or fungal spores. It is the most common form of allergy, affecting up to 20 per cent of the population. Symptoms such as itchy conjunctivitis, runny nose, stuffiness, sneezing and headache occur when pollen or spores come into contact with moist mucous membranes lining the eyes, nose and sinuses. This triggers the release of histamine and other powerful chemicals that cause inflammation and swelling. Hay fever may also make other allergic conditions such as asthma or eczema worse. Hay fever symptoms vary from month to month, and can last from February to October, depending on which pollens are causing the allergy.

February–May	hazel, elder and birch pollen
April, May	plane tree pollen
June–August	grass pollens
August–October	mould and fungal spores in damp weather

Only one in 20 hay fever sufferers escapes allergic eye problems altogether – usually it is those allergic to the pollen of oil-seed rape. Conjunctivitis tends to be worse in those allergic to tree pollens.

Hay fever seems to run in families. It tends to strike first between the ages of six and 20, with symptoms peaking in the late teens and early 20s. Symptoms often disappear after five to 15 years so have usually improved by middle age.

Prevention
There are several things sufferers can do to help prevent hay fever symptoms.

- Check pollen forecasts and stay indoors when levels are highest, as well as between 7–9 am and 3–7 pm when pollen is most likely to be just above ground level.
- Avoid city centres and other areas of high traffic density.

- When going out is unavoidable, dabbing petroleum jelly just inside the nostrils to trap pollen and wearing sunglasses to protect the eyes are sensible precautions.
- When possible, change clothes and shower after going outside and wash your hands before touching your eyes.
- Avoid pets that have been outdoors and carry pollen on their fur.
- Keep house windows and doors shut, especially bedroom windows at night.
- Vacuum the home and dust regularly, and use a negative ionizer indoors to settle airborne pollen.
- Keep car windows and doors shut, and consider buying a car with an integral pollen filter.
- Avoid gardening or mowing the lawn, barbecues, picnics and cut grass.
- Avoid exposure to cigarette smoke and chemical fumes (e.g. paint, solvents).

Treatment

Treatments often work best if started early in the season before pollen counts become too high. Those available include eye drops, nasal sprays and oral antihistamines. A study by the Drug Safety Research Unit suggests that the oral antihistamines loratadine and fexofenadine (prescription only) are around three times less likely to cause sedation than cetirizine and acrivastine.

As preventatives, some practitioners recommend chewing lumps of honeycomb as a chewing gum throughout winter and late spring (but not for anyone who is allergic to bee products). The B group vitamins (e.g. Brewer's yeast) may also be started in spring. High-dose vitamin C and bioflavonoids such as quercetin (found in citrus fruits, blackcurrants and rosehips) have a natural antihistamine action and help to damp down inflammation. *See also* **Bee products** – bee pollen, and **Yerba maté**.

On the herbal front, Luffa Complex containing seven plant extracts is effective in relieving hay fever symptoms in 75 per cent of cases, with 56 per cent claiming to have been either fully or nearly freed of allergic symptoms. Supplements containing extracts of the traditional Chinese herbal remedy for allergy, perilla frutescens, reduce sneezing and runny nose due to hay fever, with 85 per cent of those taking them finding them effective. Garlic powder tablets can also have an anti-allergy action.

Acupressure can also be helpful if nasal symptoms start: press on the top end of the web between your thumb and index finger – at the highest point of the muscle, just before you can feel the bones meet. Press and rub firmly for one minute, then repeat on the other side.

Headache

Tension headaches are commonly linked with stress, as blood flow to the brain is affected by tension in neck and scalp muscles, as well as high levels of the stress hormone epinephrine (formerly adrenaline). A tension headache usually feels like severe, continuous pressure applied on both sides of the head, which may centre over the top of the skull, the back of the head or above both eyes. Some tension headaches feel like a tight, constricting band, while others are more like a non-specific ache.

Migraine – in which pain is more severe and usually only felt on one side of the head or which is definitely worse on one side – is often misdiagnosed as a tension headache. It is important to consult a doctor about a recurrent headache that may be migraine.

Tension headache is often brought on by feelings of excess pressure, relief of stress (e.g. at the end of a long, trying week), physical fatigue, lack of sleep, missed meals and extreme emotions such as anger and excitement.

Treatment

Massage is often effective, as gentle manipulation of muscles in the neck, shoulders and back will relax taut muscles. This can be combined with relaxing aromatherapy oils such as chamomile, geranium, lavender or peppermint.

To avoid muscle tension, try not to stoop when standing or sitting. Keep a straight back and shoulders, with the abdomen lightly pulled in. Shoulders should be circled from time to time, and arms should not be folded tightly; let them hang loosely from the shoulders and shake them regularly. Avoid clenching fists; hold hands loosely with the palms open and fingers curled lightly and naturally. Don't clench or grind teeth; keep your mouth slightly open and try to relax upper and lower jaws.

Herbal remedies that help to reduce stress and promote relaxation and relief of tension include valerian (often combined with lemon balm and hops) and kava kava. Guarana can help to reduce tension headache. Feverfew is effective in reducing the frequency and severity of recurrent headaches, such as migraine.

Other supplements that may be used include devil's claw, peppermint, yerba maté, 5-HTP, agnus castus (to relieve menstrually related headaches), vitamin B2 (riboflavin), calcium and magnesium which may help to reduce spasm of muscles and blood vessels.

Related entry: **Migraine**

Helicobacter pylori

Helicobacter pylori is a motile form of bacteria found in the stomachs of at least 20 per cent of 30-year-olds and 50 per cent of those over 50 in the UK. It burrows into the mucous lining of the stomach leaving a small breach in the wall through which acids can reach the stomach wall. *Helicobacter* then coats itself with a small bubble of alkaline ammonia, protecting itself from the acid attack and at the same time, irritating and inflaming the stomach lining. Although it doesn't cause symptoms in everyone, virtually all patients with duodenal ulcers are infected, plus three quarters of those with gastric ulcers. *H. pylori* infection is also associated with an increased risk of gastric cancer.

Treatment

Orthodox eradication usually involves a week's course of two antibiotics plus a drug that switches off acid production.

Several natural treatments are used to help reduce *H. pylori* infection. Manuka honey made by bees feeding on nectar from the New Zealand tea tree contains a unique antibiotic that can eradicate *Helicobacter*. It is usually taken on an empty stomach at a dose of four teaspoons, four times a day, for eight weeks. Another natural approach is to take mastic gum derived from a pistachio-like tree grown on the Greek island of Chios.

Interesting research also provides preliminary evidence that cranberry juice can help to stop *Helicobacter pylori* sticking to cells in the stomach lining due to the unique anti-adhesin compounds it contains. This may help to flush *Helicobacter* from the stomach so they are expelled more easily.

Eating live bio yoghurt or supplements containing cultures of probiotic bacteria (e.g. *Lactobacillus acidophilus*, *Lactobacillus bifidus*) has also been shown to inhibit growth of *Helicobacter pylori* as well as maintaining overall intestinal health.

Note:
● Recurrent intestinal symptoms should always be reported to a doctor.
● Diabetes sufferers should consult a doctor before using a honey treatment.

See also **B12, Bilberries, C**

Herpes simplex

Eight out of ten people show antibody evidence of infection with the *Herpes simplex* viruses that cause cold sores, but studies suggest that only 20–40 per cent of those exposed develop clinical symptoms.

Cold sores are most commonly acquired during childhood, between the ages of six and 18 months. Primary infection in childhood can cause extensive, painful ulceration of the mouth (herpetic gingivostomatitis). Kissing is the main mode of infection and should be avoided from the first sign of a cold sore appearing until it is fully healed.

Treatment
Echinacea is known to increase the proliferation and activity of immune cells responsible for fighting infections and is

often used to reduce herpes recurrences. A typical regime is to take 25 drops echinacea tincture in water as soon as possible at the beginning of an attack. Repeat every two hours for four doses, then continue four times a day until symptoms resolve. Avoid trigger factors such as stress and ultraviolet light (e.g. sunbeds).

The essential amino acid L-lysine can suppress herpes virus growth and may speed ulcer healing, neutralize pain (sometimes within 24 hours) and reduce recurrences. Supplements of the amino acid L-lysine have been shown to reduce the frequency of herpes recurrences. In field trials involving over 1500 sufferers, more than 80 per cent reported that recurrences were either prevented or decreased in frequency. When sores did occur, their severity and healing time were both greatly reduced. Not all clinical studies have shown significant results, however, and supplements may work best when taken together with vitamin C and zinc and when following a diet low in L-arginine – an amino acid needed by the herpes virus to replicate. Chocolate, nut and grain intake should be limited while more vegetables should be eaten. Lysine supplements should not be taken long term in high doses as they may increase cholesterol levels and the risk of atherosclerosis.

A double-blind study in which 200 mg vitamin C plus bioflavonoids were taken three or five times daily (starting within 48 hours of initial symptoms) found that blisters developed in only 26 per cent of treated patients compared with 100 per cent in those receiving a placebo. The average interval from onset to complete healing was also significantly reduced in those taking vitamin C.

Olive leaf extracts have a powerful anti-viral action, and a comparative trial of three products conducted by the Herpes Viruses Association (olive leaf extract versus the cactus,

Opuntia streptacantha, and a combined lysine pollen and propolis capsule) found that olive leaf extracts were the clear winner. Out of 45 members taking part, 78 per cent of those using olive leaf extracts were pleased with the results in treating and preventing attacks.

Applying the contents of a vitamin E capsule to a cold sore regularly can also reduce pain – usually within eight hours.

See also **Damiana, Elderberry, Goldenseal, Grapefruit seed, Iron, Lapacho, Oregano, Sarsaparilla, Siberian ginseng**

Hiatus hernia

A hiatus hernia forms when part of the stomach pushes up – or herniates – into the chest through a natural weakness in the diaphragm. In many cases, it causes no problems and symptoms only occur when the hernia affects the valve mechanism between the stomach and oesophagus so that acid is regurgitated and refluxes upwards, sometimes as far as the mouth. This causes a condition known as gastro-oesophageal reflux disease (GORD) whose main symptom is heartburn. Heartburn is partly due to acid irritation of delicate tissues lining the lower oesophagus, and partly to painful spasm of underlying muscles in the wall of the oesophagus. Hiatus hernia can also cause symptoms of coughing, shortness of breath, palpitations or hiccoughs due to extra pressure in the chest. In severe cases, bleeding and anaemia can occur. These symptoms often mimic those of angina or heart attack and it is estimated that 20 per cent of patients admitted to coronary care units have GORD rather than heart disease.

Treatment

To help reduce symptoms of hiatus hernia, excess weight should be lost, and over-filling the stomach avoided. Eating and drinking little and often throughout the day is recommended. Stooping, bending, late-night eating and lying down after eating should all be avoided. It also helps to follow a relatively bland diet without hot, acid, spicy, fatty or pastry foods and to avoid tea, coffee, alcohol and acidic fruit juices. Loose clothing should be worn, especially around the waist. It might also help to elevate the head of the bed by about 15–20 cm.

Traditionally, eating bitter, green leafy vegetables such as endive, lettuce and artichoke (also available as supplements) are recommended for relieving symptoms due to hiatus hernia. Live bio yoghurt and probiotic supplements containing digestive bacteria (e.g. *Lactobacilli*) are also helpful. Evening primrose and flax seed oil provide essential fatty acids which help to reduce inflammation, while aloe vera gel is widely used to relieve intestinal symptoms including dyspepsia. Start with a small dose (e.g. 1 teaspoon) and work up to around 1–2 tablespoons per day to find the ideal dose.

Colloidal silicol gel is also worth trying. Herbalists frequently recommend marshmallow root preparations to relieve hiatus hernia symptoms; however, diabetics on hypoglycemia medication should monitor blood sugar levels closely if taking these as some studies have suggested that they may lower blood sugar levels.

HIV and AIDS

The Human Immunodeficiency Virus (HIV) which can cause acquired immune deficiency syndrome (AIDS) is transmitted through contact with infected body fluids such as blood, urine, semen, breast milk and saliva.

The virus is readily transmitted sexually, and in the West at least one in seven people diagnosed with HIV is thought to have caught the infection through heterosexual intercourse. Practising safer sex and using a condom plus nonoxynol-9 spermicide helps to reduce the risk of contracting HIV sexually. In one study, only one in ten partners of HIV-positive people who used condoms became HIV positive themselves, compared with 12 in 14 partners infected where condoms were not used.

HIV selectively invades a type of immune cell known as a T-helper lymphocyte (also known as T4 or CD4 cells) in which it multiples and, in some cases, destroys the cells or stops them working properly. T4 cells are essential for regulating the activity of other immune cells, and are especially important for triggering the production of antibodies from B lymphocytes.

Treatment

Anti-viral drugs are given to help reduce viral replication. A number of supplements may also be advised to help boost immunity, but should only be taken under medical supervision. These include:

- vitamin E and selenium which together increase production of antibodies

- other antioxidants such as vitamin C, carotenoids and zinc which are important for healthy immune function and to reduce inflammation

- co-enzyme Q10 which increases oxygen uptake and energy production in cells, and is often helpful for overcoming fatigue

- the amino acid N-acetylcysteine, which helps to stimulate immunity, reduces production of excess mucus, and is thought to interfere with viral replication (as is turmeric)

- omega-3 fish oils, which help to reduce weight loss and also improve immune function.

Other immune stimulants include reishi, shiitake, maitake, astragalus, cat's claw, echinacea, goldenseal and lapacho. Two or more of these taken in rotation may be recommended to obtain the maximum benefit. Nutritional advice should be sought from a qualified medical herbalist.

See also **B12, Catuaba, Elderberry, Turmeric**

Homocysteine levels – raised

A raised level of the amino acid homocysteine damages artery walls to trigger atherosclerosis and is now recognized as an important risk factor for coronary heart disease and stroke. Normally, homocysteine levels are tightly controlled by three different enzymes that convert homocysteine to cysteine – a safe end product that promotes cell growth. Two of these three enzymes depend on adequate intakes of folic acid, vitamins B6 and B12 for optimal activity. When these nutrients are lacking, homocysteine levels rise. Genetic mutations also affect enzyme activity and an estimated one in ten people inherits levels of homocysteine that triple the risk of cardiovascular disease. One in 160,000 inherits extremely high homocysteine levels with 30 times the risk of premature heart disease. After the menopause, women seem less able to process homocysteine so levels build up to increase the risk of osteoporosis and coronary heart disease.

Treatment

High levels of homocysteine can be reduced by taking folic acid supplements (400–650 mcg per day) plus B6 and B12.

Although diet should always come first, synthetic forms of folic acid found in supplements and fortified foods (e.g. breakfast cereals) are more bioavailable than those found in natural food sources (e.g. green leafy vegetables) which are in the less easily absorbed polyglutamate form.

See also **Choline**

Hormone replacement therapy – natural

Hormone replacement therapy aims to restore oestrogen levels to the normal, pre-menopausal state. This relieves the signs and symptoms of oestrogen deficiency and postpones long-term consequences such as osteoporosis and coronary heart disease. Although hormone replacement therapy (HRT) is the medical treatment of choice to reduce menopausal symptoms and the risk of post-menopausal osteoporosis, a large number of women are unable, or unwilling, to take it. For these, a number of alternative options are available.

Black cohosh (*Cimicifuga racemosa*) has been prescribed in Germany for over 40 years. Several comparison studies have shown standardized extracts of black cohosh to be at least as effective as standard HRT (conjugated oestrogens) in relieving hot flushes, vaginal thinning and dryness. It outperformed diazepam and oestrogen HRT in relieving low mood and anxiety. It probably does not protect against heart disease or osteoporosis, however. No side effects have been reported and the only contra-indications are pregnancy and lactation. Because it does not stimulate oestrogen-sensitive tumours (and may even inhibit them) black cohosh may be used in women with a history of breast cancer.

Other popular herbal alternatives include red clover and soy extracts which contain natural plant hormones known as phytoestrogens of which isoflavones are the most widely studied (*see* **Isoflavones**).

See also **Dong quai, Liquorice, Maca, Oats, Pfaffia, Sage, Sarsaparilla, Siberian ginseng, Wild yam**
Related entry: **Menopause**

Hypertension

When blood pressure (BP) is measured, two readings are taken: the higher reading is the pressure in the system as the heart contracts and pushes blood into your circulation and is known as systolic pressure; the lower reading is the pressure in the system when your heart rests between beats and is known as diastolic pressure. These two pressures are recorded one over the other. A young, healthy adult has a resting BP of around 120/80 mmHg (as measured against a column of mercury to give a unit of mmHg). BP naturally tends to rise with age, and a healthy 50-year-old may have a BP of around 150/90 mmHg.

Significant high blood pressure, or hypertension, is diagnosed when your BP is consistently above 160/95 mmHg. A systolic blood pressure of 140–160 mmHg and diastolic values of 90–95 mmHg are sometimes referred to as mild, or borderline hypertension and also require regular monitoring and treatment.

One of the main causes of high blood pressure is hardening and furring up of the arteries (atherosclerosis). This naturally occurs with increasing age and comes on more quickly in those who smoke, are diabetic or overweight. Other factors that increase blood pressure include an abnormally raised blood fat level, drinking too much alcohol, excessive salt intake, stress, lack of exercise and the side effects of some drugs. Some research suggests that high BP is linked with lack of essential fatty acids (such as those found in evening primrose oil), and the minerals calcium and magnesium. High blood pressure also runs in some families, so it is even more important to have regular checks if there is a family history.

Some people with hypertension feel dizzy, tired or suffer from headaches but most people feel relatively well even when their blood pressure is dangerously high. If not corrected, prolonged hypertension can damage blood vessels in the brain, heart, kidneys and eyes to cause serious complications, including kidney failure, impaired eyesight, heart attack and stroke. A man in his early 40s is 30 times more likely to have a stroke if he has hypertension than a man with normal blood pressure.

Treatment

The aim of blood pressure treatment is to reduce diastolic BP to below 85 mmHg and/or systolic BP to below 140 mmHg. Sometimes two or even three different types of drug are needed to achieve this goal.

Some lifestyle changes can help to improve high blood pressure. These include:

- regular exercise (e.g. walking, cycling, swimming, gardening) for at least 30 minutes, five times a week and preferably every day
- quitting smoking: cigarettes damage artery linings, cause spasm and constriction of vessels, and raise blood pressure
- losing any excess weight – just losing half a stone can significantly reduce a raised blood pressure
- avoiding excess alcohol intake; a maximum of no more than two or three units of alcohol per day, and regular alcohol-free days is recommended (1 unit = 1 small glass wine *or* half a pint of beer *or* 1 shot of spirits *or* 1 measure of liqueur wine)
- avoiding stressful situations and taking time out to relax.

In addition to the above, a low-fat diet is recommended with plenty of fresh fruit and vegetables for protective vitamins, minerals, antioxidants, fibre and potassium, which helps to flush excess sodium from your body. Not adding salt during cooking or at the table will lower systolic blood pressure by a modest amount, and if everyone who was hypertensive did this it is estimated that the incidence of stroke would be reduced by as much as 26 per cent, and coronary heart disease by 15 per cent. Against this, however, a study involving over 11,000 US adults found that, after adjustment for age and sex, the mortality rate from any cause was highest among people who reported the lowest sodium intake, and lowest among the group with the highest sodium intake. Perhaps the best compromise is to use a low-sodium salt that also contains potassium, magnesium and beneficial trace elements such as selenium.

A daily dose of 100 mg Co Q10 has been found to significantly reduce blood pressure compared with a placebo. Garlic powder tablets are widely prescribed in Europe to reduce hypertension, and in one study where 600–900 mg garlic powder tablets were taken daily for up to six months, systolic blood pressure (BP) fell by an average of 8 per cent.

Transcendental Meditation has been shown to significantly reduce blood pressure within 3 months.

A number of other supplements have a beneficial effect on the circulation, including: **Calcium, Evening primrose oil, omega-3 Fish oils, Ginger, Green tea, Gynostemma, Hawthorn, Magnesium, Maitake, Olive leaf, Olive oil, Potassium, Reishi, Selenium, Siberian ginseng, Tribulus terrestris, Yerba maté.**

Related entry: **Atherosclerosis**

Hypotension

Low blood pressure is not routinely treated in the UK unless it causes recurrent symptoms such as dizziness. A study of over 10,000 civil servants suggested that persistent low blood pressure – sometimes known as hypotension syndrome – can also be associated with tiredness, headaches, anxiety, depression and minor psychological dysfunction. This is probably related to reduced blood circulation and supply of oxygen, glucose and other nutrients to the brain.

Treatment

Ginkgo supplements would be expected to reduce the above symptoms but would not raise the underlying blood pressure. Increasing intake of dietary table salt (sodium chloride) is the approach most usually suggested as this encourages fluid accumulation in the circulation. *Panax ginseng*, butcher's broom and liquorice can raise blood pressure but should not be taken long term except under the supervision of a medical herbalist.

In older people, low blood pressure can occur when getting up quickly from a sitting or lying position. This is known as postural hypotension and may be remedied by getting up slowly and, for example, sitting on the side of the bed for a minute or two to adjust before standing.

Immunity

In order to function properly, the body's immune cells need a plentiful supply of vitamins, minerals and immune boosters. These help them to produce communication chemicals that control their activity, and to make powerful disease-fighting substances.

There are several ways to help maintain healthy immune function to increase natural protection against diseases such as influenza.

- Getting regular, good nights' sleep; this is a time of relaxation, regeneration and rejuvenation in which growth hormone and other vital substances involved in healing and fighting disease are secreted.

- Eating a wholefood diet providing plenty of fresh fruit and vegetables – these supply vitamins, minerals, antioxidants and certain non-nutrient substances (phytochemicals) that help to prevent cancer and boost immune function.

- Eating a low-fat diet with less omega-6 polyunsaturated fatty acids derived from vegetable oils and more omega-3 polyunsaturated fatty acids derived from oily fish; ideally, a balanced intake of omega-3s and omega-6s is needed, but the average adult currently eats seven times more omega-6 fats than omega-3s. For those who don't like eating fish, taking an omega-3 supplement is recommended. Evening primrose oil capsules supply important essential fatty acids, too.

- Avoiding excess stress which puts the body's systems on red alert; in the long term, this depletes the adrenal glands, interferes with the body's ability to fight disease and increases susceptibility to infections.

- Taking regular exercise.

● Taking a good vitamin and mineral supplement to act as a nutritional safety net and guard against deficiencies (research involving 96 elderly people showed that those taking multivitamins for one year had better immune function, mounted a better response to influenza vaccination, and had half as many days ill compared with those not taking them).

High-dose vitamin C with bioflavonoids helps to protect against viral infections, while sucking zinc lozenges reduces symptoms of the common cold. Many herbal remedies are also known to boost immune function. Some act as adaptogens, helping the body to cope with the stress. Adaptogens work best when low immunity and fatigue are due to an underlying problem such as poor or irregular diet, hormone imbalance, stress or excess consumption of coffee, nicotine or alcohol. When adaptogens are used together with vitamin C and the B complex, results are often impressive.

Where low immunity is linked with excess stress, an adaptogenic supplement such as Siberian ginseng (*Eleutherococcus senticosus*) or Korean ginseng (*Panax ginseng*) will help to boost general resistance. Many of us are selenium-depleted due to low selenium levels in the soil on which crops and livestock are produced. Taking a selenium/antioxidant supplement will significantly improve antibody production and, when combined with vitamin E, can increase antibody production by up to thirty times.

Other popular immune-boosting supplements include **Echinacea**, which increases the number and activity of white blood cells that fight viral infections, **Arginine, Astragalus, Ashwagandha, Bee products** – propolis, **Cat's claw, Co-enzyme Q10, Garlic, Glutamine, Goldenseal,**

Gotu kola, Green tea, Guarana, Lapacho, Maitake, Probiotic supplements, Reishi, Selenium, Shiitake, Schisandra, Wheatgrass and **Yerba maté**. These may be used in rotation for maximum benefit.

Impotence

Erectile dysfunction affects as many as one in ten men. It is important to seek medical advice as, in the vast majority of cases, appropriate investigations and treatment are successful in restoring potency.

Treatment

Stress, overwork and tiredness are among the commonest causes of loss of sex drive and impotence. Taking time out for rest, relaxation and plenty of sleep are important. Reducing alcohol intake to no more than one or two units per day and making an effort to cut back or quit smoking are also important. Smoking cigarettes lowers sex hormone levels and can also reduce rigidity of erections. A regular exercise programme is also recommended as brisk physical activity increases secretion of hormones important for sexual function.

Extracts from the ginkgo biloba tree (usually taken to improve memory) improve blood flow to the peripheries as well as the brain, and have been shown to strengthen erections. Clinical studies in Paris involving 262 men found that extracts from a Brazilian tree, muira puama, were as effective in treating erectile dysfunction as yohimbine – a pharmaceutical drug that is licensed for treating impotence in the USA.

Taking a good vitamin and mineral supplement will help to guard against nutritional deficiencies, while evening primrose oil provides essential fatty acids and natural sterols that can normalize sex hormone balance. Extracts from the bark of a Brazilian tree, catuaba, promote erotic dreams, increase sexual desire and improve erections

See also **Arginine, Cayenne, Damiana, Ginseng, Grapeseed, Maca, Pfaffia, Pine bark, Siberian ginseng**

Indigestion

Indigestion (or dyspepsia) is a discomfort or burning felt centrally in the upper abdomen, while heartburn is felt behind the chest bone.

Treatment

Those who are prone to discomfort after eating should avoid consuming excess fat, pastry, spicy dishes, chocolate, acidic fruit juices, coffee or alcohol as much as possible, as these are the commonest culprits. Eating little and often throughout the day to avoid over-filling the stomach is recommended, as well as taking care not to stoop, bend or lie down immediately after eating. It also helps to wear loose clothing, especially around the waist, and to avoid late-night dining. Elevating the head of the bed by about 15–20 cm is an excellent trick if recurrent heartburn is linked with hiatus hernia (in which part of the stomach slips up through the diaphragm into the chest). Other useful measures for those with recurrent symptoms include losing any excess weight and stopping smoking.

Short-term symptoms of heartburn may be treated with antacids (containing calcium carbonate) available over the counter. More powerful drugs that temporarily switch off stomach acid production (e.g. cimetidine, ranitidine, famotidine) are also available over the counter but should not be used long-term without seeking medical advice.

Liquorice (DGL form) is widely used to soothe indigestion. Other supplements that many people find helpful include probiotic bacteria (e.g. *Lactobacilli*), aloe vera juice, colloidal silicol gel and vitamin B complex.

Note: it is estimated that around one in ten people regularly taking antacids – especially those over the age of 40 – could have a more serious underlying problem of stomach cancer which needs to be diagnosed and treated as early as possible. A doctor should be consulted if symptoms last more than a week or if they keep recurring, as further investigations and treatment may be needed. A peptic ulcer might need to be excluded, for example, or tests carried out for a stomach infection with *Helicobacter pylori* (*see* separate entry).

See also **Cayenne, Ginger, Glutamine, Peppermint, Sage, Turmeric, Yerba maté**

Infertility

See **Conception**, and **Sperm count – low**

Inflammatory bowel disease

See Crohn's disease and Ulcerative colitis

Influenza

Influenza is a viral disease that attacks the respiratory system. Infection spreads rapidly through airborne droplets (coughs, sneezes) so that small outbreaks tend to occur in different areas.

Symptoms start off similar to those of a cold with cough, sore throat and runny nose, which then become significantly worse. Chills, fever, headache, loss of appetite, fatigue and muscle aches and pains set in, often lasting for seven to ten days. Tiredness, weakness and depression may last for several weeks after.

For most healthy people, flu is a nasty experience but is not life-threatening. Sometimes, however, complications – including pneumonia, inflammation of the heart (myocarditis) and febrile fits – can occur. Some people are more at risk of complications than others. These include the elderly – especially those living in residential homes where the virus spreads rapidly – and those with:

- chronic lung disease, including asthma, bronchitis and emphysema
- heart disease
- kidney failure
- hormone problems such as sugar diabetes

- low immunity due to drugs (e.g. steroid tablets) or disease (e.g. cancer, AIDS).

Anybody who falls into any of the above groups should consider protecting themselves with an annual flu vaccination which offers 70–80 per cent protection against infection. Immunization is not routinely recommended for healthy, fit adults, however.

For prevention, *see* **Echinacea, Elderberry, Goldenseal, Lapacho, Olive leaf, Perilla frutescens, Shiitake, Siberian ginseng.**

Treatment

Resting in bed and staying warm are important, but the room must be well ventilated. Those who live alone should arrange for someone to check on them regularly and do any essential shopping. Painkillers such as ibuprofen or paracetamol will help to relieve the aching and also keep a fever down. Drinking plenty of warm fluids and eating simple, soothing foods such as soup, yoghurt or scrambled eggs on bread are recommended. Sucking ice cubes will be cooling and will also relieve a sore throat. Steam inhalations can ease congestion. If you have chest pain or difficulty in breathing, medical advice should be sought immediately.

Supplements to consider include high-dose vitamin C plus other antioxidants such as vitamin E and selenium (which together increase antibody production), grapeseed or pine bark extracts. Sucking lozenges containing zinc gluconate may shorten the duration of a sore throat.

Nasal congestion can be relieved by plain steam inhalation, but adding essential oils such as menthol, eucalyptus, cinnamon, or pine will bring immediate relief.

Elderberry extracts contain anti-viral compounds that have been shown to reduce the severity and duration of influenza infections, as do olive leaf extracts. Other supplements used to treat influenza include echinacea and Siberian ginseng (*Eleutherococcus senticosus*) which, according to Russian research, reduces the incidence of colds, flu and other respiratory infections by 40 per cent in those taking it regularly.

Note: if flu symptoms develop in the elderly, or in someone with lung, kidney, heart or other serious problems, a doctor should be contacted straight away. In some cases, an anti-viral drug may be needed to reduce the risk of complications. These ideally need to be taken within 24 hours of the onset of symptoms. Prevention through immunization is by far the best protection, however (see above).

See also **Olive leaf, Reishi**
Related entry: **Immunity**

Insect bites and stings

Biting insects are attracted to our individual body scents with some proving more attractive to them than others. The injected venom of biting and stinging insects can contain a cocktail of over 100 chemicals which trigger rapid inflammation and pain.

Prevention

- Covering up as much exposed skin as possible is important, especially from dusk onwards when biting insects become more active.

- Spraying a repellent inside the openings of clothes for extra protection or wearing impregnated wrist and ankle bands can help.

- If walking in long grass, always tuck trouser legs into socks and boots.

- Sunscreens containing insect repellent are worth trying for a useful double action.

- Muslin screens fitted inside windows so that they can still be opened during the day are useful.

- Scenting the home with essential oils that repel insects such as lavender, peppermint and eucalyptus has been shown to be effective.

- Brewer's yeast is an excellent source of B group vitamins and is sometimes taken to reduce the incidence of insect bites.

- There have been claims that taking very high-dose vitamin B1 (thiamin) supplements can repel biting insects, but it takes several weeks to work and is probably not that effective.

- Natural insect repellents include garlic powder tablets taken every day, and applying diluted citronella, lemon, eucalyptus or tea tree essential oils to the skin. These strong aromas make it less easy for mosquitoes and midges to find a host.

Note: if travelling to areas where malaria or other insect-born diseases are endemic, seek medical advice about appropriate prevention and treatments.

Treatment

If a bee leaves its sting and poison sac lodged in your skin, remove it gently by scraping with a fingernail or a sterile needle – don't grasp with fingers or tweezers or you may force more poison into the wound. Wash the affected area with soap and water and, as bee stings are acid, apply a little baking soda mixed with water. Wasp stings and gnat bites are alkaline, so apply a little wine vinegar or lemon juice to relieve pain.

Treatments to reduce itching and swelling include:

- a drop of neat lavender oil applied directly to a bite or sting, and repeated every five minutes up to a maximum of 10 drops
- an ice pack (e.g. bag of frozen peas) wrapped in a clean cloth and applied for two to five minutes at a time
- arnica cream
- antihistamine creams (consider tablets if seriously affected)
- local anaesthetic cream or an anti-inflammatory cream (e.g. 1 per cent hydrocortisone).
- a drop of chamomile oil applied three times a day for two days
- aloe vera gel.

Oral supplements to reduce symptoms include bromelain, vitamin C and bioflavonoids such as quercetin for their anti-inflammatory actions.

Note: if someone develops symptoms such as faintness, collapse, swelling or difficulty in breathing after being stung, urgent medical help must be sought immediately by dialling 999. If they have been stung in the mouth or throat, give them ice cubes to suck while waiting for help to arrive. Anyone who has a severe allergy to bites or stings may need to carry a pre-filled syringe of adrenaline with them at all times to be injected immediately if an allergic reaction occurs.

Insomnia

Most people need less sleep as they get older. While the average adult sleeps for between seven and eight hours a night, those over the age of 70 often only need five hours. Sleep architecture also changes, so that by the age of 70, most people get no stage 4 (really deep) sleep at all and spend more time in the shallower stages of sleep. It is therefore common for older people to wake several times during the night, although they may not recall this the following morning. So because their expectations dictate that they need a certain amount of sleep, many people think that they suffer from insomnia when, in fact, they are getting all the sleep they need. Those who feel fit and refreshed during the day are probably getting all the sleep they need and should make use of the new-found hours by developing a hobby that can be indulged at any hour, such as painting or writing memoirs.

Having said that, many elderly people do suffer from insomnia and the tell-tale signs to look out for include difficulty in getting off to sleep, waking unusually early in the morning and not being able to get back to sleep at all, feeling tired and listless during the day, yawning a lot, and feeling unusually irritable or snappy. Insomnia can also occur as part of a depressive illness.

Treatment

Napping during the day should be avoided as should over-indulgence in substances that interfere with sleep such as caffeine (coffee, tea, chocolate, colas), nicotine, alcohol and rich or heavy food – especially close to bedtime.

The simplest sedative is to sprinkle a few drops of lavender essential oil on a cotton wool pad near your pillow or to invest in a lavender-scented pillow. Herbal preparations containing valerian, hops and lemon balm are helpful in promoting sleep, especially if it is an overactive mind that is causing the problem. Extracts from the root of *Valeriana officinalis* are widely used to relieve anxiety, reduce muscle tension and promote sleep. If anxiety is at the root of a sleep problem kava kava may be helpful and can be taken as needed.

A number of vitamin and mineral deficiencies can interfere with sleep, so taking a multi-supplement that includes calcium, magnesium and B group vitamins is worthwhile. 5-HTP is another supplement option that may suit some people by boosting levels of serotonin in the brain.

Regular exercise during the day is important, but vigorous exercise in the evening should be avoided as it may compound the problem.

See also **Ashwaghanda, Hawthorn, Kava kava, Pfaffia, Rhodiola, St John's Wort, Yerba maté**

Intermittent claudication

Leg pain on exercise due to peripheral vascular disease is known as intermittent claudication.

Treatment

Standardized gingko supplements can help intermittent claudication as they open up small blood vessels to improve peripheral perfusion. A randomized, placebo-controlled, double-blind study of over 100 sufferers looked at the effects of taking 120 mg daily for six months. Significant differences between those who took ginkgo and those on inactive placebo were noted after two and four months. By six months, pain-free walking distance in those taking gingko had increased by 50 per cent with no side effects.

An interesting Tibetan preparation, Padma 28, contains a complex mix of 20 Tibetan medicinal herbs but surprisingly contains no ginkgo biloba. Padma 28 is currently undergoing clinical trials as it has previously been shown in a pilot clinical trial to increase pain-free walking distance in over half of patients. No one seems to have investigated the combined effects of ginkgo and Padma 28 which would seem to be a logical next step.

See also **Carnitine, E, Garlic, Grapeseed, Gynostemma, Olive oil, Pine bark**

Irritable bladder

Irritable or unstable bladder, in which there is a frequent and often urgent need to pass small volumes of urine (with no signs of infection) is a common and annoying problem. It is due to over-activity of the detrusor muscle in the bladder wall which contracts involuntarily as the bladder fills. A variety of triggers have been suggested, including psychological stress, drinking excessive or insufficient fluids, allergy, tight trousers, drinking acidic juices, tea, coffee or alcohol, eating spicy foods, the presence of bladder stones or weak pelvic floor muscles.

Treatment
It can be difficult to treat but referral for bladder training can achieve the return of normal voiding patterns by teaching sufferers to resist the urge to pass urine. A variety of herbal extracts can help, including chamomile and valerian, but it is best to consult a medical herbalist for individual advice.

Irritable bowel syndrome

Irritable bowel syndrome is the most common condition to affect the gut. At least a third of the population are affected at some time during their life, even if only mildly. Overall, 15 per cent of people are affected badly enough to consult their doctor.

According to the Rome II Criteria, in order to diagnose Irritable Bowel Syndrome, there must be at least 12 weeks (which need not be consecutive) in the preceding 12 months of abdominal discomfort or pain characterized by two of the following three features:

- it is relieved with defecation; and/or
- its onset is associated with a change in frequency of stool; and/or
- its onset is associated with a change in form (appearance) of stool.

The following symptoms also cumulatively support the diagnosis of IBS:

- fewer than three bowel movements a week
- more than three bowel movements a day
- hard or lumpy stools
- loose or watery stools
- straining during a bowel movement
- urgency (having to rush to have a bowel movement)
- feeling of incomplete bowel movement
- passing mucus (white material) during a bowel movement
- abdominal fullness, bloating or swelling.

IBS is not a condition that should be self-diagnosed, as similar symptoms can occur in other more serious bowel problems needing medical or surgical treatment.

Treatment

Once diagnosed with IBS, it is worth trying probiotic supplements containing friendly digestive bacteria (e.g.

Lactobacilli) which replenish the bowel with healthy bacteria and often improve symptoms of IBS. In one study of 100 patients with symptomatic IBS, patients given *Lactobacillus plantarum* showed a 75 per cent improvement in symptoms compared with only 30 per cent in those receiving drug treatment (e.g. mebeverine) alone. When mebeverine (which is available over the counter) and probiotic bacteria were taken together, improvement increased to 90 per cent.

Recent research involving 279 people with symptoms compatible with IBS, also showed that Cynara artichoke supplements produced an overall reduction in IBS symptoms of 71 per cent within an average of ten days.

Brewer's yeast is used medicinally to treat acute diarrhoea, acne, pre-menstrual symptoms and to prevent candida proliferation. Diarrhoea prevention has been shown in double-blind, placebo-controlled studies involving critically ill patients and in people taking penicillin. Oral intake of fermentable yeast can cause flatulence however, so although it may be helpful in reducing diarrhoea in some people with IBS, in others it may make symptoms such as bloating worse.

Many people find aloe vera juice helpful, while psyllium can help to overcome both diarrhoea and constipation.

See also **Glutamine**

Jet lag

Jet lag is a disturbance of the body's 24-hour sleep-wake biorhythms due to flying across several time zones, especially in an eastward direction which shortens the traveller's day. Jet lag is most likely to affect people over 30 who normally follow an established daily routine, causing symptoms of general disorientation, fatigue, poor memory, insomnia, headaches, irritability, poor concentration, decreased mental ability and reduced immunity.

Prevention/treatment

If flying east it can help to try going to bed earlier than usual for several nights before traveling. Conversely, if flying west, staying up later than usual for several nights before leaving can help. On the flight it is advisable to drink plenty of fluids, avoid alcohol, only eat light meals and sleep as much as possible. High-dose antioxidants should be taken (vitamin C, 1–3 g with bioflavonoids a day; vitamin E 400 IU a day) before, during and after travelling. Also, high-strength vitamin B complex (50–100 mg) should be taken twice a day during the flight and for the first two days after arrival.

Guarana is widely used to reduce the effects of jet lag when it is taken before, during and after a long-haul flight. On arrival, herbal sleep preparations containing natural extracts of valerian (*Valeriana officinalis*), lemon balm (*Melissa officinalis*) and hops (*Humulus lupulus*) will help. Alternatively, essential oils of lavender promote relaxation, and rosemary or lemon will stimulate and keep you awake.

See also **Siberian ginseng**
Related entry: **Economy-class syndrome**

Joint pains

Painful, inflamed joints due to sports injury or arthritis can be helped by a number of supplements.

Glucosamine sulphate improves the quality and quantity of synovial fluid – the joint's oil – for a better internal cushioning effect. Research published in *The Lancet* showed that glucosamine sulphate is an effective and potentially disease-modifying treatment for osteoarthritis of the knee. It can be taken together with vitamin C (an antioxidant that damps down inflammation) or with green-lipped mussel extracts (which prevents inflammatory cells moving into joints). Raw extracts of New Zealand green-lipped mussels (*Perna canaliculus*) contain glycoproteins that damp down inflammation in arthritic joints. They work by preventing white blood cells from moving into the joints, where they would have released powerful chemicals making pain and swelling worse. Extracts produce significant reductions in pain and stiffness and have been shown to outperform non-steroidal anti-inflammatory drugs (NSAIDs) such as ibuprofen and indomethacin. In a trial of 86 patients, 67 per cent of those with rheumatoid arthritis and 35 per cent of those with osteoarthritis benefited. If the joint has damaged ligaments or cartilage (e.g. from a sports injury) glucosamine can be combined with chondroitin to boost joint repair.

MSM-sulphur is worth considering, and extracts from the root tuber of devil's claw (*Harpagophytum procumbens*), bromelain and boswellia have significant anti-inflammatory and analgesic properties to treat painful, inflamed joints. Omega-3 fish oils (e.g. found in cod liver oil) are also beneficial. Choose a cod liver oil product described as high strength or extra high strength for the most effective anti-inflammatory action.

Related entry: **Arthritis**

Keratosis pilaris

Keratosis pilaris is a roughness of the skin, which feels like sandpaper, commonly on the upper arms and legs. It is associated with atopic eczema.

Treatment

Plenty of moisturizing emollients should be used to soothe and rehydrate the skin. Applying a generous amount on the upper arms at night then placing a bandage on top will improve penetration. Aqueous cream should be used to cleanse the skin rather than soap, and cotton rather than woollen or nylon clothes should be worn. It is best not to get too hot, and scratching should be avoided at all costs.

Essential fatty acids found in omega-3 fish oils help to reduce inflammation and was shown in a double-blind study to improve scaling and itching. As lack of vitamin A can also cause scaly skin with raised, pimply hair follicles, taking cod liver oil, which is rich in both omega-3 essential fatty acids and vitamins A and D, may help. Evening primrose oil may reduce itching. Avoiding cows' milk products for a trial period under the supervision of a nutritionist is also worth trying. Patch testing will help to identify any common allergens that may be causing a reaction.

Kidney stones

Kidney stones are due to the precipitation of insoluble salts in the urinary tract to form solid lumps. Nine out of ten kidney stones contain calcium, usually combined with oxalate. Paradoxically, a study of over 90,000 nurses showed that women with a good dietary calcium intake of above 1100 mg from food sources had half the risk of developing kidney stones as those with intakes of less than 500 mg per day. This is because calcium-rich foods bind oxalates in the gut so that less is absorbed. Calcium supplements are best avoided, however, except under medical supervision. Oxalate-rich foods such as beans, beets, celery, blueberries, chocolate, grapes, spinach and strawberries should also be avoided. Vegetarians have a lower risk of kidney stones and eating meat seems to increase the risk although this can be offset by eating more fruit and vegetables. A low-sodium diet should be followed and a good fluid intake maintained. Various studies have shown that drinking water, milk, coffee, tea, beer, wine or orange juice is associated with a reduced risk of kidney stone formation, while drinking apple and grapefruit juice significantly increases the risks for reasons that remain unclear.

Magnesium supplements can reduce stone formation, especially when taken with vitamin B6. A blend of terpene essential oils that help to dissolve kidney stones is available on prescription only (called Rowatinex); according to the manufacturer, this dissolves at least 50 per cent of kidney stones within eight weeks.

See also **Bilberry**

Leg ulcers

Leg ulcers are a painful and unpleasant condition that greatly reduce mobility and quality of life. They may be due to a number of conditions, including poor blood supply (arterial insufficiency) and poor venous drainage. They are especially common in people with diabetes.

Treatment

Some research has suggested that leg ulcers may be associated with low zinc levels – especially if senses of taste or smell are reduced (another possible sign of zinc deficiency) – so zinc supplements may be helpful. In addition, antioxidant supplements such as vitamin C and vitamin E will help to reduce inflammation and promote healing.

Garlic powder tablets, ginkgo biloba extracts and a blend of over 20 Tibetan herbs known as Padma 28 can also improve circulation through tiny blood vessels in the base of the ulcer. Ginkgo should not be combined with prescription drugs or regular blood-thinning agents such as aspirin, however. Oily fish such as salmon, sardines, mackerel and herrings should be included in the diet and intakes of fatty and sugary foods should be cut down.

Aloe vera gel and Gotu kola extracts may be used externally to improve healing of chronic ulcers; however topical treatments should only be used with the guidance of the doctor or nurse in charge of dressing the ulcer.

See also **Bee products – Manuka honey; Myrrh**

Leukoplakia

Leukoplakia produces areas of white, boggy skin in the mouth that resemble patches of grey-white paint and are usually painless. As this condition is considered premalignant (can develop into a cancer) it is usually kept under close medical supervision or even removed under anaesthetic.

Treatment

At least eight studies have shown that betacarotene, an antioxidant carotenoid, can reverse oral leukoplakia lesions, although other studies have not been conclusive. Antioxidants in general appear to be beneficial and, in one study, vitamin E supplements (800 IU a day) taken for 24 weeks caused regression of oral leukoplakia (pre-cancerous lesions) in 67 per cent of patients. In another study, a combination of 30 mg of beta-carotene, 1 g vitamin C and 800 IU of vitamin E taken daily for nine months, helped 55 per cent of patients who experienced either complete or partial clinical resolution of lesions.

When olive leaf extracts (1 g, three times a day) were taken by 67 people with dental problems including leukoplakia, 60 experienced full recovery. Spirulina algae are also worth trying – in a trial in which 44 people with leukoplakia took 1 g a day for one year, over half the lesions either vanished or significantly reduced in size while those receiving a blue-green placebo experienced no change in their lesions. There is no reason why antioxidants, olive leaf and spirulina extracts should not be taken together.

Libido – low

Low sex drive is common and affects as many as one in five adults at any one time. Those most at risk include stressed executives, new parents and post-menopausal women.

Treatment
A number of supplements have natural prosexual actions:

● Oyster extracts owe their aphrodisiac reputation to their high zinc content, which is important for maintaining testosterone levels and for both male and female fertility.

● Chicken egg extracts have been found to enhance sex drive in males, although the exact way in which they work is not understood. After nine days' incubation, the fertilized eggs have reached a critical stage of pre-embryonic development and contain a variety of high molecular weight substances which, when freeze-dried and consumed, are thought to increase the effects of testosterone in the body. Clinical trials involving male volunteers with low sex drive found that they significantly increased sex drive within three weeks compared with an inactive placebo

● Catuaba – known as the tree of togetherness – is a Brazilian tree whose powdered bark acts as a sexual stimulant and aphrodisiac in both men and women. Erotic dreams are usually experienced within 5–21 days of taking extracts regularly, followed by increased sexual desire. It also improves peripheral blood flow which may be another mechanism for boosting sexual performance, and has been used to combat extreme exhaustion.

- Muira puama – popularly known as potency wood – is another Brazilian tree whose powdered bark contains hormone-like substances that enhance sexual desire and improve impotence. Researchers are unsure how it works but it is thought to stimulate sexual desire both psychologically and physically, through a direct action on brain chemicals, through stimulating nerve endings in the genitals and by boosting production/ function of sex hormones, especially testosterone.

- St John's Wort is effective in treating low sex drive associated with mild to moderate depression.

Note: if low sex drive continues for longer than three months, medical advice should be sought. In around 5 per cent of cases low libido may be linked with high levels of prolactin hormone, which needs further investigation and treatment.

See also **Arginine, Ashwagandha, B3, Foti, Ginseng, Maca, Pfaffia, Phenlyalanine, Sarsaparilla, Schisandra, Tribulis terrestris, Tyrosine**

Lichen planus

Lichen planus is an inflammatory skin disease associated with intensely itchy, raised, purple lesions – usually on the inside of the wrists and lower legs, although they can occur anywhere. Papules often have a fine, white, lacy pattern on the surface, and in 50 per cent of cases, painful lacy white streaks or ulcers form on mucous membranes such as the mouth or genitals. The exact cause is unknown, but it is thought to be related to an abnormality of a type of immune cell known as T-lymphocytes. A similar rash can occur as a side effect of certain drugs (eg gold, penicillamine, antimalarial therapy). The prognosis is good as symptoms usually clear within two years, although recurrences can appear. Mucosal lesions need regular inspection as they may be pre-malignant.

Treatment

Where treatment is needed, potent steroids or immune modifying drugs may be tried. Aloe vera pulp or gel is often helpful when applied to skin or vaginal lesions. Omega-3 fish oil supplements have a useful anti-inflammatory action. A medically qualified herbalist might suggest herbs that support immune function such as echinacea or cat's claw (*Uncaria tomentosa*).

Lichen sclerosus et atrophicus

Lichen sclerosus et atrophicus (LSA) is an inflammatory skin condition that can affect the anal and genital regions. It is thought to affect around one in 300 people, and while it can affect men, women or children, it is most common in females. Affected skin usually becomes thinned, crinkly and ivory coloured (like cigarette paper), and when active may have a purple-red border. Itching, soreness and pain are often present. Medical diagnosis is important to rule out other skin conditions with a similar appearance, and long-term lesions need regular review.

Treatment

Unfortunately, there is no cure, although symptoms often improve with time. Some researchers have had good results from treating LSA with evening primrose oil (applied locally and taken orally).

Liver problems

For liver problems, it is always advisable to seek medical or herbal advice about appropriate supplementation. Those most likely to be recommended include antioxidants (e.g. vitamins C, E, carotenoids, selenium, grapeseed or pine bark extracts), milk thistle, Cynara artichoke, dandelion root and liquorice.

Lupus

Lupus is an inflammatory disorder that affects many systems in the body. The most common form is known as systemic lupus erythematosus (SLE) and it is nine times more common in women than men, the usual age of onset being between 20 and 40. It often produces a characteristic butterfly-shaped red rash across the nose, cheeks and forehead. The palms may also redden and the joints become inflamed. These visible changes reflect the widespread inflammation of blood vessels (vasculitis) occurring throughout the body. Most people develop extreme tiredness, and around half suffer from muscle aches and fever. The most serious problems occur if the nervous system or kidneys become involved. A mild form, chronic discoid lupus, can occur in which only the skin is affected.

The exact cause of SLE is unknown but it is linked with abnormalities of the immune system such as increased production of antibodies aimed against the membranes found in body cells. Latest research suggests that these may be triggered by a viral infection that causes excess death of lymph cells. As these lymph cells break up, other immune cells mistake their disintegrating membranes for foreign bodies and start to attack them.

Treatment

SLE sufferers may require treatment with drugs that damp down over-active immune changes. The outlook is good, with remissions often lasting for long periods of time. Some women with severe SLE experience infertility or recurrent miscarriages, but for many women fertility is normal.

It is advisable to avoid taking the oral contraceptive pill and HRT, which can trigger flare-ups, and to reduce intake of red meat. Aim to eat a mainly vegetarian diet and avoid caffeine, alcohol, sugar and tobacco.

Extracts of the herb milk thistle which helps to support liver function might be recommended. Flaxseed, evening primrose, omega-3 fish or hemp seed oils containing essential fatty acids with anti-inflammatory actions are worth trying, and high-dose vitamin C is important as an antioxidant, to damp down inflammation and promote tissue repair. B group vitamins, vitamin E, carotenoids and selenium also help to maintain healthy tissues.

See also **Echinacea**

Macular degeneration

Age-related macular degeneration (AMD) affects around 20 per cent of people aged over 65 and is due to deterioration of the part of the retina involved in fine vision for reading and recognizing faces.

Treatment

The macula of the eye contains two carotenoids, lutein and zeaxanthin (which can be made from lutein). People with macular degeneration have, on average, 70 per cent less lutein and zeaxanthin in their eyes than those with healthy vision and poor dietary intake is thought to cause breakdown of this vital part of the retina. Lutein and zeaxanthin are found in sweetcorn, carrots and other yellow-orange fruit and vegetables, and in spinach and other dark-green leafy vegetables. Those who eat the most carotenoids have at least a 60 per cent lower risk of developing AMD than those with low intakes, partly because of their antioxidant activity, which neutralizes harmful chemical reactions involved in light detection, and partly because their yellow colour filters out potentially harmful, visible blue light.

Lycopene, a carotenoid pigment found in tomatoes is also beneficial – those with the lowest intakes have more than double the risk of developing macular degeneration. Bilberry extracts contain antioxidant blue-red pigments with a similar action and can also increase blood flow to the retina.

Zinc supplements have been found to reduce visual loss in people with AMD compared with a placebo, while extracts of ginkgo biloba have been shown to produce a significant improvement in long-distance visual acuity AMD sufferers.

Supplements containing carotenoids, bilberry or other micronutrients important for eye health (e.g. vitamins C, E, selenium) are readily available and highly recommended. Powerful antioxidants such as grapeseed and pine bark extracts may also be recommended.

Memory – poor

Poor memory is a common complaint, particularly as a result of tiredness, not eating or skipping meals, and with increasing age.

Treatment

Eating a cereal breakfast has been found to improve memory in healthy adults, increasing the speed at which new information can be recalled, and improving concentration and mental performance. This is partly because it boosts glucose levels at a crucial time of the day, and partly because fortified breakfast cereals are a good source of vitamin B1 (thiamine) which improves mood and clarity of thought.

Double-blind, placebo-controlled trials have shown two other supplements can boost memory: firstly, ginkgo biloba extracts significantly improve short-term working memory within just two days – probably by improving blood circulation to the brain; secondly, phosphatidylserine (related to choline) has also been shown to improve all cognitive functions, including learning, recall, recognition and concentration, by providing nutrients needed to synthesize brain neurotransmitters. It seems to work by increasing glucose metabolism within brain cells and speeding transmission of messages from one neurone to another. Ginkgo and phosphatidylserine may be taken together.

Other types of memory loss might also benefit from these supplements. They should not be taken during pregnancy, but poor memory associated with the third trimester of pregnancy may benefit from essential fatty acid supplements.

See also **Alpha lipoic acid, Arginine, B6, Gotu kola, Olive oil, Reishi, Rhodiola, Sage, Siberian ginseng**

Menopause

The menopause is a natural phase in a woman's life when her fertility draws to a close. It usually occurs between the ages of 45 and 55 with an average of 51 years. The menopause is dated from a woman's last period, but the process really starts five to ten years before as the ovaries slowly run out of egg follicles. As a result, levels of oestrogen (oestradiol, oestrone plus oestriol) start to fall until too little is produced to maintain the monthly menstrual cycle.

Some women quickly adapt to lower levels of oestrogen and notice few – if any – problems. Others find it harder to lose their oestrogen and experience unpleasant symptoms that last for between one and five years – occasionally longer. Surveys suggest that one in four women has few problems, and half only notice mild symptoms while a quarter suffer quite badly.

The short-term symptoms of oestrogen withdrawal vary but commonly include hot flushes, night sweats, headaches, tiredness and mood swings. In time, symptoms such as vaginal dryness, urinary problems, thinning and loss of elasticity of skin occur. In the long term, oestrogen withdrawal also increases the risk of a number of potentially serious problems such coronary heart disease, stroke and osteoporosis.

Hot flushes are experienced by around 80 per cent of women around the menopause. They can be triggered by a number of factors, including heat, increased humidity, alcohol, caffeine and spicy foods. *See also* **Fibre.**

Treatment

Supplements containing isoflavones (oestrogen-like plant hormones) are often beneficial in reducing hot flushes. Phytoestrogens are plant hormones with a similar structure to human oestrogens but which are 500–1000 times less active. They can both damp down high oestrogen states (by competing for the stronger natural oestrogens at oestrogen receptors) and also provide a useful additional hormone boost when oestrogen levels are low (as they are at the menopause).

The most widely researched phytoestrogens – known as isoflavones – can significantly reduce the number of hot flushes experienced per day by 45 per cent within 12 weeks, have beneficial effects on the circulation to reduce the risk of coronary heart disease, and increase bone density in the lumbar spine to help protect against spinal osteoporosis. They may also reduce the risk of breast and prostate cancer. In Japan, blood phytoestrogen levels are as much as 110 times higher than those typically found in the West and do not appear to produce any long-term ill effects. Because phytoestrogens are so much weaker than natural oestrogens, there is no evidence that they need to be balanced by progesterone.

Black cohosh (*Cimicifuga racemosa*) has been prescribed in Germany for over 40 years. Several comparison studies have shown standardized extracts of black cohosh are at least as effective as standard HRT (conjugated oestrogens) in relieving hot flushes, vaginal thinning and dryness, although it probably does not protect against heart disease or osteoporosis. No side effects have been reported and the only contraindications for its use are pregnancy and lactation. Because it does not stimulate oestrogen-sensitive tumours (and may even inhibit them) black cohosh may be used in women with a history of breast cancer under medical supervision. Vitamin and mineral supplements containing boron are also important.

Related entries: **Hormone replacement therapy – natural; Osteoporosis**

Migraine

Migraine is a severe form of headache in which the pain is usually only felt on one side of the head or is definitely worse on one side.

Treatment

One of the most effective alternative treatments for migraine is the common garden herb feverfew (*Tanacetum parthenium*). This contains parthenolide which inhibits release of a neurotransmitter, serotonin, in the brain circulation to neutralize blood flow changes linked with symptoms. Clinical trials have found that, in 70 per cent of patients taking the herb, it either prevented or lessened the severity of headaches as well as related symptoms of nausea and vomiting. Trials on 60 migraine sufferers also found that those taking feverfew experienced significantly fewer attacks and less nausea and vomiting.

See also **B2 (riboflavin), Ginger, Ginkgo biloba, 5-HTP, Magnesium, Yerba maté**

Miscarriage

Sadly, of all pregnancies that are advanced enough to be recognized by the mother, around one in seven fails to progress beyond the first 20 weeks. Reasons often remain unknown and a specific, recurrent abnormality is only diagnosed in 5 per cent of cases.

Prevention

The chance of successfully becoming a parent after a miscarriage is still high at 60–70 per cent. A couple who have experienced one or more miscarriages are usually advised to follow a preconceptual care programme which includes stopping smoking (if applicable), avoiding alcohol, unnecessary drugs and foods that pose a risk of *Listeria* or toxoplasmosis infection (such as unpasteurized soft cheeses, blue cheeses, pâté).

Taking a vitamin and mineral supplement especially designed for pregnancy is also helpful. Where no specific cause for miscarriage is found, a future pregnancy may be prepared for in the normal way. Waiting at least three months before trying for pregnancy again is usually advised, in order to allow for both physical and emotional recovery.

See also **Selenium**
Related entry: **Conception**

Molluscum contagiosum

Molluscum contagiosum is a harmless viral infection that forms multiple, shiny, pearly, white lumps that may have a central dimple. As its name suggests, they are contagious with close contact as, when broken, an infectious, cheesy fluid is released. Many people are naturally immune, however. Lesions usually disappear within 18 months, but can be more troublesome in some children, especially those with eczema – possibly because scratching encourages their spread.

Treatment

Treatment involves disrupting the architecture of lesions – e.g. by freezing with liquid nitrogen. If freezing is not suitable, dermatologists suggest applying betadine paint daily, assuming there is no allergy to iodine.

Alternatively dilute tea tree oil may be applied to the lesions twice a day using a cotton bud to gently irritate the lesions. Emollient bath preparations can help to reduce itching. Evening primrose oil drops should be given (by mouth) and an evening primrose oil moisturizing body cream can also be used. An echinacea formula designed for children may help to boost immunity against this annoying viral infection. Some doctors have started prescribing the antacid drug cimetidine to treat the infection following the observation that it disappeared quickly in those prescribed cimetidine for excess acid production.

Morning sickness

Morning sickness affects 70 per cent of pregnant women. Its cause is not fully known, but it is thought to be linked with raised levels of oestrogen hormone, low blood sugar, or possibly increased secretion of bile. Another possibility is that it is triggered by increased production of an intestinal hormone.

Symptoms tend to start before the sixth week of pregnancy and have usually disappeared by the fourteenth week, although a few women suffer for longer. Excessive sickness (hyperemesis) causes dehydration, salt imbalances and a harmful build-up of ketones in the blood. Signs to watch for include weakness, dizziness and passing urine that is dark and scant.

Treatment

It is important to keep sipping water and sugary drinks. Ginger has excellent anti-emetic properties, so drinking ginger tea and ginger beer (the fizz seems to help), or chewing crystallized ginger or taking ginger tablets can all be helpful. Some practitioners also recommend treatment with vitamin B6 but this is best used under medical supervision. Stimulation of the PC6 acupuncture point in the wrist is effective and acupressure bands available from chemists make this easier. If problems continue, regular assessment by a doctor or midwife is important.

Motion sickness

Motion or travel sickness can be triggered while travelling by car, sailing at sea or riding on other forms of transport such as a horse, camel or elephant. It can also be a major problem for weightless astronauts in space. Susceptibility to travel sickness is present in everyone, but we all have a different sensitivity. One in three people is highly susceptible to motion sickness, a further third only suffer during fairly rough conditions while another third only react under prolonged, violently rough conditions. Very young children seldom suffer from motion sickness. The worst age seems to be around ten years old.

Motion sickness is caused by excessive and repetitive stimulation of motion-detecting hair cells in the inner ear. This triggers motion sickness when the brain receives conflicting messages from the eyes that do not match the degree of movement detected by the inner ears. This is especially likely to happen when travelling in a closed space such as a car, where you tend to focus on a nearby object. Your eyes tell your brain the environment is stationary, while your balance organs say it is not. If there is good visual evidence of the head's position – as in cycling or skiing for example – motion sickness does not occur.

Treatment

Travel sickness tablets containing the antihistamine cinnarizine can control symptoms for at least eight hours per dose with most children remaining alert or only slightly drowsy.

Ginger can help with the symptoms of motion sickness: try drinking ginger tea or ginger beer, chewing crystallized ginger or taking ginger tablets. Stimulation of the PC6 acupuncture point in the wrist is effective and elasticated wrist bands or the newer disposable acupressure plasters may be used on children.

Ensure that children sit high enough in the car so that they can see out of the window (in an appropriate child's car seat if applicable) and play 'I Spy' games that encourage them to look into the distance. Try to discourage them from focusing on near objects when in a car, such as reading a book. Only supply light meals, allow fresh air to circulate in the car, and stop to stretch legs frequently. A few drops of Bach rescue remedy under the tongue often work wonders if they start feeling unwell.

Mouth ulcers

Mouth ulcers linked with stress may be cold sores due to the *Herpes simplex* virus or aphthous ulcers which have been linked with hypersensitivity to a common mouth bacterium, haemolytic streptococcus. Recurrent mouth ulcers can also occasionally be a sign of coeliac disease (dietary sensitivity to gluten), inflammatory bowel diseases, SLE or other immune problems. It is therefore important to seek medical advice for a proper diagnosis.

Researchers in Norway have suggested that some unexplained mouth ulcers may be linked with a detergent, sodium lauryl sulphate (SLS) found in most brands of toothpaste. As it is a detergent, it is possible that SLS dries out the protective mucous membranes in the mouth so that irritants or infection can trigger ulceration. They found that when people with recurring mouth ulcers switched to using an SLS-free toothpaste, their incidence of mouth ulcers reduced by 70 per cent.

Treatment

Severe lack of vitamin C can lead to mouth ulcers as part of scurvy, although this is now rare in developed countries. Even so, a vitamin C supplement will help by reducing inflammation, and assisting in the formation of collagen during the healing process. Mouth ulcers have also been linked with a lack of other vitamins (B2, B3, B6, B12, folic acid) and mineral iron, so it is worth taking a multi-supplement providing around 100 per cent of the RDA for as many micro-nutrients as possible.

Applying aloe vera hydrogel has been shown to reduce healing time from ten days to between five and six days, and to rapidly improve discomfort within minutes of application. Sucking lozenges made from liquorice (DGL form) also has a soothing and anti-inflammatory action. Olive leaf extracts have a powerful antibiotic effect and in one study of people with mouth problems, including ulceration, the quickest improvement was seen in those who took olive leaf extracts (1 g) three times a day.

Other natural approaches include colloidal silicic acid, or mouthwashes containing myrrh. When feeling run down, it is worth taking a herbal adaptogen such as Siberian ginseng (*Eleutherococcus senticosus*) or an immune stimulant such as echinacea. *See also* **Sage.**

It is also advisable to avoid smoking and maintain good oral hygiene.

Note: any mouth ulcer or area of soreness that lasts for longer than three weeks should be checked by a doctor to exclude a mouth cancer.

Multiple sclerosis

Multiple sclerosis (MS) is a progressive, degenerative condition affecting the nervous system, whose effects vary from mild to severe. Many people have minimal disability, but others may develop visual difficulties, clumsiness, slurred speech, problems with walking, and loss of bowel or bladder control.

Some research suggests that levels of an essential fatty acid (linoleic acid) are low in people with MS, especially during a relapse, and taking high-dose evening primrose oil (2–3 g a day) may help. Also eating more nuts, seeds and oily fish and using extra-virgin olive oil for cooking, and linseed (flaxseed) oil for dressings is recommended.

Supplements containing selenium, magnesium, manganese and high-dose vitamin B12, C and E may be recommended to help relieve stiffness and spasm, and to strengthen muscles while improving co-ordination. A vitamin B complex supplement is generally taken to help improve nerve function, and an A to Z-style vitamin and mineral formula plus extra antioxidants might be helpful too.

The herbs most commonly recommended include black cohosh, echinacea, ginseng, St John's Wort and valerian. Ginkgo opens up small blood vessels and improves circulation to muscles and nerves and is often helpful, while echinacea has a beneficial effect on the immune system and may also be suggested. However, it is always advisable to consult a trained herbalist for the most appropriate treatment.

Mercury has been implicated in worsening symptoms. Chelation therapy to remove mercury from the body, plus replacement of mercury fillings is therefore advocated by some practitioners but this should only be done by a dentist who is experienced in removing mercury fillings.

Myalgic encephalitis (ME)

See **Chronic fatigue syndrome**

Myasthenia gravis

Myasthenia gravis is usually considered to be an auto-immune disorder in which weakness affects a variety of muscle groups and responds to treatment with anticholinesterase drugs.

Treatment

Some doctors feel that mercury toxicity or allergy play a role in the development of myasthenia gravis and recommend that silver/black dental amalgams are removed from the mouth. A dentist who specializes in the removal of these fillings should be consulted, however, as special techniques are needed for their safe elimination.

Herbal remedies used to help relieve symptoms include astragalus (often in combination with ginseng) and reishi mushrooms.

Nail problems

Nails are made of a hard, fibrous protein called keratin which is designed to strengthen the tips of fingers and toes and protect them from damage. They grow at a rate of up to 5 mm per month. Some people have strong, thick, nails which if not cut, can grow up to 30 cm in length.

Fungal nail infection (onychomycosis)

This can, unfortunately, be difficult to eradicate as the nail plate is composed of a hard, fibrous matrix through which fungal hyphae can easily penetrate.

Treatment

Treatment is aimed at prevention of fungal penetration of a newly emerging nail. This is successful as long as treatment continues but if topical applications are not used regularly, the new uninfected nail quickly becomes contaminated and the benefit of previous treatment is lost. Treatment then has to start all over again, continuing until the last section of infected nail has grown out.

Many people have had success in clearing nail and skin fungal infections by applying neat tea tree essential oil, but this must be done at least once daily and should ideally be left on for at least an hour before washing off. Jurlique's Nail Oil, which combines tea tree oil with other natural anti-fungal agents and nail-nourishing ingredients such as spilanthes, golden rod, walnut and ivy in a safflower oil base is also worth trying.

White patches in fingernails

These are common and there are many theories regarding their cause. They have been variously attributed to lack of calcium, zinc, thyroid hormones or vitamins A and B6. The most likely cause is minor damage to nail beds which affects the way in which the nail plate is laid down – perhaps nutritional deficiencies contribute to poor healing.

Treatment
It's worth trying an A to Z-style vitamin and mineral formula plus evening primrose oil to see if this helps, although it takes at least three months for fingernails to grow through completely. Garlic powder tablets have been shown to improve blood flow to capillaries at the base of the nails by 55 per cent which will improve nutrient flow to the area. Ginkgo also improves peripheral circulation to nails.

Soft, brittle nails
This is another common problem which may be hereditary or it may be linked with deficiency of certain nutrients.

Treatment
Avoid prolonged immersion in water. A vitamin, mineral and herbal supplement designed to strengthen hair, skin and nails is worth taking. Ginkgo improves circulation to nail beds, while evening primrose oil is also helpful in strengthening nails, especially when combined with calcium. *See also* **Kelp, Manganese, Silicon.**

Ridges in nails
These are believed to result from fluctuating blood flow during times of stress or illness, and can also relate to a lack of B group vitamins.

Treatment

Biotin in particular is known to strengthen keratin, and studies suggest that supplements can increase nail thickness by at least a quarter.

In-growing toenails

This is a common problem that can be prevented: trim toenails straight across, avoid picking them, wear comfortable shoes and walk barefoot at home as much as possible. Some people suggest cutting a small V in the centre of the nail's leading edge, but this can tend to catch on socks or tights.

Treatment

The foot should be bathed in a warm, diluted antiseptic solution for 15–20 minutes. After softening the flesh, carefully tuck a small wisp of cotton wool under the ingrowing corner of the nail using a blunt pair of scissors or a tiny screwdriver. This acts as a cushion which pushes the tender flesh away from the nail and allows it to grow out normally. The old piece of cotton wool should be removed each day, and another wisp tucked in, slightly larger if necessary. The cotton wool helps to lift the nail edge away from the flesh it is digging into and encourages it to grow out properly. Adding a few drops of St John's Wort oil to the affected area will soothe pain and encourage healing. Calendula cream will also help in the healing of inflamed tissue.

Medical advice should be sought as soon as possible by diabetics, or if the toe becomes infected.

Nosebleeds

Nosebleeds are common and are linked with fragile, poorly supported blood vessels in the lining of the nose. These easily become damaged by picking fingers, inflammation, and vigorous blowing or sneezing, causing them to rupture and bleed.

Treatment

Most nosebleeds are easily stopped by:

1. sitting slightly forward, mouth open (some doctors recommend leaning backwards but this makes blood trickle down the throat which tastes horrible!)
2. pinching the lower (soft) part of the nose for 15 minutes, while breathing through the mouth
3. releasing the nostrils slowly, to check whether bleeding has stopped.

It is best to avoid touching or blowing the nose again for a few hours.

Extracts of horsechestnut help to strengthen connective tissue surrounding veins and may help to prevent recurrent nosebleeds. Vitamin K may be suggested if deficiency is thought to contribute to prolonged bleeding times.

Note: if bleeding does not stop after 20 minutes, or if it seems torrential, seek medical advice.

Osteoporosis

Osteoporosis is a bone-thinning disease which is largely preventable. Bone is a living tissue made up from a network of collagen fibres filled with mineral salts. These minerals – of which the most important is calcium phosphate – are constantly broken down and replaced as part of a carefully balanced remodelling process. Osteoporosis develops when this balance is lost, so that not enough new bone is made to replace that which is absorbed. As a result, bones become thin, brittle and fracture more easily.

Treatment

Vitamin D is essential for the absorption of dietary calcium and phosphate in the small intestine and for their deposition in bone. While dietary intake should always come first, studies in older people suggest that taking 1.2 g calcium phosphate plus 800 IU vitamin D daily can potentially reduce the incidence of hip and other non-vertebral fractures by up to 30 per cent. Other micro-nutrients that are also important for bone health include boron, vitamin C, copper, silica, strontium, vitamin K, folic acid, magnesium, manganese and zinc.

Some bone-building supplements also contain plant hormones (isoflavones) that mimic the beneficial action of oestrogen to increase bone mineralization. Essential fatty acids found in fish, evening primrose and flaxseed oils also help to increase calcium deposition in bone.

Regular exercise is important for its bone-strengthening effects.

Palpitations

Palpitations are an unpleasant awareness of the heartbeat, or a sensation of having rapid, missed or unusually strong heartbeats. They are felt quite normally after exercise, in periods of increased stress, or after a sudden scare. They can also be brought on by a high intake of caffeine. Palpitations can sometimes be a sign of an over-active thyroid gland, an abnormal heart rhythm or a chest problem (such as hiatus hernia) that needs treatment.

Treatment

If no serious medical causes are found for palpitations, it might be helpful to take kava kava if they are linked with anxiety, or valerian if linked with stress.

Try switching to caffeine-free versions of tea, coffee and cola, avoid excess alcohol, nicotine and over-the-counter cough and cold preparations containing theophylline or pseudoephedrine which can also trigger attacks.

Note: if palpitations are persistent, recurrent, or are accompanied by chest pain, shortness of breath, dizziness or faintness, always seek immediate medical advice.

Pancreatitis

Pancreatitis is an inflammation of the pancreas gland. Eight out of ten cases of pancreatitis are linked with gallstones or alcohol, while the remaining cases are usually attributed to the side effects of some drugs, infection, raised blood fat levels or injury. Some researchers believe that unexplained pancreatitis may result from lack of antioxidants, which are important for reducing free radical attack, and inflammation.

Treatment

In one small study of 28 patients, vitamins C and E, beta carotene and selenium helped to alleviate pancreatitis, while in a large study of over 300 patients with acute pancreatitis, those receiving selenium were significantly less likely to develop serious complications.

Green tea extracts (which contain powerful antioxidant catechins) have also been shown to reduce the severity of pancreatitis, while lack of magnesium has also been linked with it. Olive oil (now available in capsules as OleoMed) appears to increase production of pancreatic enzymes and, in studies with people who were either healthy, or had pancreatitis, was at least as effective as giving pancreas enzyme therapy.

Alcohol and caffeine should be avoided and a low-fat, low-sugar, high-fibre diet providing plenty of fruit and vegetables (similar to that suggested for diabetics) should be followed as much as possible.

Chromium and niacin (vitamin B3) are essential for production of Glucose Tolerance Factor (GTF) which interacts with the pancreatic hormone insulin to regulate the uptake of glucose by cells. Low levels of chromium have been linked with poor glucose tolerance and diabetes.

Chlorella supplements have a useful detox effect while probiotic supplements help to maintain general digestive health and discourage intestinal infections.

Panic attacks

Panic attacks affect one in 20 people on a regular basis and seem to be more common in women than men. In situations or periods of extreme stress, breathing patterns can change so that quick, irregular, shallow breaths are taken to draw in more oxygen. This in turn means that more carbon dioxide – a waste acidic gas – is blown off. If hyperventilating continues, so much carbon dioxide may be exhaled that the blood loses its acidity and becomes too alkaline. This causes symptoms of dizziness, faintness and pins and needles, which in turn heighten anxiety and panic so that breathing becomes even faster, causing even more carbon dioxide to be blown off, and triggering a panic attack.

People who habitually hyperventilate can experience a frightening number of physical symptoms, including chest pain, palpitations, visual disturbances, numbness, severe headache, insomnia and even collapse. Medical diagnosis of these symptoms is important to avoid missing a more serious problem.

Treatment

When panic begins rising, the classic advice is to breathe in and out of a paper bag to re-inhale some of the lost carbon dioxide – alternatively, breathe in and out of cupped hands. Concentrate on breathing slowly, deeply and quietly, holding a few breaths for a count of three if possible.

Valerian is one of the most calming herbs available and can help to relieve anxiety, muscle tension and promote calmness. Kava kava is also widely used to combat mild anxiety as it promotes feelings of relaxation and calm. In a trial involving 101 patients suffering from generalized anxiety, tension and panic attacks, kava kava produced an improvement in most patients within two months.

Students whose panic attacks are associated with exam nerves should always test any herbal remedies well in advance of the exam period to ensure that they do not cause sleepiness or affect concentration. A bottle of rescue remedy should be kept to hand, and five drops added to a glass of water when needed. It should be sipped slowly, every three to five minutes, keeping the liquid in the mouth for a while. Alternatively, five drops may be placed directly on your tongue when panic rises.

See also **Kelp**
Related entry: **Stress**

Parkinson's disease

Parkinson's disease is a neurological condition associated with low levels of a neurotransmitter, dopamine, in some parts of the brain. It is associated with a combination of tremor, rigidity and slowness of movement. Fine movements in particular are made difficult.

Although a number of complementary treatments are used to help slow the disease's progression, few have been clinically evaluated.

Treatment

Medical treatment consists of giving an amino acid, levodopa, which is converted into dopamine within the central nervous system. A co-enzyme, NADH, is needed for levodopa to work properly, and some researchers have claimed that taking NADH supplements alone can improve Parkinson's disease in some people. In one study it was shown to help four out of five sufferers, especially those who were younger and more recently diagnosed. This remains controversial, however.

Antioxidants such as vitamins C and E are sometimes prescribed by physicians to reduce the free radical attack thought to be associated with neurological damage. In one study involving over 5000 people, those with the highest intakes of vitamin E were the least likely to develop Parkinson's disease. Other powerful antioxidants that may be recommended include co-enzyme Q10, grapeseed or pine bark extracts. Ginkgo biloba, which improves blood flow to the brain, may also help.

Periodontitis

See **Chronic fatigue syndrome**

Period problems

Painful periods (dysmenorrhoea) are due to cramping of uterine muscles. Some women suffer more than others – possibly because they make more of the chemicals (prostaglandins) that trigger muscular spasm. Another theory is that some women have an unusually narrow cervical outlet from the womb making cramping more likely before they have experienced pregnancy and childbirth. It is important to have full investigations to find the cause of symptoms as around one in ten women suffers from endometriosis, in which womb lining cells are found elsewhere in the body – most usually in the abdominal cavity. Because these cells remain sensitive to the monthly hormone cycle, they swell and bleed into surrounding tissues once a month to produce pain, inflammation and scarring. Period pains can be severe in endometriosis and may be linked with nausea, vomiting and diarrhoea.

Treatment

Dysmenorrhoea seems to be significantly worse in women with a low intake of dietary fish oils, so it is worth eating more sources of omega-3 essential fatty acids (oily fish, flaxseed and evening primrose oils) which have a beneficial effect on the types of prostaglandins produced. Taking omega-3 fish oil supplements has been shown to significantly improve painful periods in teenage girls. Taking magnesium supplements for six cycles has also been found to reduce back pain and lower abdominal pain associated with menstruation – especially on the second and third days – probably due to its muscle relaxant effect.

Heavy periods (menorrhagia) have been linked with a lack of essential fatty acids (such as those found in evening primrose and flaxseed oils) vitamins A, C, K, and minerals iron and zinc.

See also **Bilberry, Black cohosh, Dong quai, Maca, Muara puama, Myrrh, Wild yam**
Related entry: **Endometriosis**

Peripheral vascular disease

See **Intermittent claudication**

Peyronie's disease

Peyronie's disease affects around one in 250 men, and occurs when some of the spongy, erectile tissues of the penis are replaced with fibrous scar tissue. Why this happens is unknown. As the fibrous area does not expand during erection, the penis curves – often dramatically – towards the area of rigidity during erection, which may be painful.

Treatment

Some specialists have reported success in reducing pain and lumpiness using the anti-oestrogen drug, tamoxifen. When intercourse becomes difficult, surgery to either remove the fibrous tissue, or insert a wedge from the opposite side of the penis, may be recommended. In advanced cases, implantation of a penile prosthesis may be necessary to maintain erections.

Treatment with vitamin E tablets (at least 200 mg a day) is sometimes recommended as vitamin E helps to maintain tissue elasticity. This is controversial however.

Phlebitis

Phlebitis – more properly known as thrombophlebitis – is the inflammation of a vein with formation of a blood clot within the affected segment. It often occurs after a minor injury such as a knock, and is frequently a complication of varicose veins. Swelling, redness and tenderness are often accompanied by fever and feeling unwell.

Treatment

Usually the condition resolved with bandaging for support, anti-inflammatory drugs and sometimes – if infection is suspected – antibiotics. Eating more oily fish (such as salmon, sardines, herrings, mackerel) or taking omega-3 essential fatty acid supplements will have a thinning effect on the blood and reduce clot formation.

Garlic powder tablets also have beneficial effects on the circulation, and for anyone who is not taking prescribed blood-thinning agents, ginkgo is also worth considering, or the Tibetan herbal blend, Padma 28, which helps to improve blood flow through the peripheral circulation.

Antioxidants (e.g. selenium ACE, pycnogenol, grapeseed extracts) will reduce inflammation while extracts of horse chestnut (*Aesculus hippocastanum*) can strengthen tissues surrounding blood vessels and reduce discomfort of varicose veins. Co-enzyme Q10 increases oxygen uptake of cells and can also reduce leg discomfort. It is worth consulting a qualified naturopath for help in selecting those supplements most likely to help.

Applying aloe vera gel or evening primrose oil to affected skin may help to improve the cosmetic appearance.

See also **Bilberry**

Piles

See **Haemorrhoids**

Polymorphic light eruption (PLE)

See **Sun allergy**

Postnasal drip

Postnasal drip occurs when excess nasal fluids trickle down the back of the throat and is often a sign of long-term irritation of the sinuses.

Treatment

Exposure to cigarette smoke and industrial fumes should be avoided as much as possible. Some nutritionists recommend cutting out dairy products to reduce mucus production. If this works, and a dairy-free diet is continued for more than a week or two, a calcium supplement should be taken to guard against osteoporosis. Other foods that are said to promote mucus production and which might, therefore, be worth avoiding, are red meat, wheat and excess refined carbohydrates.

Mucus dispersion can be boosted by supplements containing N-acetyl cysteine (NAC) – an amino acid that boosts levels of a powerful antioxidant (glutathione) in the respiratory tract. NAC has a pronounced mucus-dissolving action and studies show that it can significantly reduce mucus production and associated cough in chronic respiratory conditions such as bronchitis, emphysema and sinusitis. It may also be helpful for ear infections and glue ear. It should not be taken by anyone who has peptic ulcers.

Related entry: **Catarrh – excess**

Post-viral fatigue syndrome

See **Chronic fatigue syndrome**

Pre-menstrual syndrome

Pre-menstrual syndrome (PMS) is a common and distressing problem affecting as many as one in two women. More than 150 symptoms have been described as forming part of the PMS complex which, for diagnosis, should start within the two weeks before a period and cease promptly when bleeding occurs.

Four main sub-groups of PMS are recognized. These are PMS-A, in which the main symptoms are **A**nxiety, irritability and insomnia; PMS-C, with sugar **C**ravings, increased appetite, headache and fatigue; PMS-D with **D**epression, forgetfulness and confusion plus PMS-H (for **H**yper-hydration) with fluid retention, weight gain, bloating and breast tenderness. PMS-A and PMS-H are most common and subtypes can co-exist.

Treatment

Some research suggests that progesterone can't work properly when blood sugar levels are low. Nibbling regular carbohydrate snacks every three hours can help to reduce symptoms.

Magnesium is a co-factor in essential fatty acid metabolism, helping to stabilize blood sugar levels, and interacting with vitamin B6 to help reduce the effects of excess oestrogen. Magnesium and vitamin B2 are needed to convert B6 into its active form.

Both zinc and magnesium are essential for the interaction of sex hormones with cell receptors and to switch on the genes that they regulate. Magnesium, zinc and B6 are also needed for prostaglandin balance to reduce cyclical breast pain. PMS has therefore been linked with nutritional factors such as lack of dietary magnesium, vitamin B6, zinc, as well as defects of essential fatty acid metabolism, excess sugar, caffeine or alcohol.

Evening primrose oil is especially helpful in reducing low mood, sugar cravings and cyclical breast pain. It contains hormone-building blocks that help to even out hormonal imbalances, but needs to be take at doses of up to 3 g a day for at least three months before an effect may be noticed.

Vitamin B6 is helpful for fatigue and emotional symptoms such as depression and irritability, while magnesium supplements can reduce symptoms of irritability, depression, anxiety/tension, bloating, tiredness and headaches.

Vitamin D and calcium appear to reduce headache, negative emotions, fluid retention and pain. Each supplement tends to help around two out of three women, but must be taken for at least three months to assess the effects.

A recent randomized, placebo-controlled trial of 170 women found that agnus castus extracts significantly reduced irritability, mood changes, headache and breast fullness.

A pilot study involving 25 women with severe PMS found St John's Wort effective in reducing the incidence of crying, low mood and nervous tension.

When over 800 women took a magnesium supplement (Magnesium-OK) that also included other vitamins and minerals (e.g. B6, zinc) results showed that symptoms of irritability improved in 73 per cent, depression in 66 per cent, anxiety/tension in 66 per cent, tiredness and headaches in 48 per cent, and 50 per cent had less bloating.

See also **Black cohosh, Flaxseed oil, Hempseed oil, 5-HTP, Liquorice, Maca, Muira puama, Pfaffia, Red clover, Wild yam**

Prostate problems

The prostate is an intimate male gland, the size and shape of a large chestnut. It lies just beneath the bladder, wrapped around the urinary tube (urethra). There are four main problems that can affect the prostate gland:

- prostatitis, in which the gland becomes infected or inflamed
- prostatodynia, in which prostate pain occurs with no obvious cause

- benign prostatic hyperplasia (BPH) in which the gland slowly enlarges
- prostate cancer.

Prostatitis

Inflammation of the prostate gland is thought to affect 30 per cent of men at some point between the ages of 20 and 40 years. Symptoms vary and may include:

- feeling unwell, sometimes with chills or fever
- aching around the thighs, genitals or lower back
- deep pain between the scrotum and anus
- pain and difficulty on passing water
- passing water more frequently
- pain on ejaculation
- discharge from the penis which may be watery or stained with blood or pus.

Prostatodynia

Prostatodynia literally means prostate pain. It is an unpleasant condition whose symptoms can include:

- discomfort in the lower abdomen, scrotum, testicles, groin
- a urinary flow that is often abnormally slow
- difficulty in urination.

No sign of infection or inflammation is found with prostatodynia and it is thought to be linked with spasm of the prostate gland and/or pelvic floor muscles and prostate engorgement.

BPH

After the age of 45, the number of cells in the prostate often increases and the gland starts to enlarge in what is known as benign prostatic hyperplasia (BPH). The result is that the urethral passage is squeezed, causing interference with urinary flow. Half of all 60-year-old men are affected and by the age of 80, four out of five men have evidence of BPH. The exact cause is unknown, but it is thought to be linked with the action of a prostate enzyme, 5-alpha reductase, which converts the male hormone, testosterone, to a more powerful hormone, dihydrotestosterone (DHT). DHT seems to trigger division of prostate cells so their numbers increase. The fact that the prostate gland is wrapped round the urinary passage is something of an evolutionary design fault, as enlargement of the gland can cause:

- straining or difficulty when starting to pass water
- a weak urinary stream which may start and stop mid-flow
- discomfort when passing water
- having to rush to the toilet
- passing water more often than normal, especially at night
- dribbling of urine or even urinary incontinence
- a feeling of not emptying the bladder fully.

Prostate cancer

Prostate cancer is one of the most commonly diagnosed male malignancies. Studies suggest that 10–30 per cent of men aged between 50 and 60, and 50–70 per cent of men aged 70 to 80 have evidence of prostate cancer when cells are examined under the microscope. Overall, however, only around one in ten men develops significant prostate cancer symptoms. The cause of prostate cancer is unknown, but seems to be linked with increasing age – perhaps because the gland enlarges as the years progress. Some research suggests that prostate cancer is linked to diet – eating green vegetables is protective, while a diet high in animal (saturated) fats and red meat increases the risk.

Unfortunately, there are few symptoms of early prostate cancer as nine out of ten tumours arise on the outside of the gland and do not interfere with urinary flow. If obstructive symptoms do occur, they are similar to those caused by BPH (see above).

Treatment

Several natural treatments and dietary changes can help to maintain prostate health and reduce the risk of prostate symptoms occurring. The same measures can also be used to help to treat prostate problems once they have been medically evaluated and a satisfactory diagnosis made.

Saw palmetto fruit extracts help to relieve urinary discomfort, improve urinary flow and ensure better bladder voiding. In particular they reduce urinary frequency and encourage shrinking of the central part of the prostate gland to improve urinary flow through the prostatic urethra. They are often combined with nettle root or pumpkin seed.

Once BPH is diagnosed, medical management often includes a frustrating period known as 'watchful waiting' in which no medications are advised, and patient and doctor wait to see if symptoms worsen. At this stage, a man has little to lose by trying a standardized extract of saw palmetto berries to see if it helps.

Extracts from the pollen of certain plants, including rye, have been shown in studies to reduce prostate pain due to chronic, non-infective prostatitis or prostatodynia and also improve symptoms of BPH. The researchers also concluded that complications should be suspected in men whose symptoms fail to respond to pollen extract within three months.

A double-blind placebo-controlled study of 60 patients with BPH showed that the flower pollen extracts improved prostate symptoms by 69 per cent compared with only 29 per cent for those taking a placebo.

Note: It is important not to self-diagnose prostate symptoms, as in some cases a possible prostate cancer may need to be excluded.

Healthy eating for a healthy prostate gland

- Follow a diet low in saturated (animal) fat.
- Eat at least five servings of fresh fruit or vegetables per day for vitamins and minerals, especially the antioxidants.
- Eat more Japanese-style foods: weak plant hormones found in soy products, rice, and green or yellow vegetables (e.g. broccoli, Chinese leaves, kohlrabi) seem to discourage prostate gland enlargement and protect against both BPH and prostate cancer.
- Eat a high-fibre diet – this binds male hormones in the gut that have been flushed out through the bile, reduces their reabsorption and may help to prevent prostate enlargement.
- Eat foods that are rich in mineral zinc (seafood – especially oysters, whole grains, bran, pumpkin seeds, garlic and pulses). Zinc is important for prostate health and controls its sensitivity to hormones.
- Eat more tomatoes and tomato-based foods as these contain lycopene and other carotenoids that seem to protect against prostate cancer.
- Eat more nuts and seeds (including evening primrose oil, flaxseed or hempseed supplements) for essential fatty

acids needed to make prostaglandins – hormone-like substances important for prostate health.

- Consider taking an antioxidant supplement containing vitamin C (at least 300 mg a day) and vitamin E (at least 40 mg a day) which may help to protect against prostate cancer.
- Consider taking a supplement containing around 15 mg zinc per day.

Other herbal supplements that may help include extracts of African prune (*Pygeum africanum*) and nettle root.

See also **Lapacho, Pfaffia, Pumpkin seed, South African star grass**
Related entry: **Benign prostatic hyperplasia**

Psoriasis

Psoriasis is an inflammatory disease in which new skin cells are produced at a rate of around ten times faster than normal. As a result, they push up to the surface faster than the dead cells they are designed to replace can fall away from the body. Live cells accumulate and form characteristic raised, red patches covered with dead cells forming fine, silvery scales. Psoriasis symptoms vary and can include the appearance of bright red, scaly patches that vary in size from a few millimetres to extensive plaques covering most of the body. In some cases, sterile pustules form – usually on the palms and soles – while in others, flaky scalp, thickening and pitting of the nails, and/or a form of arthritis known as psoriatic arthropathy develop.

Treatment

Psoriasis has been linked with abnormalities in essential fatty acid metabolism and EFAs found in fish oils (e.g. EPA and DHA) have an anti-inflammatory effect which has been shown to damp down psoriasis lesions. A study of 80 people with psoriasis, taking a dose of 1122 mg a day of EPA and 756 mg a day of DHA significantly reduced psoriasis lesions within four to eight weeks. Itching decreased most rapidly, followed by scaling then redness with over 65 per cent of people showing marked improvement.

Aloe vera gel is also noted for its wound-healing and anti-itching properties. Taking it by mouth may be beneficial, too.

Other topical treatments that can improve psoriasis include Dead Sea mineral salts/mud, mahonia ointment (made from the Oregon grape extract), gotu kola and Zambesia Botanica – a cream made from the African Kigelia tree. Some practitioners advise taking milk thistle and artichoke (*Cynara scolymus*) extracts to improve liver function, which seems to improve the rate at which new skin cells are produced.

It might also be worthwhile trying to avoid foods that are high in saturated fats, red meats, dairy products, cheese, eggs, gluten and refined sugars. However, if a restricted diet is to be continued for more than a few weeks, nutritional advice should be sought. Smoking and alcohol can trigger flare-ups and should be avoided.

A case control study looked at selenium intakes and serum selenium levels in 59 people with psoriasis and found that, compared with similar controls, selenium status was insufficient in those with psoriasis. In males with chronic disease, selenium levels were inversely correlated to the severity of disease. Increasing selenium intake may therefore help to reduce the severity and progression of psoriasis.

See also **Alpha-lipoic acid, D, Echinacea, Gotu kola, Milk thistle, Oregano, Red clover, Sarsaparilla, Zinc**

Raynaud's syndrome

Raynaud's is a condition where small arteries in the fingers and toes are overly sensitive to cold. They respond by constricting down and cutting off blood flow to the digits. This causes the fingers to go white, along with numbness and tingling. As a sluggish blood flow returns, the digits go blue, then when circulation becomes normal they turn bright red. The condition can cause pain and burning sensations. Fingers are affected more than toes and it seems to strike more females than males. When associated with other specific diseases, it is known as Raynaud's phenomenon.

Possible causes of Raynaud's include:

- arterial diseases (e.g. atherosclerosis, blood clotting disorders)
- connective tissue diseases (e.g. rheumatoid arthritis, scleroderma, lupus)
- prescribed drugs (e.g. beta-blockers, ergotamine).

Raynaud's can also be triggered by frequent use of pneumatic drills or chain saws and may be referred to as vibration white finger. Occasionally typists and pianists may suffer, too.

Treatment

General self-help measures include keeping hands and feet as warm as possible, stopping smoking (as this further constricts small arteries) and avoiding sudden or extreme changes in temperature.

Eating more oily fish or taking omega-3 fish oil supplements can help to reduce blood stickiness while garlic powder tablets and gingko biloba extracts can improve blood flow to the peripheries. Ginger has a natural warming effect and recent trials suggest that a supplement combining ginkgo, ginger and garlic was helpful in relieving symptoms. It is also worth taking a vitamin and mineral supplement that includes magnesium.

Vitamin E is an antioxidant that helps to protect polyunsaturated fatty acids in cell membranes from free radicals – including those in the blood vessels that constrict during Raynaud's – and in one trial, around 80 per cent of sufferers taking vitamin E (400 IU) found it helpful. Magnesium is also advised for its beneficial effects on the circulation.

See also **Cayenne, Co-enzyme Q10, Garlic**

Restless legs syndrome

Restless legs, or Ekbom's syndrome, is surprisingly common and affects most people at some time in their life. Around one in 20 people experiences it on a regular basis.

Restless legs syndrome is associated with an unpleasant creeping sensation in the lower limbs, sometimes accompanied by twitching, pins and needles, burning sensations or even pain, along with an irresistible urge to move the legs. It tends to occur during periods of tiredness, and typically an hour after settling down to rest, when leg twitching or jumping can affect sleep. The exact cause is unknown but it is thought to be associated with poor oxygenation of tissues. It seems to be a form of nerve irritation linked with fatigue, anxiety, stress and smoking, but can also occur in pregnancy, diabetes, kidney problems, chronic respiratory illness and stroke.

Treatment

Eating a light snack before going to bed might help, and alcohol and caffeine, which may worsen symptoms, should be avoided. Supplements containing iron and folic acid will help to improve haemoglobin concentration, while co-enzyme Q10 encourages oxygen uptake in cells.

As restless legs are linked with reduced circulation of blood, extracts of ginkgo biloba leaves and garlic tablets are often recommended to improve blood flow through small vessels in the legs. The Tibetan preparation Padma 28, which contains a complex mix of 20 Tibetan medicinal herbs, is also beneficial in opening up blood flow through the peripheries. High-dose vitamin E helps to stabilize cell membranes and has also been suggested as a treatment, while magnesium supplements are also often effective.

Other options include topical preparations containing horsechestnut extracts. It may take a month or two for supplements to show benefits and during this time, acupuncture and magnet therapy are worth trying.

Rheumatoid arthritis

Rheumatoid arthritis (RA) is an inflammatory disease in which the synovial membranes lining some joints become thickened, inflamed and produce excess synovial fluid leading to redness, stiffness, swelling and pain. Inflammation gradually spreads to involve the underlying bone, which becomes worn and distorted. Usually, RA affects the smaller joints in the hands and feet but can also occur in the neck, wrists, knees and ankles. People suffering from RA often feel unwell and may notice weight loss, fever and inflammation in other parts of their body such as the eyes. RA affects around 1 per cent of the population, with three times as many women affected as men. A quarter of sufferers develop symptoms before the age of 30, but most new cases occur within the 40–50 age group.

RA was thought to be linked with an over-active immune system attacking the joint linings following a viral infection. New research suggests, however, that RA may be the opposite – the result of an underactive immune system that leads to a build-up of a type of immune cell (T-lymphocyte) that attacks the joints leading to inflammation and damage. Another theory is that RA is triggered by a previous infection – 80 per cent of RA patients have antibodies to the Epstein-Barr virus which causes glandular fever.

Treatment

Avoiding cold draughts and keeping as warm as possible in winter are both important. Sufferers of RA should immerse their hands in hot, soapy water first thing in the morning and throughout the day. Frequent hot baths/showers are also soothing. Some people find hot or cold compresses helpful.

In four trials, fish oil supplements helped to relieve joint tenderness and fatigue in patients with rheumatoid arthritis. One study found that after 14 weeks of taking fish oil supplements, patients with rheumatoid arthritis had reduced neutrophil leukotriene B4 production (a marker for inflammation). Most double-blind trials report a decrease in morning stiffness, swelling, the number of painful joints, and overall pain, with the result that many people are able to reduce the dose of painkillers needed.

Extracts of New Zealand green-lipped mussel (*Perna canaliculus*) help to reduce inflammation in joints and can reduce the pain and swelling in osteoarthritis (possibly by up to 35–45 per cent) and rheumatoid arthritis. They contain substances known as glycoproteins, which are thought to work by preventing white blood cells from moving into the joints, where they would release powerful chemicals making pain and swelling worse. Some evidence suggests that extracts can outperform non-steroidal anti-inflammatory drugs such as ibuprofen and indomethacin.

Other supplements that may be helpful include: **B3, Bromelain, CMO, Devil's claw, Evening primrose oil, Flaxseed oil, Hempseed oil, Histidine, Maitake, Nettle, Olive leaf, Olive oil, Sarsaparilla, Selenium, Wild yam**

Related entry: **Arthritis**

Rhinitis

Persistent nasal congestion is commonly due to inflammation and swelling of the mucous membrane lining the nose.

Treatment

One of the simplest and most effective ways of relieving this is with steam inhalation which loosens mucus so that it can drain away more easily. Fill a bowl with hot water, cover your head with a tea towel and lean over the bowl to trap and inhale the hot vapours (taking care not to burn yourself). Adding decongestant essential oil blends will improve efficacy.

Supplements containing the amino acid N-acetyl cysteine help to dissolve excess mucus but should not be taken by anyone who has peptic ulcers. Yerba maté may also help.

Related entry: **Catarrh – excess**

Rosacea

Rosacea (medically known as acne rosacea) is an inflammatory skin condition in which the face flushes easily and small pimples appear along with fine, dilated capillaries (telangiectasia). The cause is unknown, although it is thought to be due to abnormal sensitivity of blood capillaries. It has also been linked with overuse of corticosteroid creams in the treatment of other skin conditions and with infection of sebaceous glands with a skin mite, *Demodex folliculorum*.

Rosacea usually starts with temporary facial flushing after drinking alcohol, eating spicy food, consuming hot drinks or entering a warm room. If the condition is allowed to progress without treatment, the skin becomes permanently red and pustules start to appear. In severe cases, there is a persistent eruption on the forehead and cheeks, with redness, puffiness and prominent blood vessels. The eyes may be affected to cause conjunctivitis and inflammation of the eyelids (blepharitis). In some people – especially older males – the skin on the nose becomes thickened and red due to enlargement of sebaceous glands.

Rosacea affects around 1 per cent of the population. Symptoms can occur in the teens, but most sufferers are fair-skinned females aged 30–50. Some estimates suggest as many as one in ten middle-aged women is mildly affected. It tends to recur over a five-to-ten-year period then may improve.

Treatment

Avoid factors that may trigger flare-ups of rosacea such as stress, hot liquids, spicy foods, alcohol, vigorous exercise, heat and exposure to sunlight – use a non-greasy high protection cream (SPF 15 or higher) or apply a product that reflects and blocks out ultra-violet rays with titanium dioxide or zinc oxide. Sometimes cutting out tea, chocolate, cheese, yeast extract, eggs, citrus fruits and wheat can be beneficial.

Lack of vitamin A and B group vitamins, especially B2, B3 and B6 is often present in rosacea sufferers. A vitamin B-complex supplement might be helpful, but this must contain vitamin B3 in the form of nicotinamide rather than niacin, as niacin can itself cause flushing.

Interestingly, some researchers believe that people with rosacea have a reduced production of hydrochloric acid in the stomach and that replenishing levels with supplements containing betaine hydrochloride reduces symptoms although the mechanism is unknown.

High-dose vitamin C is useful for its anti-inflammatory actions as well as its beneficial effects on collagen production and, together with zinc, can improve skin healing.

Topical application of natural anti-parasitic agents such as oregano, lavender or tea tree oil is helpful in many cases. If stinging is severe when applying these neat, they may be diluted first with a little olive or hemp seed oil. Aloe vera gel applied twice a day can reduce inflammation and a special range of skin care products containing vitamin K and designed for use in rosacea is also available.

Note: if rosacea is suspected it is important to seek medical advice as scarring can develop if the condition is left untreated.

See also **Grapeseed**

Scars

Scars are formed as a part of the body's natural healing process in which damaged areas of skin are replaced by collagen-rich scar tissue. This is initially pink but eventually shrinks to form a much paler scar.

Treatment

High-dose vitamin C is needed for collagen formation and will encourage scars to heal, while evening primrose oil helps to improve tissue suppleness. Rosa mosqueta oil is an exceptionally rich source of the essential fatty acid GLA, which is also found in evening primrose oil. When applied to scar tissue, anecdotal evidence suggests that it is highly effective in improving the cosmetic appearance. Vitamin E tablets help to reduce inflammation and encourage healing and vitamin E cream may be rubbed in to soften new scar tissue.

The herb gotu kola may also be used externally to improve healing of wounds, chronic ulcers and excess scar tissue. It seems to act directly on fibre-producing cells to improve the quality and texture of the underlying tissues.

The appearance of scars – even those that are 20 years old – can be helped by a medically proven treatment, Cica-Care. This is an adhesive gel sheet that is applied to scarred skin and helps to flatten, soften and fade red and raised scars.

Seasonal affective disorder

Seasonal affective disorder (SAD) is form of depression that comes on when exposure to natural sunlight is reduced. It affects an estimated 5 per cent of the population, with another 10 per cent experiencing a milder form known as sub-syndromal SAD. Shift workers are particularly susceptible to SAD.

Symptoms include winter tearfulness and depression, lethargy, sleepiness, carbohydrate cravings and a general slowing up. SAD is diagnosed when someone has experienced three winters of symptoms (November to March), two of which are consecutive, with remission during the summer months. In sub-syndromal SAD symptoms appear from January to March.

Treatment

Eating the right types of food can provide a natural energy boost while the wrong types of food can lead to fatigue. Research shows that eating fatty foods for breakfast can cause tiredness, sluggishness and poor concentration throughout the morning. Following this up with a fatty lunch causes below-par functioning all day.

Foods to avoid include:

- fatty, sugary snacks – doughnuts, pastries
- fatty, salty snacks – crisps, pork pies, salami, pizza
- cakes, biscuits and confectionery.

Foods that give a boost, that can 'pep you up', are also those that are recommended for healthy eating. They include:

- crusty whole-grain bread, especially those with added nuts and seeds
- whole-grain cereals – porridge, brown rice, pearl barley, oatcakes, unsweetened breakfast cereals
- root vegetables
- cruciferous plants – broccoli, cauliflower, Chinese leaves
- legumes – lentils, kidney beans
- fresh or dried fruit.

Aim to drink plenty of fluids during the day – especially mineral water or herbal teas – and eat little and often rather than having three traditional large meals a day. Reduce intakes of alcohol, salt and caffeine and consider taking a vitamin and mineral supplement plus CoQ10 which can boost energy levels.

Regular brisk exercise will also boost energy levels, lift depression and help to maintain a healthy weight.

Using a light box that emits bright, fluorescent light similar to natural daylight can help, especially if the box is set up near the bed and timed to come on with increasing brightness to simulate a natural dawn.

St John's Wort (*Hypericum*) is an effective herbal treatment for mild to moderate depression. Trials involving St John's Wort found it was just as effective in treating SAD when used alone as when combined with light box therapy.

See also **5-HTP**

Sciatica

See **Backache**

Shaving rash

Sycosis barbae – or barber's itch – is a bacterial infection of hair follicles. Unfortunately, shaving can perpetuate the folliculitis by nicking off the tops of healing pustules and encouraging hair to grow back into the skin. If not treated adequately it can lead to small, white scars.

Treatment
Usual advice for men with frequent recurrences is to grow a beard, clip facial hair short with nail scissors (and go for a designer look) or to use a depilatory cream designed for facial hair once the infection has cleared with antibiotics.

Soothing creams or lotions containing calendula, evening primrose, aloe vera or silicol gel applied topically can help. Tea tree oil is a useful skin antiseptic with a gentle action.

A supplement such as Siberian ginseng, propolis or echinacea that can boost general immunity may also help, and antioxidants will reduce inflammation.

Shingles

Shingles can affect anyone who has previously been exposed to the chicken pox virus, *Varicella zoster*. During the initial attack of chickenpox, the virus enters the nervous system and lies dormant in the roots of most sensory nerves. The virus can stay in this latent state for years without causing problems, but can occasionally reactivate, travelling back down the nerve to cause an attack of shingles localized to the area of skin supplied by that nerve.

Shingles is contagious as the fluid-filled blisters are teeming with viral particles which means that other people – particularly children – who are not immune to the virus may develop chickenpox if exposed to the blister fluid. Adults who have never had chickenpox should avoid contact with anyone who has either chickenpox or shingles. This is especially important for non-immune pregnant women as the chickenpox virus can cause serious birth defects known as *Varicella* syndrome particularly during the first three months of pregnancy. If a non-immune pregnant woman is exposed to chickenpox or shingles, it is vital to seek immediate medical advice as treatment with *Varicella-zoster* immunoglobulin and/or anti-viral drugs may be needed.

Treatment

Several supplements can help in the treatment of shingles. Antioxidants such as high-dose vitamins C, E or olive leaf extract are usually taken to help reduce inflammation. (Vitamin E might also help to reduce any pain – perhaps by stabilizing the nerve cell membrane – while olive leaf extracts also have a powerful anti-viral action.) Herbal extracts that boost immunity against viral infections include echinacea, cat's claw, goldenseal or reishi. Topical treatments that are traditionally applied to the rash include tea tree oil and aloe vera gel.

One in ten people with shingles subsequently develops post-herpetic neuralgia with unpleasant burning, shooting or gnawing pains for several months or even years afterwards. Axsain cream – a prescription-only treatment containing capsaicin, derived from chilli peppers (cayenne), may help. When rubbed sparingly into the skin, it sinks in to relieve post-herpetic neuralgia by blocking the passage of pain messages. St John's Wort (*Hypericum*) can help to relieve the depression that, not surprisingly, often accompanies post-herpetic neuralgia, but should not be taken together with prescribed anti-depressant drugs. A high-lysine diet can also help.

Related entry **Herpes simplex**

Smoking – quitting

Stopping smoking is one of the most powerful preventive health measures a smoker can take. Research shows that smokers are five times more likely to suffer a heart attack in their 30s and 40s than non-smokers, and that smoking-related illnesses kill 40 per cent of smokers before they reach retirement. Non-smokers therefore tend to live at least six years longer than smokers.

Risks are directly related to the number of cigarettes smoked per day – for example, the increased risk of death due to carcinoma of the bronchus is approximately equal to the number of cigarettes smoked per day (i.e. two a day doubles the risk, 20 a day increases the risk 20-fold). Stopping smoking can reduce the risk of a heart attack by as much as 50–70 per cent within five years. Within ten years, quitting halves the initial risk of lung cancer and reduces the risk of a variety of other cancers (including mouth, throat, bladder) to virtually normal. Twenty years after stopping smoking, the associated risks can be considered similar to those in non-smokers.

Quitting

Unfortunately, quitting smoking is easier said than done as nicotine is highly addictive, but here are some ideas.

- Nicotine replacement therapy, which helps to wean smokers off the drug slowly, can be more effective than willpower alone. A controlled trial of smoking cessation involving 400 participants found that 26 per cent of those using nicotine inhalers were smoking-free after four months compared with only 9 per cent using a placebo. After two years, the equivalent figures were 9.5 per cent and 3 per cent.

- Hypnosis helps one in three smokers to quit.

- Taking regular brisk exercise stimulates the release of brain chemicals that can also curb nicotine cravings.

- Wild oats (oatstraw, also known as *Avena sativa*) have been used to reduce cravings, and are also a good source of B group vitamins which are needed in extra amounts during times of stress.

- Sucking an artificial cigarette or herbal sticks available from chemists can help when there is an urge to smoke. Alternatively, try home-made carrot and celery sticks, apple slices, sunflower seeds or liquorice roots.

St John's Wort and kava kava are both helpful for reducing cravings when giving up smoking. Antioxidants are important to help protect against the damaging effects of free radicals liberated while smoking.

See also **N-acetyl cysteine, Pine bark**

Sore throat

More than one in four adults develops a sore throat each year, and it is one of the most common reasons for people to visit their doctor. At least seven out of ten sore throats are due to a viral infection, however, and as antibiotics only work against bacteria, they are ineffective for viral sore throats. Sometimes, a persistent sore throat is due to infection with haemolytic streptococcal bacteria, and a swab will identify when antibiotics are needed.

Treatment

All but the most severe sore throats can be self-treated. Medical advice is usually only needed if a sore throat has lasted for longer than five days, is severely painful or accompanied by swelling, fever, hoarse voice, or difficulty in swallowing or breathing.

In a randomized trial, over 700 patients with sore throats received either a ten-day course of antibiotics, no treatment, or an antibiotic prescription to be used only if symptoms were no better after three days. Researchers found no difference in the incidence of complications between the three groups and less than a third of those given postdated prescriptions decided to use them. Those given antibiotics immediately were more likely to return to the surgery next time they had a sore throat, however, rather than treating themselves appropriately at home.

At the first sign of a sore throat, 1 g vitamin C should be taken three times a day, and lozenges containing zinc gluconate should be sucked. Products containing echinacea, garlic and/or propolis are also effective.

Slippery elm or liquorice (DGL form) lozenges will help to soothe a sore throat, while steam inhalations are helpful at night to ease dryness and improve sleep. Eucalyptus, myrrh and olive leaf extracts are also helpful. *See also* **Sage**.

Sperm count – low

There is some concern that male sperm counts are falling, possibly due to increased exposure to environmental oestrogens.

Treatment

It takes an average of 100 days for a primitive sperm cell to mature and be ejaculated. An estimated 40 per cent of sperm damage occurring during this time is due to free radicals. Antioxidants neutralize free radicals and vitamin C (500 mg twice a day) has been shown to increase sperm count by 34 per cent, reduce sperm clumping by 67 per cent and reduce the number of abnormal sperm by 33 per cent. High-dose vitamin E (600 mg a day for three months) also improves sperm function – especially the binding of sperm to egg. In one study, 21 per cent of men taking vitamin E successfully fathered a child.

Zinc (15 mg a day) seems to prevent premature release of chemicals in the sperm head needed to drill through the egg during fertilization.

Alcohol, even in moderate amounts, is linked with 40 per cent of male infertility, so men planning to father a child should ideally try to avoid it altogether. In one study of men with low sperm counts, half returned to normal values within three months of avoiding alcohol completely.

Wearing tight, bikini-type briefs – especially those made from man-made fibres – can reduce sperm counts by as much as 20 per cent, sperm motility by as much as 21 per cent and semen volume by up to 12 per cent due to the damaging effects of excess heat and static electricity. Loose, cotton boxer shorts should be worn instead.

See also **Arginine, Astralagus, Carnitine, Co-enzyme Q10, Lecithin, Selenium**
Related entry: **Conception**

Splits in fingers

Painful splits in fingers are similar to chilblains and are thought to be triggered by reduced circulation, such as when small arteries go into spasm on exposure to cold. This reduces the flow of oxygen and nutrients to tissues.

Treatment

Evening primrose oil supplements should be taken and aloe vera gel applied to help soothe itching. Hands should also be massaged with an intensive care moisturizing cream

Supplements containing garlic, ginkgo and ginger help to improve circulation to the fingers and have a natural warming action. Inflammation may be reduced by taking vitamin C with bioflavonoids, and/or omega-3 fish oils.

Regular exercise is important, and gloves should always be worn when going out in cold weather. Applying 'artificial skin' type lotions that dry to cover and protect lesions will help. Some people find tissue glue (similar to superglue) helpful.

Related entry: **Chilblains**

Stress

Stress is a modern term used to describe the symptoms of excess pressure in daily life. A certain amount of pressure is beneficial and helps to generate the energy and reserves needed to meet life's challenges. Once pressure falls outside the range with which we feel comfortable, however, it can lead to the unpleasant physical and emotional symptoms associated with distress. Excessive or long-term pressure is harmful to health and can worsen pre-existing conditions such as eczema, asthma, psoriasis and irritable bowel syndrome. Long-term stress also lowers immunity and increases the risk of high blood pressure, heart attack and probably even cancer.

Stress can cause a number of physical and emotional symptoms such as:

- anxiety and panic
- insomnia
- fatigue
- sweating
- palpitations
- nausea and diarrhoea
- dizziness
- headache
- inability to concentrate or make decisions
- irritability
- loss of sex drive and sexual problems
- loss of concentration
- over-reliance on food, cigarettes, alcohol or drugs.

Treatment

To help reduce the effects of stress, healthy foods should be eaten, little and often, to keep blood sugar levels up – never skip meals, particularly breakfast.

It is important to concentrate on breathing slowly and deeply when anxious to prevent overbreathing (hyperventilation) which can trigger a panic attack. Excess caffeine and nicotine should be avoided as these mimic the body's stress response – tea and coffee intake should therefore be limited to three cups a day (or better still, switch to de-caffeinated brands). Sugar, salt and saturated fat intake should be cut, along with processed or convenience foods. Alcohol intake should ideally be limited to a maximum of one or two units per day.

A good multi-nutrient supplement should be taken, and it is also a good idea to consider taking additional vitamins C and B complex as these are quickly used up during stress reactions and may make anxiety and irritability worse.

Valerian and lemon balm can promote feelings of calm while kava kava is excellent for reducing anxiety. Adaptogenic herbs such as Ashwagandha, Gynostemma, Korean, American or Siberian ginsengs support adrenal function and help the body adapt to stressful situations. Rescue remedy, is useful when there are feelings of rising panic.

See also **Adaptogens, Hawthorn, Lemon balm, Liquorice, Maitake, Muira puama, Oats, Pfaffia, Yerba maté**
Related entry: **Panic attacks**

Stye

A stye is a bacterial infection causing a small abscess at the edge of the eyelid. Despite its size, usually only a single sebaceous gland draining into one of the eyelash follicles is affected.

Treatment
The affected eyelash should be gently removed so that pus can drain away – don't squeeze the area or infection may spread. Then bathe the eye regularly with an infusion of

chamomile, eyebright (*Euphrasia*) or marigold (*Calendula*). Applying a recently used camomile teabag as a compress works well.

An antioxidant supplement will help to reduce inflammation. Recurrent styes are not usually hereditary but may suggest low immunity. Taking echinacea and a vitamin and mineral supplement could help. If infection spreads or is associated with conjunctivitis, seek medical advice.

Sun allergy

Sun allergy, known as polymorphic light eruption (PLE), affects up to 20 per cent of people and is especially common in young women. Symptoms include an itchy, raised red rash, blisters and the development of scaly plaques that appear within hours of sun exposure. Only skin directly exposed to the sun is affected, such as the backs of hands, lower arms, face and the V of the neck.

PLE is linked with sensitivity to UVA rays, rather than UVB. Some drugs and cosmetics can also sensitize skin to sunlight to trigger a light-sensitive rash. As UVA light is not filtered by glass it is still possible to develop PLE while sitting in a car or by a house window in the sun.

Treatment

Cover up with loose cotton clothes as much as possible, apply a broad-spectrum sunscreen which filters out both UVA and UVB light (check before buying as some sun blocks only filter out UVB rays and will be ineffective) and avoid, as far as possible, exposure to sunlight between 10 am and 4 pm when UVA rays are at their most intense.

Antioxidant supplements, especially those containing selenium and carotenoids, may help to protect the skin. Aloe vera gel is soothing when applied to the skin rash.

Swollen ankles

Some people find that their ankles swell in hot weather as this encourages dilation of the blood vessels under the skin as part of the body's cooling mechanism. However, this makes it easier for fluid to escape into the tissues. When the body is less active than normal (e.g. when travelling), this will contribute to swelling as the pumping action of leg muscles helps to draw fluid away from the ankles.

Treatment

An increase in the level of physical activity wherever possible is helpful, as is raising the feet when sitting down. Light support stockings/tights can help but are uncomfortable in hot weather.

A natural approach to mild swollen ankles is to take extracts of a diuretic herb such as dandelion. A low-fat, low-salt, high-fibre diet should be followed, including plenty of fluids to prevent dehydration. Over-indulgence in alcohol should be avoided.

A medical check-up should be arranged to investigate the cause of persistent swollen ankles.

Note: Dandelion should not be taken during pregnancy or by anyone who has kidney problems.

Systemic lupus erythematosus (SLE)

See **Lupus**

Taste – loss of

Taste and smell sensation are closely linked. Loss of taste sensation – ageusia – is common after a bad cold when taste buds and smell receptors in the nose become blocked. Long-term problems may result from loss of taste buds with increasing age. One of the most common, reversible causes of ageusia is zinc deficiency. This is easily tested by obtaining a solution of zinc sulphate (*see* **Zinc**).

Treatment

If needed, take 10–15 mg zinc twice a day and retest after two weeks. This is best done under the supervision of a nutritionist as higher doses of zinc should ideally be taken together with other nutrients such as vitamin E, selenium and copper. Dietary sources of zinc include red meat, seafood, especially oysters, brewer's yeast, whole grains, pulses and eggs. Smokers should do their utmost to quit – *see* **Smoking – quitting**.

Thyroid gland – underactive

The thyroid gland in the neck produces iodine-containing hormones that help to regulate the body's metabolism. Around one in 100 people develops an underactive thyroid gland, a condition known as hypothyroidism. Symptoms include lack of energy, a general slowing down, muscle weakness, cramps, increasing weight, feeling the cold, dry skin, brittle hair, thickening of the ankles, slow pulse, heavy periods and a deepening voice which may seem slurred. Sometimes the thyroid gland swells to produce a swelling in the neck known as a goitre.

Most cases of hypothyroidism are due to an autoimmune condition in which, for some reasons, the immune system makes antibodies aimed against the thyroid gland. Other cases result from treatment of an overactive thyroid gland or, in some parts of the world, from severe dietary deficiency of iodine, selenium or zinc. Smoking cigarettes has also been linked with an increased risk of developing hypothyroidism.

Treatment

Thyroxine replacement therapy is carefully titrated until blood tests result in stable thyroid function tests. The aim is to restore the level of thyroid-stimulating hormone (TSH – secreted by the pituitary gland in an attempt to kick-start the thyroid) to well within the normal range. Total thyroxine concentration is also measured although the normal range is wide (58–174 mmol/L). Some endocrinologists believe that complete well-being is only restored when thyroxine is towards the upper limit of normal, and the TSH level is slightly suppressed. However this is something that needs to be medically tailored to individual needs, minimizing the risk of side effects while at the same time optimizing the body's metabolic rate so that problems such as weight gain are reduced.

Following a diet free from sugar and refined foods can improve thyroid function. A vitamin and mineral supplement including iodine, selenium and zinc is also recommended.

Siberian and Korean ginsengs help the body to adapt to stress, and medical herbalists often recommend one or the other to complement thyroid treatments.

Kelp may be suggested as a naturally rich source of iodine where an underactive thyroid is thought to be linked with low iodine intake. Only small amounts of cabbage, cauliflower, spinach, Brussel sprouts, broccoli, turnips, soy and other beans should be eaten as these contain substances known as goitrogens (goitre forming) that interfere with the action of iodine and can make symptoms worse.

See also **Oats, Selenium**

Thyroid gland – overactive

An overactive thyroid gland – known as hyperthyroidism or thyrotoxicosis – affects an estimated 2–5 per cent of women at any one time. The commonest cause is Grave's disease, an autoimmune condition in which thyroid-stimulating antibodies bind to thyroid cells and trigger over-production of thyroid hormones.

The symptoms of an overactive thyroid gland include weight loss, increased appetite, anxiety, irritability, restlessness, tiredness, weakness, rapid pulse and palpitations, sensitivity to heat, diarrhoea, period changes and loss of sex drive. The thyroid gland may also become enlarged (goitre). Extra symptoms may occur in Grave's disease due to the production of other antibodies that cause inflammation and swelling at the back of the eyes so they seem bulge, or which affect the skin to cause vitiligo in which there is a patchy loss of skin colour.

What triggers auto-antibody production in Grave's disease is unknown, but factors such as food allergy, hypersensitivity to mercury in dental fillings and stress have been suspected. Other causes of thyrotoxicosis include the development of overactive nodules in the thyroid gland, viral inflammation of the gland (thyroiditis) and excess production of thyroid stimulating hormone (TSH) from the pituitary gland in the brain.

Treatment

Several natural treatments are helpful in combination with orthodox treatment for thyrotoxicosis. These include calming herbs such as valerian or kava kava to help reduce the anxiety and nervousness. Avoid iodized salt, and stimulants such as coffee, tea and other caffeinated drinks which speed up the metabolism. Try eating more cabbage-related vegetables (e.g. broccoli, Brussel sprouts, cabbage, cauliflower, kale) which suppress thyroid hormone production — they contain fluorine which blocks iodine receptors in the thyroid gland.

Because vitamins and minerals are used up more quickly by the increased metabolic rate, a good A to Z-style vitamin and mineral supplement should be taken, plus evening primrose oil.

Siberian and Korean ginsengs help the body adapt to stress and medical herbalists often recommend one or the other to complement thyroid treatment. *See also* **B3**.

Note: medical advice should be sought before taking supplements.

Tinnitus

Tinnitus is a constant, unpleasant, ringing, buzzing, hissing or whistling sensation in one or both ears. Its causes are ill understood, but it may be related to abnormal blood flow to the inner ear in some cases, or to damage to the inner ear in others.

It is important to rule out treatable causes such as a build-up of wax in the ears or side effects associated with some drugs, especially high-dose aspirin or quinine.

Treatment

Unfortunately, tinnitus is often difficult to treat. Dietary changes such as reducing intakes of salt, refined sugar and carbohydrates, meats, saturated fats and increasing intakes of fruit and vegetables have helped some sufferers, as has losing excess weight. In severe cases, a specialist may recommend a tinnitus masker that plays a random mixture of sounds at differing frequencies (white noise) to help block out noise.

Extracts of ginkgo biloba improve circulation to the brain and have been found helpful in some cases. In one double-blind, placebo-controlled study of 103 patients, those taking gingko showed significant improvements in symptoms compared with those taking a placebo. In another study, 12 out of 33 patients receiving ginkgo extracts had complete resolution of symptoms, and in another five, symptoms were reduced. Some studies have found no benefits however – response seems to be a very individual thing.

Other supplements that may be suggested include garlic powder tablets, B group vitamins, especially B12, magnesium and zinc for their importance in nerve health.

An acupressure technique worth trying is to massage the area one finger's width in front of the ear at the top of the cheekbone. *See also* **Zinc**.

Tiredness all the time

Tiredness all the time, and lack of energy, are common problems, yet only around one in five cases is linked with an identifiable medical cause such as anaemia, underactive thyroid gland, immune disorders or abnormalities of the internal organs. Many cases are undoubtedly linked with stress, overwork, lack of exercise, dietary deficiencies or mild depression.

Treatment

A low-fat, high-fibre diet should be followed with plenty of fresh fruit and vegetables, and at least half the daily energy intake should ideally be in the form of unrefined carbohydrates such as whole-grain cereals, wholemeal bread, wholewheat pasta and brown rice.

While diet should always come first, it is worth taking an A to Z-style multivitamin and mineral supplement. Preliminary evidence suggests that B vitamin status, especially pyridoxine (vitamin B6), is low in some people with chronic fatigue and it is worth adding in a vitamin B complex to see if this helps.

If lack of energy is due to stress, an adaptogen such as Siberian or Korean ginseng may be helpful in supporting adrenal gland function.

If fatigue is linked with low mood, St John's Wort is often effective. A pilot study involving 20 women in their 20s and 30s with young children found significant improvement in fatigue after taking 300 mcg St John's Wort three times a day for six weeks. Evening primrose oil has also been shown to benefit 70–80 per cent of people suffering from long-term fatigue.

Other supplements useful for lack of energy include: **Essential fatty acids** (high-dose evening primrose, omega-3 or flaxseed oils); **Co-enzyme Q10**; **Kelp** or other iodine sources (needed for production of thyroid hormones, and often lacking in the diet due to lower intakes of iodized salt, fish etc); **Alpha-lipoic acid; Bee products – royal jelly; Biotin, Gotu kola, Iron, Magnesium, Muira puama, Oats, Pfaffia, Reishi, Rhodiola, Schisandra, Siberian ginseng, Wheatgrass, Yerba maté.**

As a more gentle, buffered caffeine substitute, guarana is useful for a short-term energy boost. Adequate sleep and time for rest and relaxation should also be ensured.

Lack of energy can be a presenting sign of a number of different medical conditions so if it is persistent or troublesome, always seek advice from your doctor.

Related entry: **Chronic fatigue syndrome**

Ulcerative colitis

Ulcerative colitis is an inflammatory bowel disease in which the lining of the bowel (colon and rectum) becomes inflamed and ulcerated. It affects around one in 1000 people and is most common in those aged between 20 and 40. Women are more frequently affected than men.

The main symptom is blood-stained diarrhoea which may also contain pus and mucus. In severe attacks fever, abdominal pain and feelings of being quite unwell can also occur. Attacks tend to come on every few months although some sufferers find that their symptoms are infrequent while others have continuous problems.

The exact cause of ulcerative colitis is unknown but hereditary factors, poor circulation of blood to the gut and abnormal immune function have been suggested. Avoiding foods that seem to provoke attacks can reduce symptoms. Some people find that they are sensitive to dairy and wheat produce, or that following a gluten-free diet is beneficial, but no foods consistently provoke symptoms in all sufferers.

Treatment

Essential fatty acids from oily fish seem to be the most effective complementary treatment. In a small, randomized, double-blind, placebo-controlled trial, those taking fish oil extracts (equivalent to EPA 3.2 g and DHA 2.4 g daily) for six months showed significant improvements compared with those taking an inactive placebo. There was also a significant reduction in the circulating numbers and cytotoxic activity of natural killer cells that have been implicated in disease severity. *See also* **Flaxseed** and **Hempseed** oils.

A group of people given psyllium husk fibre supplements during remission were found to have significantly greater improvement than those not taking them. Evening primrose oil, colloidal silicol gel, aloe vera or probiotic supplements containing *Lactobacilli* species are also helpful in many cases.

Folic acid supplements have been shown to reduce the risk of developing colon cancer by 28 per cent in almost 100 patients who had had ulcerative colitis for at least eight years. Avoiding dairy products, refined sugars and yeast may help, but this should be done under specialist supervision as a number of vitamin and mineral deficiencies can arise as a result of inflammatory bowel disease. Boswellia resin has also been found to be helpful.

Over 80 per cent of ulcerative colitis sufferers are non-smokers, and some people develop the condition when giving up smoking – especially middle-aged men. Treatment with nicotine patches or gum may help mild to moderately active ulcerative colitis, possibly by altering blood flow through the intestines or by altering the levels of inflammatory chemicals (cytokines) present. Nicotine does not seem to be as effective a treatment as prednisolone, however, and is unhelpful in maintaining remission. In one study, nearly 10 per cent of those trying nicotine patches or gum had to stop treatment due to side effects (e.g. contact dermatitis, nausea, light headedness, shakiness). Medical advice should be sought before trying nicotine replacement products. Also, do not start smoking as this will increase the risk of a number of potentially serious illness, such as chronic bronchitis, hypertension, coronary heart disease, stroke and cancer.

See also **Glutamine, Liquorice, Probiotic supplements**

Ulcers – leg

A leg ulcer is an open sore on the skin that can be difficult to heal. The usual cause is a result of poor blood supply to the area (e.g. a blocked artery) or poor drainage from it (e.g. venous stasis, commonly due to varicose veins). Poor circulation results in poor healing, and an ulcer may be triggered by a mild injury or even just a scratch.

Treatment

In the early stages, treatment consists of compression hose or stockings to prevent blood pooling in the veins of the lower leg. Sufferers are also encouraged to lose weight, to spend less time standing, and to keep their legs elevated above the waist when sitting down to reduce fluid accumulation. The ulcer is dressed with a variety of specialized powders, granules, pastes and coverings depending on whether it is infected, wet or dry. Most dressings work by helping to separate fluid and bacteria from the ulcer surface to encourage formation of granulation (healing) tissue. Although many leg ulcers eventually heal using this approach, as many as 70 per cent recur within a year.

The latest option for treating leg ulcers due to venous stasis is an endoscopic surgical procedure to examine the leg veins from the inside and clip off those that are damaged. This forces pooled blood to find a new route through the leg and helps to open up a new circulation to encourage rapid healing. Tissue growth factors may also be applied to hasten healing in diabetic leg ulcers.

Research suggests that leg ulcers are often associated with low zinc levels. It may be worth taking a good vitamin and mineral supplement containing around 100 per cent of the recommended daily amount of as many nutrients as possible, including zinc. In addition, vitamin C (1000 mg a day) and high-dose vitamin E (at least 400 IU per day – equivalent to 267 mg) will damp down inflammation and promote healing.

Garlic powder tablets and ginkgo biloba supplements improve blood flow through tiny blood vessels which will improve blood circulation in the base of the ulcer and encourage healing.

Oily fish (such as salmon, sardines, mackerel, herrings) should be included in the diet, or fish oil supplements should be taken to help thin the blood and promote healing of leg ulcers.

Gotu kola extracts used externally have been shown to significantly improve healing of wounds and chronic ulcers. It is thought to act directly on fibre-producing cells to improve the quality and texture of the underlying tissues. Aloe vera gel has also been shown to promote healing of chronic leg ulcers when applied directly.

Manuka honey is sometimes also applied to wounds to help treat or prevent infections. Honeys absorb fluid due to their high concentration of natural sugars. This osmotic effect makes it difficult for bacteria to thrive. Manuka honey also releases natural antiseptics, hydrogen peroxide and gluconic acid which inhibit many common skin bacteria, especially *Staphylococcus aureus*. In the case of leg ulcers, the honey is applied on absorbent dressings under medical supervision, to draw fluid out of the infected area. The natural sugars have an extra beneficial action of stimulating tissue growth and feeding new cells. Dressings are changed three times a day.

Note: topical treatments should only be used under medical supervision.

Vaginitis

Vaginitis is an inflammation of the vagina and, usually, the vulva. This may be due to a bacterial, viral or fungal infection, to allergy, a skin disease such as eczema or psoriasis, or to lack of oestrogen. Symptoms, which may include local pain, soreness, itching, discharge and painful intercourse, should be checked by a doctor – preferably in a genito-urinary medicine clinic – for a diagnosis.

Treatment

Cotton rather than synthetic underwear should be worn, and tight clothing avoided, as becoming hot and sweaty makes itching worse. Soap, shower gel and bubble bath should be avoided; fragrance-free bath additives, especially those designed to treat eczema are preferable – a doctor or pharmacist can advice on the wide range available. A replenishing wash containing lactic acid (Lactacyd) is also helpful and will soothe the vulval area as well as discouraging infection.

A vaginal gel containing concentrated soy extracts (PhytoSoya) has hydrating properties and, as well as improving lubrication, can also reactivate natural secretions to overcome dryness.

Evening primrose oil is helpful in reducing itching and scaling associated with eczema and may be taken by mouth and applied locally to affected areas. Aloe vera pulp or gel is often helpful when applied to vaginal lesions and has a soothing, anti-inflammatory action. Omega-3 fish oil supplements may also be taken by mouth.

Varicose eczema

Varicose, or stasis, eczema is usually associated with varicose veins and oedema. It occurs when blood circulation through tissues in the lower leg is compromised and may progress to venous ulceration.

Varicose eczema causes dry, scaly, flaky, discoloured skin around the ankle.

Treatment

It is important to control ankle swelling by wearing elasticated support stockings or tights which must be properly fitted by a pharmacist. Stockings or tights need to be put on first thing in the morning before getting out of bed for best results.

Regular exercise, such as walking, is important. Standing still for long periods of time should be avoided, and feet should be elevated as often as possible.

Gently massaging the skin daily with a moisturizing cream containing urea helps to stimulate the circulation and improve scaliness. A variety of emollient bath preparations are also available on prescription or over the counter.

Evening primrose oil (massaged directly into affected skin) and taken orally often reduces itching although it can take a few months for a noticeable improvement to occur. Aloe vera gel applied to the skin will help to reduce inflammation. Extracts of horse chestnut (*Aesculus hippocastanum*) help to strengthen tissues surrounding blood vessels and reduce leakage of fluid. This can also improve the symptoms and appearance of varicose veins. Garlic powder tablets or ginkgo biloba supplements help to improve blood flow through the peripheral circulation and may help to reduce the risk of leg ulceration.

See also **Gotu kola, Red vine leaf**
Related entries: **Ulcers – leg, Varicose veins**

Varicose veins

Varicose veins are one of the prices we pay for walking on two legs rather than four. The long veins in the legs contain a series of valves that allow blood to flow upwards against gravity. Weak valves often give way so that blood pools in superficial veins which become dilated and twisted.

Varicose veins tend to affect more women than men. They may be hereditary or triggered by pregnancy or overweight. Symptoms include bulging, tortuous veins, aching and dragging sensations, swelling of the ankles and itching.

Treatment
Support stockings help to keep varicose veins comfortable. Other self-help measures include losing any excess weight, walking regularly and avoiding standing still for long in order to boost circulation in the legs. Feet should be elevated as often as possible.

The skin over leg varicose veins should be massaged daily with moisturizing cream. Extracts of red vine leaf, horsechestnut (*Aesculus hippocastanum*) or gotu kola can strengthen tissues surrounding blood vessels and reduce discomfort of varicose veins. Bilberry, pine bark or grapeseed extracts may also be recommended.

Omega-3 fish oil, garlic powder tablets, ginkgo biloba extracts or a Tibetan herbal blend, Padma 28, help to improve blood flow through the peripheral circulation. Co-enzyme Q10 increases oxygen uptake of cells and can also reduce leg discomfort.

Related entry: **Varicose eczema**

Warts and verrucas

Common warts are caused by infection with a skin virus – human papillomavirus (HPV) – of which over 60 different types are known. Warts usually affect areas of skin prone to injury such as the hands, elbows, face, knees and scalp. Those on the soles of the feet become flattened by the weight of the body to form painful verrucas. These tend to grow quickly and can spread through wet, macerated skin to form multiple, superficial lesions known as mosaic warts. Black threads that may form in the centre of the verruca are clotted blood vessels (capillaries) not roots as commonly believed.

Warts are highly contagious and often appear in crops, especially in children.

Treatment
Half of sufferers find that their warts naturally disappear on their own within a year without treatment – that's why many folk remedies (such as buying them for a penny, or

rubbing with a piece of meat which is then buried in the garden) often seem to work.

Applying vitamin E oil directly to the wart and covering with a waterproof plaster (repeat twice or three times a day) often seems to work, although it may take several weeks. Alternatively, tea tree and garlic oil may be mixed together and applied regularly until the wart dries. Only a tiny amount of garlic should be used at first, as some people develop a painful reaction to this treatment. Surrounding skin should be protected with petroleum jelly and the oil applied only to the area of hardened, raised skin. Cover with a plaster for 24 hours.

Taking echinacea, astragalus, goldenseal or garlic powder tablets will help to boost immunity against viral infections. High-dose antioxidants such as vitamin C, E and carotenoids may also help to reduce wart growth.

Regression of warts can be hastened by freezing (cryosurgery), painting with wart-dissolving liquids, or they can be burned off under local anaesthetic. Warts and verrucas can be frozen at home by a product called Wartner, which works in a similar way to the liquid nitrogen treatment used for cryotherapy (freeze treatment) by doctors. Only one application of the spray is needed to freeze the skin, which may sting slightly. The wart or verruca then falls off after around ten days.

Note: Genital warts should never be treated at home; always seek medical advice from a doctor or genito-urinary medicine clinic.

See also **Lapacho, Oregano**

Wind – excess

Embarrassing intestinal noises – known as borborygmi – are a common feature in irritable bowel syndrome (IBS). Bowel gases come from several different sources, including fizzy drinks (which are best avoided) and swallowing air, but most derive from bacterial fermentation of dietary fibre in the large bowel. As much as 1–2.5 litres a day may be produced and expelled.

Gases seem to pass through the gut of people with IBS more slowly than normal. Some people produce insufficient amounts of an enzyme, lactase, needed to break down milk sugar (lactose), resulting in excess wind, borborygmi and loose bowels. Lactose intolerance is relatively common and it may be present from birth or develop later in life.

Treatment

It is worth avoiding all milk-based products for a few weeks. If symptoms improve dramatically, a doctor can arrange a lactose tolerance test to confirm the diagnosis, and an appointment with a dietitian.

In the meantime, 'windy' foods such as beans, lentils, cauliflower, cabbage, broccoli, Brussel sprouts and cucumber, should all be avoided, while taking a probiotic supplement containing *Lactobacillus acidophilus* can help to improve intestinal health.

Related entry: **Bloating**

APPENDICES

Further reading

Thomas Bartram, *Bartram's Encyclopedia of Herbal Medicine,* Robinson 1998

Andrew Chevallier, *Encyclopedia of Medicinal Plants*, Dorling Kindersley 2001

Dr Stephen Davies & Dr Alan Stewart, *Nutritional Medicine*, Pan 1987

Linda Lazarides, *Nutritional Health Bible*, Thorsons 1997

Mark Mayell, *Off the Shelf Natural Health*, Bantam 1995

Dr H C A Vogel, *The Nature Doctor*, Mainstream Publishing 1990

Useful resources

The Nutri Centre
The Hale Clinic
7 Park Crescent
London WIN 3HE
Tel: 020 7436 5122
Supply most of the
supplements mentioned in
this book by mail order.

Herbalism
British Herbal Medicine
Association
Sun House, Church St
Stroud GL5 1JL
Tel: 01453 751389
Information leaflets, booklets,
compendium, telephone
advice.

The General Council and
Register of Consultant
Herbalists
18 Sussex Square
Brighton
East Sussex BN2 5AA
Tel: 01243 267126

The National Institute of
Medical Herbalists
56 Longbrooke Street

Exeter EX4 8HA
Tel: 01392 426022

Naturopathy
General Council and
Register of Naturopaths
Frazer House
6 Netherall Gardens
London NW3 5RR
Tel: 020 7435 8728

Nutritional Therapy
Doctors registered with the
British Society for Allergy
Environmental and
Nutritional Medicine have a
special interest in how diet
and environmental factors are
linked with chronic illness.
Tel: 0906 3020010
www.bsaenm.org.uk

British Association of
Nutritional Therapists
27 Old Gloucester Street
London WC1N 3XX
Send £2 plus a large (A4)
SAE for a list of registered
members.

The Nutrition Society
10 Cambridge Court
210 Shepherds Bush Road
London W6 7NJ
www.nutsoc.org.uk

Society for the Promotion
of Nutritional Therapy
BCM Box SPNT
London WC1N 3XX
Tel: 01825 872921

Institute for Optimum
Nutrition
Blades Court, Deodar Road
London SW15 2NU
Tel: 020 8877 9993.
www.ion.ac.uk

Ayurveda
Ayurvedic herbs are
available from
www.thinknatural.com, as
well as some healthfood
shops and practitioners.

Alopecia
At present, Calosol 4H to
treat **alopecia** is only
available from the Alopecia
Areata Centre in London
(Tel: 0208 741 8224).

Cancer
If you have **cancer**, it is
worth contacting:
The Bristol Cancer Help
Centre
Grove House
Cornwallis Grove
Clifton
Bristol BS8 4PG
(Helpline: 0117 980 9505)
www.bristolcancerhelp.org
*They provide an holistic
approach to healthcare to
support those with cancer
and their carers, including
information on therapies
(e.g. diet, supplements,
counselling, relaxation
techniques, affirmation and
visualization) to complement
standard cancer treatment.*

Index

NOTE: Page numbers in **bold** *refer to main discussion of a topic*